Series editor
Daniel Horton-Szar
BSc (Hons)
United Medical and Dental
Schools of Guy's and
St Thomas's Hospitals
(UMDS),
London

Faculty advisor
Marek Dominiczak
MB, PhD, MRCP (Glasg.)
FRCPath
Honorary Senior Lecturer,
University of Glasgow
Consultant Biochemist,
West Glasgow Hospitals
University NHS Trust

Metabolism and Nutrition

Sarah Benyon
BSc (Hons)
United Medical and
Dental Schools of Guy's
and St Thomas's
Hospitals (UMDS),
London

D1146902

4.95

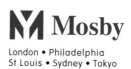

M Mosby

London • Philadelphia
St Louis • Sydney • Tokyo

Publisher	Dianne Zack
Managing Editor	Louise Crowe
Development Editors	Filipa Maia
	Marion Jowett
Project Manager	Leslie Sinoway
Designer	Greg Smith
Layout	Paul Phillips
Illustration Management	Danny Pyne
Illustrators	Sandie Hill
	Jenni Miller
	Richard Prime
	Mike Saiz
	Annette Whalley
	Amanda Williams
Cover Design	Greg Smith
Production	Gudrun Hughes
Index	Liza Weinkove

ISBN 0 7234 2990 1

Copyright © Mosby International Ltd, 1998.

Published by Mosby, an imprint of Mosby International Ltd, Lynton House, 7–12 Tavistock Square, London WC1H 9LB, UK.

Printed in Barcelona, Spain, by Grafos S.A. Arte sobre papel, 1998.
Text set in Crash Course–VAG Light; captions in Crash Course–VAG Thin.

The publisher, author and faculty advisor have undertaken reasonable endeavours to check drugs, dosages, adverse effects and contraindications in this book. We recommend that the reader should always check the manufacturer's instructions and information in the British National Formulary (BNF) or similar publication before administering any drug.

Cataloguing in Publication Data
Catalogue records for this book are available from the British Library.

Preface

Students have been known to pale at the mere mention of glycolysis; some have even passed out at the thought of the TCA cycle. Hopefully, this will no longer be the case.

This book has been written with a user-friendly approach using short blocks of text and simple, reproducible diagrams.

In Part I, I have set out the basic principles of metabolism and nutrition in order to cover the information necessary to pass the appropriate pre-clinical examinations in this subject. Chapter 1 serves as a guide on how to use this book and how to approach revision in the easiest way.

As a medical student, it is often all too easy, given the amount that has to be learned for examinations, not to question the reason behind learning something. In response to this, I have emphasized the relevance to clinical practice throughout the book in the hope of presenting a more colourful, wider viewpoint of the subject. A brief clinical assessment section has been included in Part II, which contains helpful guides to taking a basic history, examination, and details of useful tests.

Details of important metabolic and nutritional disorders are set out in Part III in a format that is useful for quick reference. These have been included to complement Part I and do not necessarily represent those disorders most often encountered in a clinical setting, as many metabolic disorders are in fact rare.

I conclude the book with a self-assessment section in which I have focused on those commonly asked examination topics. Finally, although as far as possible the book is a statement of known facts, I have tried not to oversimplify and, where there are areas of uncertainty, these have been pointed out.

Sarah Benyon

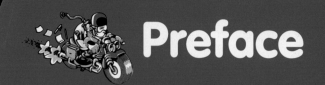

Preface

Medical education is rapidly changing. The British General Medical Council has recommended more integration of preclinical and clinical teaching.

The Crash Course series caters for the changing trends in medical curricula—the basic science titles include a clinical part which relates the content of the basic core material to clinical teaching. This book emphasises the clinical relevance of biochemistry—it will help the student retain aspects of biochemistry most important for learning clinical medicine

This text provides realistic help for students learning for examinations as they are conducted today. The reader may also be interested in looking at Crash Course *Endocrine and Reproductive Systems* which is complementary to this volume.

Crash Course is intended primarily for students. However, it will also be useful for lecturers and tutors as it provides an important insight into how students perceive today's teaching of biochemistry.

Marek H Dominiczak
Faculty Advisor

OK, no-one ever said medicine was going to be easy, but the thing is, there are very few parts of this enormous subject that are actually difficult to understand. The problem for most of us is the sheer volume of information that must be absorbed before each round of exams. It's not fun when time is getting short and you realize that: a) you really should have done a bit more work by now; and b) there are large gaps in your lecture notes that you meant to copy up but never quite got round to.

This series has been designed and written by senior medical students and doctors with recent experience of basic medical science exams. We've brought together all the information you need into compact, manageable volumes that integrate basic science with clinical skills. There is a consistent structure and layout across the series, and every title is checked for accuracy by senior faculty members from medical schools across the UK.

I hope this book makes things a little easier!

Danny Horton-Szar
Series Editor (Basic Medical Sciences)

Acknowledgements

I would like to thank all my lecturers at United Medical and Dental Schools of Guy's and St Thomas's Hospitals, especially Dr H. Thomas and Dr B. Gillham who originally taught me in my pre-clinical years. I would also like to thank my lecturers at the University of Birmingham, particularly Dr J. Davey for his encouragement and words of wisdom during my studies.

Finally, my greatest thanks to my long-suffering family who have always given me endless support, encouragement, and kindness and to whom I dedicate this book.

Figure Credits
Figures 4.21 and 11.13 adapted from *Clinical Chemistry 3e*, by Dr W. J. Marshall, Mosby, 1995

Contents

To my parents

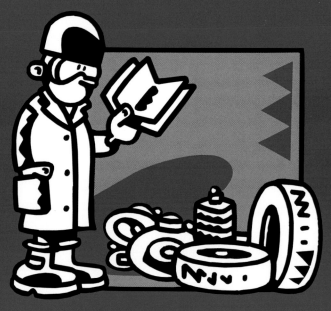

PROCESSES OF METABOLISM AND NUTRITION

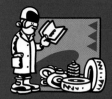

1. Overview of Metabolism

Metabolism

Metabolism is an integrated set of chemical reactions occurring in the body that enable us to extract energy from the environment and use it to synthesize building blocks that are used to make essential proteins, carbohydrates and fats. Some fundamental points to remember about metabolism:

- Each reaction does not occur in isolation but provides a substrate for the next.
- In this way, pathways are built up in which the ultimate product of each pathway forms a substrate for others, producing a continuous process.
- Many people liken metabolism to a map, the 'metabolic map', in which the pathways are like roads with 'stop-off points' (intermediates) along the way.
- Some of the roads are one way, meaning you have to travel a long way round to form some intermediates.
- Remember, when you make any journey, it is important to know where you are going but you do not need to know the names of all the places you travel through.

Metabolic pathways can be classified as either catabolic or anabolic.

Catabolism

Catabolism is the breakdown (degradation) of energy-rich complex molecules such as protein, carbohydrate, and fat to simpler ones, for example, CO_2, H_2O and NH_3. The energy released is 'captured' as adenosine triphosphate (ATP) and stored for use in synthetic, anabolic reactions.

Anabolism

Anabolism is the synthesis of complex molecules from simpler ones, for example, proteins from amino acids and glycogen from glucose. Synthetic reactions require energy which comes from the hydrolysis of ATP. Some examples of catabolic and anabolic pathways are shown in Fig. 1.1.

Examples of catabolic and anabolic pathways	
Catabolic pathways names end in 'lysis' meaning 'to break down'	**Anabolic pathways** names end in 'genesis' meaning 'to create'
glycogenolysis: glycogen breakdown proteolysis: protein breakdown lipolysis: fatty acid breakdown glycolysis: glucose breakdown	glycogenesis: glycogen synthesis protein synthesis lipogenesis: fatty acid synthesis gluconeogenesis: glucose synthesis

Fig. 1.1 Examples of catabolic and anabolic pathways.

Although sometimes difficult to realize, all metabolic pathways do have a purpose and were not just invented in an attempt to make the first year at medical school very dull! Do not get 'bogged down' remembering every single step and enzyme in a pathway, you will not be asked to regurgitate this sort of information in an exam. It is much more likely that you will have to discuss the overall functions of a cycle and in which tissues they are particularly important.

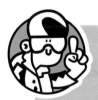

The best way to revise metabolism is to take a large piece of paper (A3 size) and draw simplified cycles of all the pathways; listing the six key criteria in Fig. 1.2 for each: purpose/function, location, site, reaction sequence, key steps; and effect of inhibition.

Key criteria for remembering a metabolic pathway	
Key criteria	**Example—glycolysis**
What is the purpose of the pathway? form a working definition of its function knowing: the substrates and products involved and any other key intermediates produced, for example, ATP or NADH	oxidation of glucose (substrate) to pyruvate (product) with the generation of energy in the form of ATP and NADH (the reduced form of nicotinamide adenine dinucleotide)
Location: particularly, tissues or cells in the body where the pathway is most important	glycolysis occurs in all cells of the body but in red blood cells it is the only energy-producing pathway
Site: where in the cell it occurs, for example cytosol, mitochondria or both	glycolysis occurs in the cell cytosol. pyruvate formed can be transported into mitochondria for addition by the TCA cycle
Sequence of events know the overall reaction sequence and the number of stages and reactions	glycolysis has 10 reactions
Pick out key steps: either those which form major control sites or those which are main 'branch points'	1. hexokinase reaction 2. phosphofructokinase reaction 3. pyruvate kinase
Effect of inhibition of the cycle	increase in [intermediates] which arise before the site of inhibition decrease in [intermediates] formed after the block

Fig. 1.2 Key criteria for remembering a metabolic pathway.

Regulation of pathways

Every metabolic pathway usually contains one reaction that is essentially irreversible and forms the 'rate-limiting' reaction of the pathway. Enzymes catalysing these reactions are subject to strict regulation to ensure that:

- The rate of the pathway is adapted to the cell's needs.
- For any molecule, its synthetic and breakdown pathways are not active at the same time as this would lead to a 'futile cycle'.

Most metabolic pathways occur in different cells and in different tissues of the body at the same time. The pathways must be carefully regulated, to ensure not only that the production of energy and intermediates is sufficient to meet the needs of the individual cell, but also to 'fit in' with the requirements of the rest of the cells in the body. The control of metabolic pathways must also be flexible enough to enable adaptation to

different environments, for example, fed state as opposed to starvation, or periods of exercise and so on. These control mechanisms must co-ordinate the pathways in all cells of the body.

Mechanisms of control

There are three main mechanisms of control of metabolic pathways; supply of substrate, allosteric control and hormonal control. Learn these now because they form the basis for control of all metabolic pathways.

Substrate supply

If the concentration of substrate is limiting, then the rate of the pathway decreases.

Allosteric control

Allosteric control may either be due to end-product inhibition, in which feedback inhibition by the amount of product may be positive (stimulate pathway) or negative (inhibit pathway), or to via the production of allosteric effectors which bind to regulatory sites on an enzyme that are distinct from the catalytic (active) site; they may increase or decrease enzymatic activity.

Hormonal control

There are two possible ways hormones such as insulin or glucagon can affect enzyme activity and thus the rate of metabolic pathways:

- Firstly by reversible phosphorylation of enzymes which may either increase or decrease their activity.For example, glucagon causes phosphorylation of both glycogen synthase and glycogen phosphorylase. Glycogen synthase is inhibited by phosphorylation whereas glycogen phosphorylase is activated. This

- ○ **Define catabolic and anabolic pathways (giving examples of each).**
- ○ **What are the key points or criteria for learning metabolic pathways?**
- ○ **Why are metabolic pathways regulated?**
- ○ **What are the three main mechanisms of control?**

ensures glycogen synthesis and breakdown are not active at the same time and is discussed fully in Chapter 2.

- Secondly, hormones can affect the rate of a metabolic pathway by induction; that is, they increase the amount of enzyme synthesized by stimulating the rate of transcription of its RNA. Similarly, under certain conditions hormones can inhibit transcription and thus the synthesis of certain enzymes—this is called repression.

BASIC PRINCIPLES OF BIOENERGETICS

Bioenergetics is the study of the energy changes accompanying biochemical reactions. It allows us to work out why some reactions occur (i.e. because they are energetically favourable) and why some do not. The direction and extent to which a chemical reaction occurs is determined by a combination of two factors:
- Enthalpy change, ΔH, which is the heat released or absorbed during a reaction.
- Entropy change, ΔS, a measure of the change in disorder or randomness in a reaction.

Neither enthalpy nor entropy change alone can predict whether a reaction can occur. Together they are used to calculate ΔG, the change in Gibb's free energy of a reaction. It is ΔG that predicts favourability and direction of a reaction since:

$$\Delta G = \Delta H - T \times \Delta S$$

where T = absolute temperature in degrees Kelvin (K) (°C + 273) and ΔG is the energy available to do work.

- If ΔG is negative, there is a net loss of energy during the reaction; making this a spontaneous, favourable, exergonic reaction.
- If ΔG is positive, there is a net gain of energy during the reaction and the reaction does not occur spontaneously; it is an endergonic reaction as energy must be added to the system to drive the reaction.
- If ΔG is 0, the reaction is at equilibrium. At equilibrium, the rate of the forward reaction is equal to the rate of the backward reaction and there is no net direction.

Be sure not to confuse exergonic and exothermic and endergonic and endothermic. Exothermic reactions release heat during a reaction and have a negative enthalpy change, $-\Delta H$. Similarly, endothermic reactions absorb heat during a reaction and have a positive enthalpy change, $+\Delta H$. However, it is not possible to predict favourability or direction of a reaction from enthalpy values. Remember only reactions with a negative ΔG occur spontaneously.

- **What are the principles behind predicting the direction and extent of a reaction?**
- **Define exothermic, endothermic, exergonic, and endergonic reactions.**

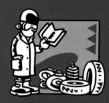

2. Carbohydrate and Energy Metabolism

An overview of glycolysis

Working definition

Glycolysis is the sequence of 10 reactions that break down one molecule of glucose (a six-carbon ring) to two molecules of pyruvate (two chains of three carbon molecules) with the net generation of two molecules of ATP and NADH (the reduced form of nicotinamide adenine dinucleotide). Therefore glycolysis provides energy and intermediates for other metabolic pathways.

Location

All the cells of the body.

Site

Cell cytosol.

Aerobic and anaerobic respiration

Unlike other metabolic pathways, glycolysis can produce ATP under either aerobic or anaerobic conditions (see Fig. 2.2).

- Under aerobic conditions, the end-product, pyruvate, enters mitochondria where it is oxidized by the tricarboxylic acid (TCA) cycle and oxidative phosphorylation to CO_2 and H_2O with the production of large quantities of energy.
- Under anaerobic conditions, pyruvate is reduced by NADH to lactate in the cytosol. This allows the continued production of ATP in cells that lack mitochondria or are deprived of oxygen. This pathway produces only a small amount of energy.

Functions and importance of glycolysis

For many tissues glycolysis is an 'emergency' energy-producing pathway when oxygen is the limiting factor. It is of the utmost importance in:

- Red blood cells because they lack mitochondria and therefore glycolysis is their only energy-producing pathway.
- Active skeletal muscle when oxidative metabolism cannot keep up with increased energy demand.

- The brain because glucose is its main fuel (it uses about 120 g/day).

Glycolysis also contributes to the synthesis of certain specialized intermediates, for example, 2,3-bisphosphoglycerate, an allosteric effector of haemoglobin. It also helps in the metabolism of other sugars, especially fructose and galactose. (Both of these topics are covered later in this chapter.)

Glucose entry into cells

Glucose is not small enough to diffuse directly into the cell—it needs help. There are two transport mechanisms that exist specifically for glucose.

Facilitated diffusion

The first mechanism, facilitated diffusion, is mediated by a family of glucose transporters present in the cell membrane. At least five have been identified and are named glut-1 to glut-5; each has a different tissue distribution (Fig. 2.1). The transporters are integral membrane proteins that bind glucose and transport it through the cell membrane into the cell. Glucose enters the cell down its concentration gradient from an area of high concentration outside the cell to an area of low concentration inside.

Distribution of some of the glucose transporters		
Transporter	**Location**	**Function**
glut-1	most cell membranes	Provides basal glucose transport to cells at a relatively constant rate
glut-2	liver β cells of pancreas	Glut-2 transporters have a lower affinity for glucose than glut-1, therefore, glut-2 are only active when there is a high blood glucose, that is, in the fed state
glut-4	muscle and fat cells	Insulin dependent: muscle and fat cells 'store' glut-4 transporters in intracellular vesicles. In the presence of insulin, these vesicles fuse with the cell membrane resulting in an increase in the number of glut-4 transporters in membrane. Therefore insulin promotes glucose uptake by muscle and fat

Fig. 2.1 Distribution of some of the glucose transporters.

Sodium–glucose cotransporter

The second mechanism requires energy to transport glucose against its concentration gradient (i.e. from a low concentration outside the cell to a high concentration inside). This method of glucose transport occurs in the epithelial cells of the intestine (for the absorption of dietary glucose), renal tubules and the choroid plexus. The movement of glucose is coupled to the concentration gradient of sodium: sodium ions flow down their concentration gradient into the cell providing the energy to transport glucose into the cell against its gradient.

Trapping glucose in the cell

Glucose may enter the cell but will not necessarily stay there. Glucose must undergo irreversible phosphorylation to 'trap' it inside the cell. Why? Well, there are two reasons, first, phosphorylated glucose molecules cannot penetrate cell membranes because there are no carriers for them (glucose-6-phosphate is not a substrate for the glucose transporters). Secondly, converting glucose to glucose-6-phosphate keeps the concentration of free glucose inside the cell low compared with outside, maintaining the concentration gradient.

Stages of glycolysis

Glycolysis can be divided into two phases: an energy investment phase and an energy generating phase.

I Energy investment phase (reactions 1–5 in Fig. 2.2)
Glucose is phosphorylated and cleaved into two molecules of glyceraldehyde-3-phosphate. This process uses two moles of ATP to activate and to increase the energy content of the intermediates (see Figs 2.2 and 2.3).

II Energy generating phase (reactions 6–10)
Two molecules of glyceraldehyde-3-phosphate are converted into two molecules of pyruvate with the generation of four moles of ATP (see Figs 2.2 and 2.3). The overall reaction can be written as:

Glucose + 2NAD$^+$ + 2ADP + 2Pi → 2NADH + 2 pyruvate + 2ATP + 2H$_2$O + 2H$^+$

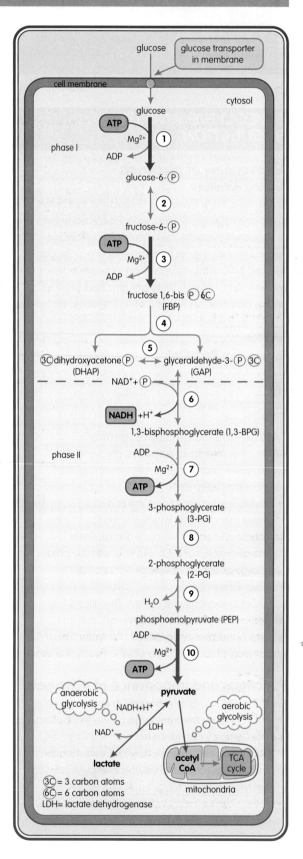

Fig. 2.2 The Embden–Meyerhof glycolytic pathway. Glycolysis takes place in the cell cytosol and consists of two distinct phases of energy investment (1–5) and energy generation (6–10). The names of the enzymes catalysing reactions 1 to 10 can be found in Fig. 2.3.

8

Stages of glycolysis		
Phase I: Energy investment phase		
Step	**Enzyme**	**Type of reaction**
1.	hexokinase: most tissues (glucokinase in liver and β cells of pancreas)	phosphorylation **irreversible regulatory step**
2.	phosphoglucose isomerase	isomerization aldose → ketose
3.	phosphofructokinase-1 (PFK-1)	phosphorylation **irreversible rate-limiting step of glycolysis**
4.	aldolase	cleavage FBP (6C) → DHAP(3C) + GAP(3C)
5.	triose phosphate isomerase	isomerization therefore phase I produces two molecules of glyceraldehyde-3-phosphate (GAP)
Phase II: Energy generating phase the following reactions occur for each molecule of glyceraldehyde-3-phosphate		
6.	glyceraldehyde-3-phosphate dehydrogenase	oxidative phosphorylation 2 NADH are generated per molecule of glucose oxidized
7.	phosphoglycerate kinase	substrate-level phosphorylation
8.	phosphoglycerate mutase	transfer of phosphate group from C3 to C2
9.	enolase	dehydration
10.	pyruvate kinase	substrate-level phosphorylation **irreversible regulatory step**
	N.B. All kinases require Mg^{2+} as a co-factor	

Fig. 2.3 Stages of glycolysis. Steps 1 to 10 refer to reactions 1 to 10 in Fig. 2.2.

Synthesis of ATP

ATP can be synthesized from ADP by two processes: substrate level phosphorylation and oxidative phosphorylation.

Substrate level phosphorylation

Substrate level phosphorylation is the formation of ATP by the direct phosphorylation of ADP, that is, the direct

The name of an enzyme can be easily worked out, if you forget it, by knowing the name of the substrate and the type of reaction involved (Fig. 2.4). For example, pyruvate is phosphorylated by pyruvate kinase.

Enzymes and the types of reactions they catalyse	
Enzyme	**Type of reaction**
kinase	phosphorylation
mutase	transfer of a functional group from one position to another in the same molecule
isomerase	conversion of one isomer into another (isomers are compounds with the same chemical formula, e.g. fructose and glucose are both $C_6H_{12}O_6$)
synthase	synthesis of molecule
carboxylase decarboxylase	addition of CO_2 removal of CO_2
dehydrogenase	oxidation–reduction reaction

Fig. 2.4 Enzymes and the types of reactions they catalyse.

transfer of a phosphoryl group from a 'high-energy' intermediate to ADP. It does not require oxygen and is therefore important for ATP generation in tissues short of oxygen, for example in active skeletal muscle. Reactions 7 and 10 of glycolysis (see Fig. 2.2) are both examples of substrate level phosphorylation. Further examples are found in Fig. 2.25.

Oxidative phosphorylation

Oxidative phosphorylation requires oxygen and is the most important mechanism for the synthesis of ATP. It involves the oxidation of NADH and the reduced form of flavin adenine dinucleotide (FADH$_2$) by the electron transport chain. This is discussed fully on p. 24.

Energy yield of glycolysis
Anaerobic glycolysis
The overall reaction can be written as:

Glucose + 2Pi + 2ADP → 2 lactate + 2ATP + 2H$_2$O

The net effect is the generation of two moles of ATP from the anaerobic oxidation of one mole of glucose (Fig. 2.5). There is no net production of NADH because it is used by lactate dehydrogenase to reduce pyruvate to lactate. It is important to remember that although anaerobic glycolysis only produces a small amount of ATP, it is an extremely valuable energy source for cells when the oxygen supply is limited.

Aerobic glycolysis
The overall reaction can be written as:

Glucose + 2Pi + 2NAD$^+$ + 2ADP → 2 pyruvate + 2ATP + 2NADH + 2H$^+$ + H$_2$O

Two moles of NADH are generated from the oxidation of one mole of glucose; each NADH is oxidized by the electron transport chain to yield about 2.5 ATP. Therefore the net effect of aerobic glycolysis is the generation of 7 ATP per mole of glucose (2 directly by

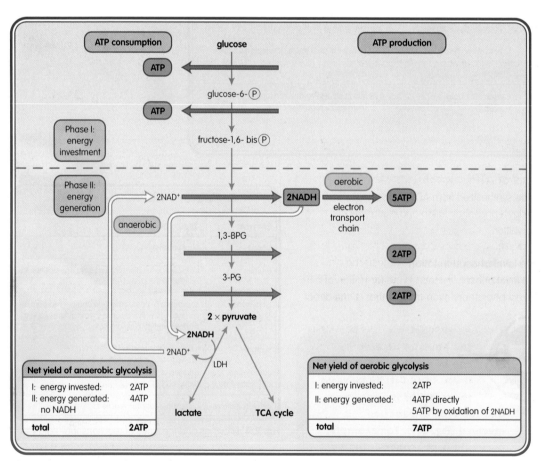

Fig. 2.5 ATP yield from aerobic and anaerobic glycolysis showing the two phases of energy investment and energy generation. (Refer to text for explanation of ATP yields.).

substrate level phosphorylation and about 5 indirectly by oxidative phosphorylation) (see Fig. 2.5).

Importance of NAD+ regeneration from NADH

NAD+ is the primary oxidizing agent of glycolysis and an important co-factor for glyceraldehyde-3-phosphate dehydrogenase (reaction 6 in Fig. 2.2). However, there is only a limited amount of NAD+ available and therefore a major problem is its regeneration from NADH, which is essential for glycolysis to continue. There are three possible mechanisms for the regeneration of NAD+:

- Firstly, under anaerobic conditions, pyruvate is reduced to lactate by lactate dehydrogenase with the simultaneous oxidation of NADH to NAD+ in the cell cytosol (see Fig. 2.2). This is a reversible reaction in which the direction is determined by the ratio of NADH to NAD+.
- Secondly, under aerobic conditions, NADH is oxidized to NAD+ by the electron transport chain in mitochondria. NADH must first enter the mitochondria either via the glycerol-3-phosphate shuttle or the malate–aspartate shuttle (Figs 2.6 and 2.7).
- Thirdly, under anaerobic conditions in yeast (alcoholic fermentation), pyruvate is decarboxylated to CO2 and acetaldehyde, which is then reduced by NADH to yield NAD+ and ethanol.

Relevance of a high concentration of lactate in the blood

If anaerobic glycolysis continues, lactate will accumulate. The concentration of lactate in the blood is normally about 1 mmol/L. A blood lactate concentration of about 5 mmol/L is regarded as high and is called hyperlactataemia; a concentration greater than this is called lactic acidosis. During lactic acidosis the blood pH may decrease from the normal range (7.35–7.45). Mild lactic acidosis may be caused by intense exercise such as sprinting, leading to increased lactate production and muscle cramps (this is covered later in Chapter 7). Severe lactic acidosis may be the result of tissue hypoxia occurring, for example, because of circulatory collapse or shock such as in myocardial infarction or massive haemorrhage.

Functions of the malate–aspartate and glycerol-3-phosphate shuttles

NADH produced by glycolysis must first enter the mitochondrial matrix before it can be oxidized by the electron transport chain to make ATP. The inner mitochondrial membrane is impermeable to NADH and there is no carrier protein present in the membrane to transport it across. Therefore, instead of transporting NADH itself across, its two 'high energy' electrons are transported into mitochondria by shuttle mechanisms. In the glycerol-3-phosphate shuttle (located mainly in brain and muscle cells), electrons are transferred from NADH to FADH$_2$ (see Fig. 2.6), which in turn donates them to the electron transport chain to generate 1.5 ATP. In the malate–aspartate shuttle (located mainly in liver and heart cells), electrons of cytosolic NADH are transferred to mitochondrial NADH (see Fig. 2.7); they are then transferred to the electron transport chain to make about 2.5 moles of ATP.

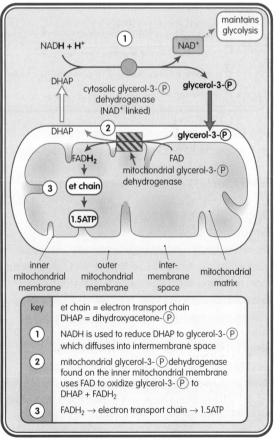

Fig. 2.6 The glycerol-3-phosphate shuttle located mainly in brain and muscle cells.

Carbohydrate and Energy Metabolism

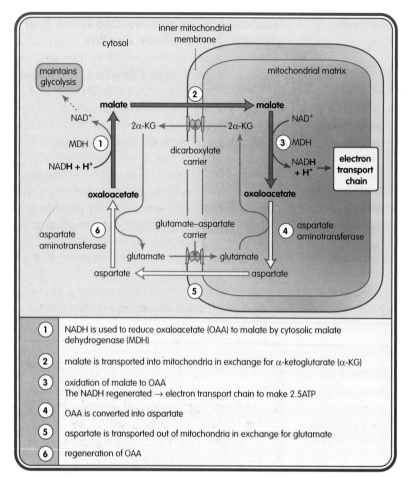

Fig. 2.7 The malate–aspartate shuttle is located mainly in liver and heart cells.
N.B. the outer mitochondrial membrane is not shown.

1	NADH is used to reduce oxaloacetate (OAA) to malate by cytosolic malate dehydrogenase (MDH)
2	malate is transported into mitochondria in exchange for α-ketoglutarate (α-KG)
3	oxidation of malate to OAA The NADH regenerated → electron transport chain to make 2.5ATP
4	OAA is converted into aspartate
5	aspartate is transported out of mitochondria in exchange for glutamate
6	regeneration of OAA

The functions of the shuttles are therefore to:
- Transport electrons from NADH into mitochondria for ATP generation by the electron transport chain.
- Regenerate NAD+ to allow glycolysis to continue.

Regulation of glycolysis
Regulation sites
Three reactions in glycolysis are essentially irreversible, namely steps 1, 3, and 10 (see Fig. 2.2) and constitute the main regulatory sites of glycolysis (ΔG is negative and exergonic for each reaction). The control of these steps and the enzymes catalysing them is now discussed.

Step 1: Hexokinase ($\Delta G = -17$ kJ/mol)
Hexokinase is controlled by product inhibition: high levels of glucose-6-phosphate allosterically inhibit it (see Fig. 2.11). Hexokinase is present in most cells and has a high affinity for glucose (Km = 0.1 mM). The enzyme is therefore most active when the concentration of glucose in the blood is low or limiting, for example, following an overnight fast or muscle during exercise.

In the liver and β cells of the pancreas, hexokinase is replaced by glucokinase, which has a lower affinity for glucose (Km = 10 mM). Glucokinase is activated by high concentrations of glucose in the blood, and by insulin; therefore it is active after a carbohydrate-rich meal. It is not inhibited by glucose-6-phosphate, which enables the liver to respond to high blood glucose levels. Therefore, dietary glucose goes to the liver to be dealt with by glucokinase before it enters the systemic circulation preventing hyperglycaemia (high blood glucose).

Step 3: Phosphofructokinase-1 ($\Delta G = -14$ kJ/mol)
Phosphofructokinase-1 (PFK-1) is the most important regulatory enzyme because it catalyses the rate-limiting step and is also the first reaction unique to glycolysis. It may be regulated in two ways:

Regulation of PFK-1 by energy levels
High ATP levels allosterically inhibit PFK-1 because they indicate an 'energy-rich' cell and therefore there is no

12

need for further energy generation by glycolysis. Increased ATP levels also lower the affinity of PFK-1 for its substrate, fructose-6-phosphate.

Citrate enhances the inhibitory effect of ATP. This is because an increased citrate level indicates an abundance of products and metabolic intermediates (e.g. pyruvate, acetyl CoA, and oxaloacetate) and therefore there is no need to break down more glucose.

Increased levels of adenosine monophosphate (AMP) allosterically activate PFK-1 because they signal that energy stores are depleted.

Regulation of PFK-1 by fructose 2,6-bisphosphate

Fructose 2,6-bisphosphate (F2,6-BP) is formed by the phosphorylation of fructose-6-phosphate catalysed by phosphofructokinase-2 (PFK-2). It is converted back again by fructose 2,6-bisphosphatase (Fig. 2.9). The properties and actions of F2,6-BP are:

- It is the most potent allosteric activator of PFK-1 and glycolysis (Fig. 2.8).
- Specifically it increases the affinity of PFK-1 for its substrate, fructose-6-phosphate and it relieves inhibition of PFK-1 by ATP.
- In the liver, it inhibits fructose 1,6-bisphosphatase, an enzyme of gluconeogenesis (the pathway responsible for making glucose that is unique to the liver; see Fig. 5.17).

Therefore the reciprocal action of F2,6-BP ensures that the glycolytic (glucose breakdown) and gluconeogenic (glucose forming) pathways are not active at the same time (see Fig. 2.8).

Regulation of fructose 2,6-bisphosphate

Since F2,6-BP is such an important allosteric activator of glycolysis, its concentration must be carefully regulated. Its concentration is controlled by hormone-dependent reversible phosphorylation of PFK-2 and fructose 2,6-bisphosphatase, the enzymes responsible for its synthesis and breakdown (see Fig. 2.9).

In the liver, an increase in the ratio of insulin to glucagon (e.g. following a meal) leads to dephosphorylation and activation of PFK-2, resulting in an increase in the synthesis of F2,6-BP and thus in the rate of glycolysis. A decrease in the ratio of insulin to glucagon, such as occurs during starvation, leads to phosphorylation and activation of fructose 2,6-bisphosphatase, decreasing the amount of F2,6-BP and the rate of glycolysis.

Step 10: Pyruvate kinase ($\Delta G = -31$ kJ/mol)

Pyruvate kinase catalyses the final step of glycolysis and is subject to both allosteric regulation and hormone-dependent reversible phosphorylation. Fig 2.10 illustrates the regulation of pyruvate kinase.

Hormonal regulation of glycolysis

Insulin, released after the consumption of a carbohydrate-rich meal, increases the synthesis and thus the amount of the enzymes glucokinase, PFK-1, and pyruvate kinase; this is known as induction. The increased synthesis of all three enzymes leads overall

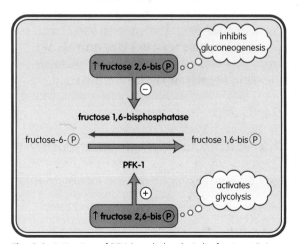

Fig. 2.8 Activation of PFK-1 and glycolysis by fructose 2,6-bisphosphate.

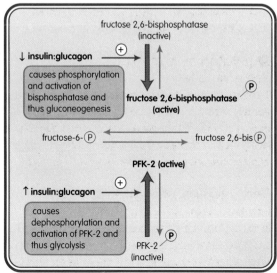

Fig. 2.9 Control of fructose 2,6-bisphosphate production by hormone-dependent reversible phosphorylation of PFK-2 and fructose 2,6-bisphosphatase.

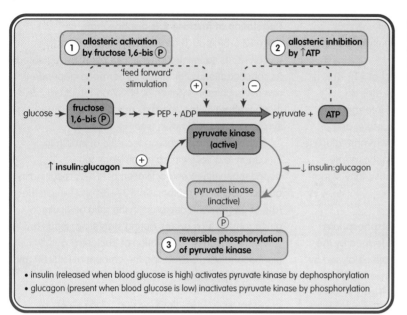

Fig. 2.10 The regulation of pyruvate kinase is carried out by allosteric activation and inhibition and also by hormone-dependent reversible phosphorylation of the enzyme.

- insulin (released when blood glucose is high) activates pyruvate kinase by dephosphorylation
- glucagon (present when blood glucose is low) inactivates pyruvate kinase by phosphorylation

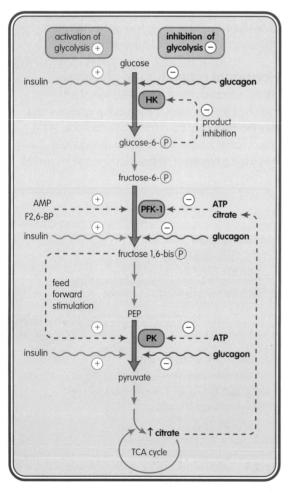

- What is the working definition of glycolysis?
- What are the main functions of glycolysis?
- Know the location and the site of the pathway.
- What is the fate of pyruvate in anaerobic and aerobic glycolysis?
- Describe the overall reaction sequence noting the three important regulatory sites.
- Know the ATP yield of anaerobic compared with aerobic glycolysis.
- What is the importance of the glycerol-3-phosphate and malate–aspartate shuttles?
- What are the main branch points of glycolysis?

Fig. 2.11 Overall regulation of glycolysis. Remember, whilst this looks very complicated, the regulation of glycolysis can be divided into allosteric control and hormonal control. Refer back to Chapter 1 for a summary of the mechanisms of control if necessary. (F2,6-BP, fructose 2,6-bisphosphate.)

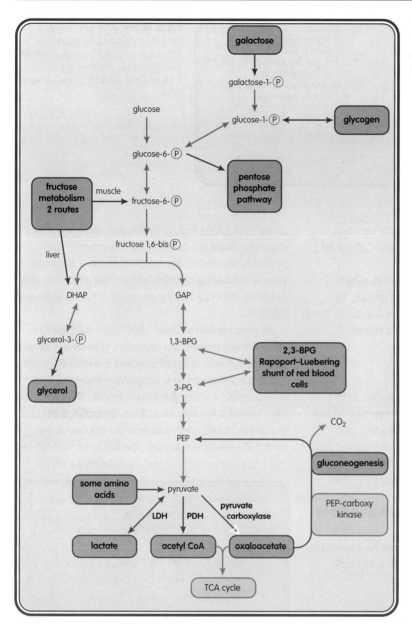

Fig. 2.12 The branch points of glycolysis, which lead off to many other pathways. All these pathways are covered later in the book.

to an increase in the rate of glycolysis. When glucagon levels are high (e.g. in starvation or diabetes), there is a decrease in the synthesis of these enzymes (repression) and therefore a decrease in the rate of glycolysis.

The overall regulation of glycolysis is mapped out in Fig. 2.11.

The branch points of glycolysis, that is, where it leads into other pathways, are shown in Fig. 2.12. This figure also illustrates how a number of glycolytic intermediates serve as 'entry points' for other sugars or substrates into glycolysis.

CENTRAL ROLE OF ACETYL CoA

Structure of acetyl CoA

Acetyl CoA is formed from co-enzyme A (abbreviated to CoA or CoASH). CoA is a large organic compound containing:

- An adenine group.
- A ribose sugar.
- Pantothenic acid (B vitamin).
- A sulphydryl or thiol group (–SH), the active group.

The thiol group (–SH) of CoA reacts with carboxyl groups

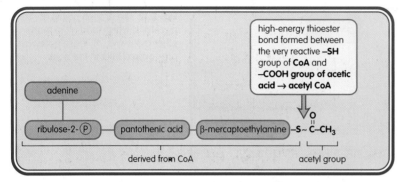

Fig. 2.13 The structure of acetyl CoA. Acetyl CoA is made by the formation of a high-energy thioester bond between the thiol group of CoA and the –COOH group of acetic acid.

(–COOH) to form acyl CoA molecules. If the carboxyl group is an acetyl group (CH_3COO^-), acetyl CoA will be formed.

Acetyl CoA is a high-energy compound, which enables it to serve as a donor of acetyl groups, for example, in fatty acid synthesis and the TCA cycle. It is a carrier of acetyl groups just like ATP is a carrier of phosphate groups.

Central role of acetyl CoA

Acetyl CoA plays a central role in metabolism, in fact, most energy-generating metabolic pathways of the cell eventually produce it. It can be formed from carbohydrate, fat, and protein. It is also the starting point for the synthesis of fats, steroids, and ketone bodies. Its oxidation provides energy for many tissues (Fig. 2.14).

Formation of acetyl CoA from pyruvate
Working definition
Pyruvate dehydrogenase (PDH) catalyses the irreversible, oxidative decarboxylation of pyruvate to acetyl CoA.

Location
Mitochondria, specifically the inner face of the inner mitochondrial membrane.

Significance
The formation of acetyl CoA is completely irreversible; $\Delta G = -33.4\,kJ/mol$. Therefore, pyruvate cannot be formed from acetyl CoA, that is, carbohydrates can be converted to fats but not vice versa. This reaction is a key point in metabolism because it means there can be no net synthesis of glucose from fatty acids (Fig. 2.15).

Pyruvate dehydrogenase
PDH is a multi-enzyme complex consisting of three enzymes E1, E2, and E3. A multi-enzyme complex is a

group of enzymes that catalyse two or more sequential steps in a metabolic pathway. As the enzymes are physically associated, the reactions occur in sequence without the release of intermediates; this minimizes side reactions. PDH requires the presence of five co-enzymes (Fig. 2.16).

The mechanism of action of PDH is a complex, five-step pathway and it is not necessary to know it in detail. Basically pyruvate is decarboxylated and then an acetyl group is transferred first to lipoate and then to CoA to form acetyl CoA. Thiamine pyrophosphate (TPP) and CoA are involved in the transfer of the two-carbon acetyl group. NAD^+, FAD, and lipoic acid are involved in the oxidation–reduction reactions. The NADH formed can be

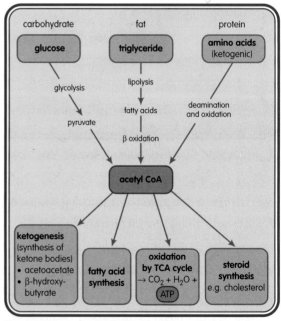

Fig. 2.14 The central role that acetyl CoA plays in metabolism The main pathways that produce and utilize acetyl CoA.

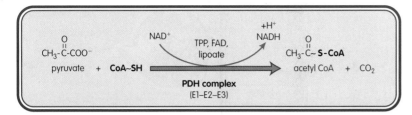

Fig. 2.15 The overall reaction describing the formation of acetyl CoA. The reaction is completely irreversible.

oxidized by the electron transport chain to generate 2.5 moles of ATP.

The control of pyruvate dehydrogenase
PDH is controlled by two mechanisms; allosteric control and reversible phosphorylation (see Fig. 2.17).

1. Allosteric control—product inhibition
NADH and acetyl CoA compete with NAD^+ and CoA for binding sites on the enzymes. NADH specifically inhibits E3 and acetyl CoA specifically inhibits E2.

2. Regulation by reversible phosphorylation of PDH
The PDH complex can exist in two forms: an active non-phosphorylated form and an inactive phosphorylated form (see Fig. 2.17). Associated with the PDH complex are two enzymes, PDH kinase and PDH phosphatase, which have important regulatory roles.

PDH kinase catalyses the phosphorylation and thus inactivation of PDH. PDH kinase is activated by the products NADH and acetyl CoA resulting in inactivation

Components of pyruvate dehydrogenase complex		
Enzyme	Name of enzyme	Co-enzymes
E1	pyruvate decarboxylase	TPP
E2	dihydrolipoyl transacetylase	lipoic acid CoA
E3	dihydrolipoyl dehydrogenase	FAD NAD^+

Fig. 2.16 Components of the pyruvate dehydrogenase complex. Note that four of the five co-factors are vitamin B derivatives.

of PDH; this is in addition to their direct, allosteric effect on the PDH complex. PDH kinase is also activated by an increase in the ATP to ADP ratio since this signifies an 'energy-rich' cell and thus a decreased need for energy production by the TCA cycle.

PDH phosphatase dephosphorylates and thus activates PDH. It is activated by insulin and Ca^{2+}, which lead to an increase in the formation of acetyl CoA.

Deficiency of thiamin
A dietary deficiency of thiamin (vitamin B_1) leads to a deficiency of the co-enzyme thiamine pyrophosphate. This results in a decrease in the activity of PDH and an accumulation of pyruvate. The excess pyruvate is converted into lactate, which may build up in the blood, leading to lactic acidosis. Vitamin B_1 deficiency can lead to:
- Beriberi, a neurological and cardiovascular disorder.
- Wernicke's syndrome, which is seen in nutritionally deprived alcoholics who are thiamin deficient. It may progress to Korsakoff's psychosis, which is an irreversible amnesic syndrome characterized by impairment of short-term memory (this is discussed further in Chapters 8 and 13).

Inherited PDH deficiency is very rare and presents with a similar lactic acidosis. The build-up of lactate may lead to severe neurological defects.

You should know thoroughly the role of acetyl CoA in metabolism because it is a common essay question.
Be able to briefly discuss the pathways that produce and utilize acetyl CoA (Fig. 2.14) and under what conditions they are particularly active. For example, ketogenesis is active at low levels most of the time, but during prolonged starvation it becomes very important!

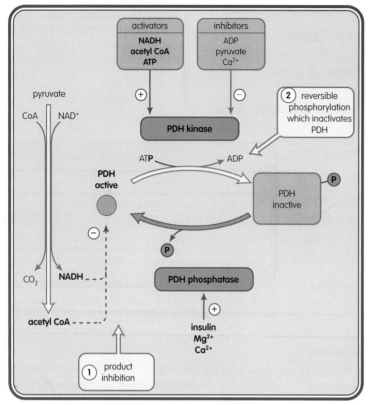

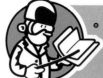

○ **Describe the role of acetyl CoA as a carrier of acetyl groups and appreciate its central role in metabolism.**
○ **What is the significance of the irreversible, oxidative decarboxylation of pyruvate to carbohydrate metabolism?**
○ **Know the location, enzyme, and co-enzymes involved.**
○ **What is the significance of the inhibition of pyruvate dehydrogenase (i.e. diverting pyruvate to lactate production)?**

Fig. 2.17 The control of PDH complex by product inhibition and reversible phosphorylation (numbers refer to text on p.17).

THE TRICARBOXYLIC ACID CYCLE

The TCA cycle is also known as the citric acid cycle or the Kreb's cycle.

Working definition

A cyclical series of eight reactions that oxidize one molecule of acetyl CoA completely to two molecules of CO_2 generating energy, either directly as ATP or in the form of reducing equivalents (NADH or $FADH_2$). The cycle is aerobic; the absence or a deficiency of oxygen leads to total or partial inhibition of the cycle.

Location

All mammalian cells that contain mitochondria (i.e. not red blood cells).

Site

All the enzymes are found free in the mitochondrial matrix, except succinate dehydrogenase, which is found on the inner face of the inner mitochondrial membrane.

Functions

- The TCA cycle provides a final common pathway for the oxidation of carbohydrate, fat, and protein since glucose, fatty acids, and many amino acids, are all metabolized to acetyl CoA or to other intermediates of the cycle (see Fig. 2.23).
- The main function of the cycle is the production of energy, either directly as ATP or as the reducing equivalents NADH or $FADH_2$, which are oxidized by the electron transport chain. Each turn of the cycle produces 10 molecules of ATP; it is therefore the main pathway for energy generation in mammals.
- The cycle provides substrates for the electron transport chain.
- The cycle is also a source of biosynthetic precursors, for example, porphyrin is synthesized from succinyl CoA or amino acids are synthesized from oxaloacetate and α-ketoglutarate.
- Some of the cycle intermediates also exert regulatory effects on other pathways; for example, citrate inhibits PFK-1 in glycolysis.

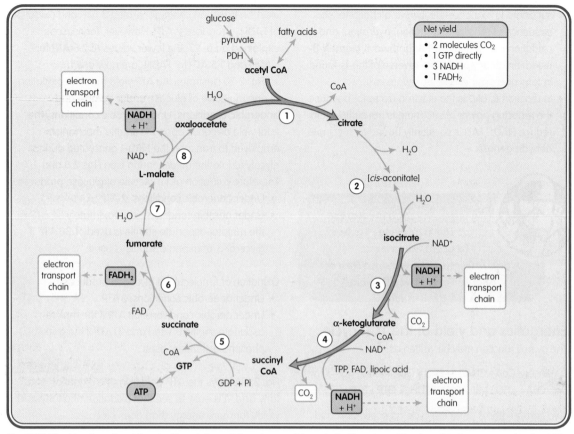

Fig. 2.18 The tricarboxylic acid cycle. Steps 1, 3, and 4 are irreversible, rate-limiting steps. Numbers 1 to 8 correspond to Fig. 2.19.

The stages of the TCA cycle	
Types of reaction	**Enzyme**
stage I: 1. condensation: 2C + 4C = 6C	citrate synthase
stage II: 2. isomerization: two steps: dehydration then rehydration	aconitase
3. oxidative decarboxylation: 6C → 5C	isocitrate dehydrogenase
4. oxidative decarboxylation: 5C → 4C	α-ketoglutarate dehydrogenase complex requires co-enzymes TPP, FAD, lipoic acid, NAD⁺, and CoA (like PDH)
5. substrate-level phosphorylation	succinyl CoA synthetase nucleoside diphosphate kinase catalyses GTP → ATP
stage III: 6. oxidation 7. hydration 8. oxidation	succinate dehydrogenase fumarase malate dehydrogenase

In summary, the cycle occupies a pivotal role in metabolism and is considered to be an amphibolic pathway, that is, it operates both catabolically (oxidation of substrates) and anabolically (synthetic reactions).

Stages of the TCA cycle

The cycle can be subdivided into three stages based on the role oxaloacetate plays as a carrier of acetyl CoA (Figs 2.18 and 2.19).

- Stage I: the attachment of acetyl CoA to the oxaloacetate carrier (reaction 1).
- Stage II: the breakup of the carrier (reactions 2 to 5).
- Stage III: the regeneration of the carrier (reactions 6 to 8).

It is important to know that:

- Steps 1, 3, and 4 are irreversible rate-limiting steps.
- The last three steps of the TCA cycle that convert

Fig. 2.19 The stages of the TCA cycle (numbers 1–8 refer to Fig. 2.18).

succinate to oxaloacetate involve a characteristic sequence of reactions: oxidation, hydration, and oxidation also found in other pathways, namely β-oxidation of fatty acids. The reverse of this is found in fatty acid synthesis so be aware of it.

- In reaction 6, FAD is the electron acceptor because the reducing power of succinate is not sufficient to reduce NAD^+. FAD is covalently bound to succinate dehydrogenase.

> To learn the intermediates of the TCA cycle it is best to use a mnemonic:
> e.g. A Certificate In Kama Sutra Should Further My Orgasm!

Energetics and yield of the TCA cycle

The overall reaction may be written as:

$$Acetyl\ CoA + 3NAD^+ + FAD + GDP + Pi + 2H_2O \rightarrow$$
$$CoA + 2CO_2 + 3NADH + FADH_2 + GTP + 3H^+$$

Two carbon atoms enter the cycle as acetyl CoA and two carbon atoms leave it as CO_2 (but they are not the same carbon atoms). There is no net consumption or production of oxaloacetate or any other intermediates of the cycle.

One molecule of ATP is generated directly by substrate level phosphorylation, reaction 5, from guanosine triphosphate (GTP). Three molecules of NADH and one of $FADH_2$ are produced for each molecule of acetyl CoA oxidized by the cycle (reactions 3, 4, 5, and 8). They are then oxidized by the electron transport chain on the inner mitochondrial membrane, generating ATP by oxidative phosphorylation. Remember, the oxidation of NADH by the electron transport chain yields 2.5 ATP and the oxidation of $FADH_2$ yields 1.5 ATP since it joins the chain further down, bypassing the first oxidative phosphorylation site (see Fig. 2.26).

Therefore the ATP yield for each molecule of acetyl CoA oxidized (i.e. per turn of cycle) is:

- 1 ATP directly by substrate level phosphorylation.
- 9 ATP indirectly by the oxidative phosphorylation of three NADH (3×2.5 ATP) and one $FADH_2$ (1×1.5 ATP) by the electron transport chain; giving a total of 10 ATP.

It was previously thought that oxidation of NADH by the

electron transport chain generated 3 ATP and oxidation of $FADH_2$ produced 2 ATP. However, for reasons explained on p. 27, the lower values of 2.5 ATP for NADH and 1.5 ATP for $FADH_2$ are now used.

Fig. 2.20 illustrates the ATP yield from the oxidation of one molecule of glucose under aerobic and anaerobic conditions. Under aerobic conditions, the total yield depends upon the shuttle mechanism employed to transport the NADH generated during glycolysis into the mitochondria (see Figs 2.6 and 2.7). Therefore oxidation of 1 molecule of glucose produces:

- Under anaerobic conditions: 2 ATP
- Under aerobic conditions: approximately 32 ATP if the malate–aspartate shuttle is used or 30 ATP if glycerol-3-phosphate shuttle is used.

Oxidation of 1 molecule of glycogen produces:

- Under anaerobic conditions: 3 ATP
- Under aerobic conditions: 33 ATP if the malate-aspartate shuttle is used and 31 ATP if the glycerol-3-phosphate shuttle is used.

Fig. 2.21 shows the ATP yield from the oxidation of a fatty acid: it is easy to see that oxidation of a fatty acid yields far more energy than does glucose.

Please note that the exact ATP yields for these processes are still a matter of debate amongst biochemists. However, it is not the exact values that are important but rather, the concepts involved.

Regulation of the TCA cycle

The TCA cycle is a central pathway of metabolism; it oxidizes acetyl CoA derived from carbohydrate, fat, and protein and provides substrates for a number of synthetic reactions. Its regulation must therefore be coordinated to satisfy the demands of other pathways in a number of tissues. PDH (see Fig. 2.15) determines whether or not pyruvate enters the TCA cycle, that is, it 'guards the door' to the cycle.

The control of the cycle itself can be considered at two levels; allosteric regulation and respiratory control.

Regulation at the level of the cycle: allosteric regulation of enzyme activities

There are three key enzymes, all of which catalyse irreversible reactions:

- Citrate synthase.
- Isocitrate dehydrogenase.
- α-ketoglutarate dehydrogenase.

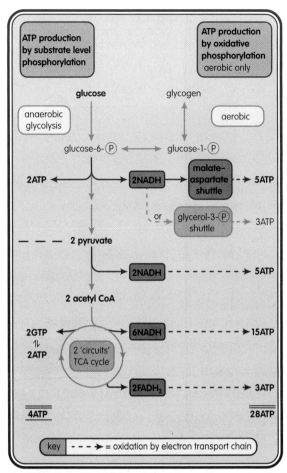

Fig. 2.20 The ATP yield from the oxidation of one molecule of glucose under aerobic and anaerobic conditions. Interestingly, the oxidation of one molecule of glycogen 'saves' an ATP molecule. The extra ATP comes from the fact glycogen is broken down into glucose-1-phosphate, bypassing the need for the first phosphorylation step of glycolysis.

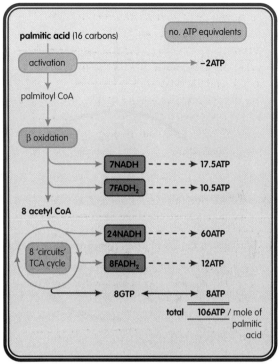

Fig. 2.21 The ATP yield from the oxidation of palmitic acid to acetyl CoA.

All are activated by Ca^{2+}, the levels of which are increased for example, during muscular contraction, thus increasing the rate of the cycle and ATP generation to cope with the increased energy demand of the muscle. The enzymes are also regulated by the ATP and NADH requirements of the cell. An increase in ATP, NADH, or the concentration of products indicates a high energy status of the cell and therefore less need for energy production by the TCA cycle, thereby inhibiting it (see Fig. 2.22).

Respiratory control

The overriding control of the TCA cycle is by respiratory control, which is governed by the activity of the electron transport chain (which oxidizes NADH and $FADH_2$) and the rate of oxidative phosphorylation (ATP synthesis).

How does this occur?

- The activity of the TCA cycle is dependent on a continuous supply of NAD^+ and FAD, co-factors for the dehydrogenases.
- The electron transport chain is responsible for oxidizing any NADH and $FADH_2$ formed during glycolysis and the TCA cycle back to their oxidized forms i.e. NAD^+ and FAD.
- As the activity of the electron transport chain is tightly coupled to the generation of ATP by oxidative phosphorylation (see Fig. 2.26), the TCA cycle is also dependent on the ADP:ATP ratio.
- Therefore, anything affecting the supply of substrates namely oxygen, ADP, or the source of reducing equivalents (NAD^+ or FAD), may inhibit the cycle.

The TCA cycle is a source of intermediates for biosynthesis

The TCA cycle, as well as being a degradative pathway for the generation of ATP, has most of its intermediates as substrates for biosynthetic pathways (remember: an

21

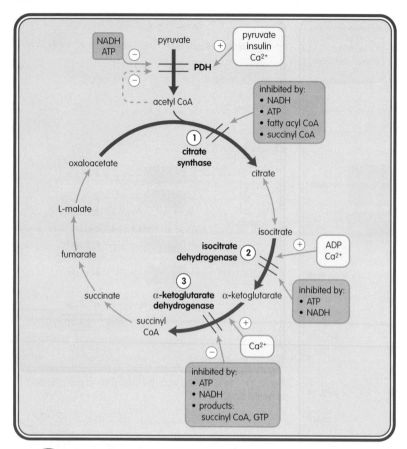

Fig. 2.22 Regulation of the TCA cycle. The three rate-limiting reactions (numbered) of the TCA cycle are all inhibited by ATP and NADH.

Remember the principle of respiratory control says that:

The rate of oxidative phosphorylation is proportional to $\dfrac{\textbf{[ADP] [Pi]}}{\textbf{[ATP]}}$

For example:

- **A low concentration of ADP or phosphate (i.e. less substrate available) leads to a drop in the rate of ATP formation.**
  As electron transport and ATP synthesis are coupled, electron transport and thus NADH and FADH2 oxidation will also decrease.
  Therefore, high ATP:ADP or NADH:NAD⁺ inhibits the TCA cycle.
- **Secondly, if the concentration of ADP increases, the production of ATP increases until it matches the rate of consumption by energy-requiring reactions such as muscle contraction or biosynthetic reactions.**

amphibolic pathway). The main synthetic pathways that use TCA cycle intermediates are:

- Lipid synthesis: both fatty acids and cholesterol are made from acetyl CoA in the cytosol. Acetyl CoA formed in the mitochondria cannot cross the inner mitochondrial membrane but citrate can. Cytosolic acetyl CoA is recovered from the breakdown of

citrate by ATP–citrate lyase (see Fig. 2.23).

- Amino acid synthesis: for example, aspartate from oxaloacetate and glutamate from α-ketoglutarate (see Chapter 5).
- Porphyrin biosynthesis: from succinyl CoA (see Chapter 6).
- Gluconeogenesis (glucose synthesis): this occurs in

the cell cytosol from oxaloacetate. However oxaloacetate cannot cross the inner mitochondrial membrane but malate can. Malate is reconverted to oxaloacetate in the cytosol (Fig. 5.17).

The intermediates that are used for synthetic reactions must be replaced for the TCA cycle to be able to continue. For example, if oxaloacetate is used to make amino acids for protein synthesis it must be reformed. The carboxylation of pyruvate by pyruvate carboxylase reforms the oxaloacetate.

$$\text{Pyruvate} + \text{ATP} + CO_2 + H_2O \leftrightarrow \text{oxaloacetate} + \text{ADP} + \text{ Pi}$$

This is an example of an anaplerotic reaction, that is, it replenishes or fills up the intermediates of the cycle.

Others include (see Fig. 2.23):

- The oxidation of odd-chain fatty acids to succinyl CoA.
- The breakdown of various amino acids.
- The transamination and deamination of amino acids to oxaloacetate and α-ketoglutarate.

The role of the TCA cycle as a source of biosynthetic precursors is a common essay question so learn it well.

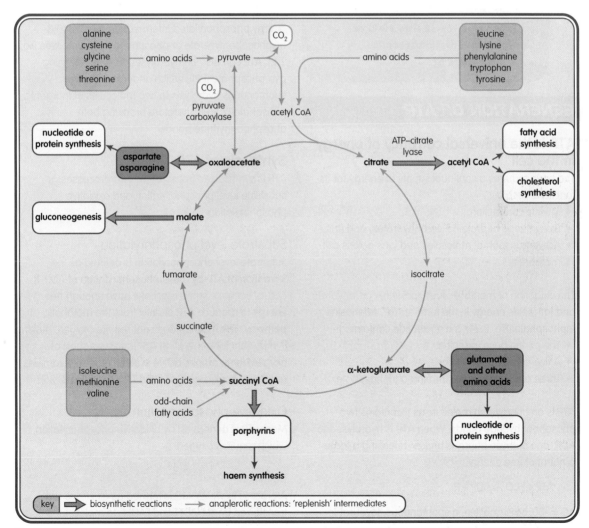

Fig. 2.23 The TCA cycle is a rich source of biosynthetic precursors which go on to form many other substances, such as porphyrins, amino acids, and fatty acids.

- **What is the working definition of the TCA cycle?**
- **Know the location, site and main functions of the TCA cycle (be able to list four).**
- **Describe the main reaction sequence noting the three important rate-limiting reactions.**
- **What is the effect of inhibition of the pathway and what does it mean to the cell and to the body as a whole?**
- **What is the energy yield of aerobic and anaerobic metabolism?**

GENERATION OF ATP

ATP is the universal currency of energy in the cell

The body requires a continual supply of energy for its functions such as:

- Muscle contraction.
- Biosynthesis of proteins, carbohydrates, and fats.
- Active transport of molecules and ions across cell membranes.

The oxidation of metabolic fuels (protein, carbohydrate, and fat) yields energy in the form of ATP. Adenosine triphosphate (Fig. 2.24) is a nucleotide containing:

- The purine base, adenine.
- A five-carbon sugar, ribose.
- Three phosphate units, forming a triphosphate.

ATP is an energy-rich molecule as it contains two phosphoanhydride bonds. When ATP is hydrolysed to ADP, one of these bonds is broken releasing a large amount of free energy:

$$ATP + H_2O \rightarrow ADP + Pi$$

$\Delta G = -30.66 \, kJ/mol$ (i.e. a spontaneous, favourable reaction)
The energy liberated is used to drive metabolic reactions

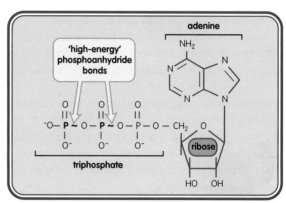

Fig. 2.24 The structure of ATP. ATP is made up of the purine adenine, the five-carbon sugar ribose, and three phosphate units linked by high-energy phosphoanhydride bonds.

and other processes. For example, in glycolysis, the hydrolysis of ATP is coupled to the formation of high-energy phosphorylated intermediates such as 1,3-bisphosphoglycerate or phosphoenolpyruvate (see Fig. 2.2). ATP can also be hydrolysed to AMP releasing pyrophosphate (PPi), which undergoes further spontaneous hydrolysis to two molecules of inorganic phosphate ($2 \times Pi$), therefore breaking both phosphoanhydride bonds.

Synthesis of ATP

ATP is synthesized from ADP by two processes; substrate level phosphorylation and oxidative phosphorylation.

Substrate level phosphorylation

Substrate level phosphorylation is defined as the formation of ATP by direct phosphorylation of ADP. It occurs because some reactions have enough free energy to produce ATP directly from the metabolic pathway. The reaction does not require oxygen, making it important for generating ATP in tissues short of oxygen, for example, active skeletal muscle. Examples are found in glycolysis and the TCA cycle (Fig. 2.25).

Oxidative phosphorylation

Most ATP is generated by oxidative phosphorylation, which requires oxygen.

Definition
A process in which ATP is formed as electrons are transferred from NADH and $FADH_2$ to molecular oxygen, via a series of electron carriers that make up the electron transport chain.

Examples of substrate level phosphorylation		
Example	**Reaction**	**Enzyme**
glycolysis	1,3-BPG + ADP ↔ 3-PG + ATP	phosphoglycerate kinase
	PEP + ADP → pyruvate + ATP	pyruvate kinase
TCA cycle	succinyl-CoA + GDP ↔ succinate + GTP	succinyl-CoA synthetase

Fig. 2.25 Examples of substrate level phosphorylation.

Location

The inner surface of the inner mitochondrial membrane in all cells that contain mitochondria.

Pyruvate from glycolysis, fatty acids via β oxidation, and some amino acids through transamination reactions provide acetyl CoA, which is oxidized by the TCA cycle to CO_2 and H_2O. During these processes high-energy electrons are donated from metabolic intermediates to the co-enzymes NAD+ and FAD to form the energy-rich reduced forms NADH and $FADH_2$. Therefore, energy is conserved as these 'reducing equivalents'.

Origin of the reduced intermediates NADH and $FADH_2$

NADH is formed via glycolysis in the cytosol and via the TCA cycle and β-oxidation in mitochondria. $FADH_2$, comes from both the TCA cycle and β oxidation in the mitochondria. NADH and $FADH_2$ donate their electrons, one at a time, to the electron transport chain. As each high-energy electron is passed down the chain it loses most of its free energy. Part of this energy is captured and used to produce ATP from ADP and inorganic phosphate.

How does this occur?

- The transport of electrons down the electron transport chain is coupled to the transport of protons across the inner mitochondrial membrane, from the mitochondrial matrix into the inner mitochondrial space (Fig. 2.26).
- This occurs at three specific 'proton-pumping' sites and thus creates an electrochemical gradient across the membrane.
- The protons are only allowed back into the mitochondrial matrix via an enzyme, ATP synthase, present in the inner mitochondrial membrane.
- The movement of protons activates ATP synthase to catalyse ATP synthesis.
- Any energy not trapped as ATP is released as heat.

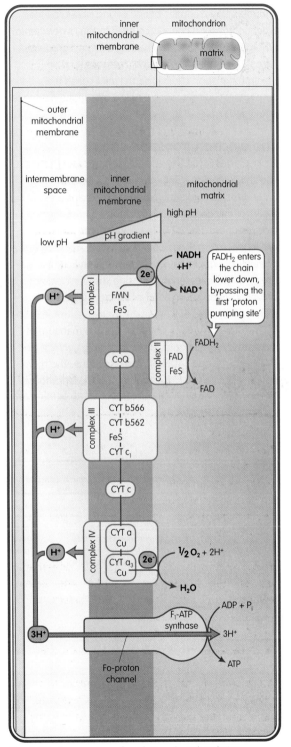

Fig. 2.26 An overview of oxidative phosphorylation showing components of the electron transport chain (refer also to Fig. 2.27).

Therefore, the oxidation of NADH and FADH$_2$ by the electron transport chain is coupled to the generation of ATP (phosphorylation) by creating a proton gradient across the inner mitochondrial membrane. (The electron transport chain is sometimes called the respiratory chain because it only works in the presence of oxygen.)

The electron transport chain
Components of the electron transport chain
The chain consists of four protein complexes (see Fig. 2.26). These are integral membrane proteins present in the inner mitochondrial membrane through which electrons pass (Fig. 2.27). The electron-carrying groups within these complexes are either flavins, iron–sulphur proteins, haem groups, or copper ions. The complexes are arranged in order of increasing standard redox potential (measured in volts) and increasing electron affinity.

The standard redox potential (Eo) is a measure of the tendency of a particular redox pair (e.g. NAD$^+$ and NADH or FAD and FADH$_2$) to lose electrons. The more negative the Eo value, the greater the tendency to lose electrons (i.e. lower electron affinity), whereas the more positive the Eo value, the more likely the redox pair is to accept electrons (higher electron affinity). Therefore, electrons flow from electron carriers with more negative Eo values to carriers with more positive Eo values, until they are passed to molecular oxygen, which has the highest Eo value.

The complexes are linked by two soluble, membrane proteins: ubiquinone (co-enzyme Q) and cytochrome c, which diffuse easily through the membrane.

The reactions within the chain
1. The oxidation of NADH or FADH$_2$ initiates electron transport down the chain.
2. Electrons of NADH are passed to complex I, whereas electrons of FADH$_2$ go directly to complex II. This is because FADH$_2$ is produced by succinate dehydrogenase, a TCA cycle enzyme, which is actually part of complex II (see Fig. 2.27).
3. Each component of the chain is alternately oxidized and reduced as electrons pass down the chain.
4. Finally, electrons are donated to molecular O$_2$, reducing it to water.

Components of the electron transport chain		
Electron carrier	**Components**	**Function**
complex I: NADH dehydrogenase	two types of redox proteins: • flavin mononucleotide (FMN) reduced by NADH → FMNH$_2$ • 1–5 iron–sulphur proteins (FeS) reduced by NADH → Fe^{3+}	enzyme catalyses the oxidation of NADH by CoQ **proton pumping site**
complex II: succinate ubiquinone reductase	TCA cycle enzyme succinate dehydrogenase FAD 1–3 iron–sulphur proteins	catalyses the oxidation of FADH$_2$ by CoQ
CoQ (ubiquinone)	quinone derivative	shuttles electrons from complexes I and II to III
complex III: ubiquinol–cytochrome c reductase	b cytochromes (b562 and b566) cytochrome c$_1$ iron–sulphur proteins	catalyses the oxidation of CoQ by cytochrome c **proton pumping site**
cytochrome c	cytochrome c	shuttles electrons between complexes III and IV
complex IV: cytochrome c oxidase	cytochromes a and a$_3$ two copper atoms	catalyses the four electron reduction of oxygen to H$_2$O **proton pumping site**

Fig. 2.27 Components of the electron transport chain. Complexes III, IV, and cytochrome c are all cytochromes and contain a haem prosthetic group. The iron atom of the haem group is reversibly oxidized and reduced, that is, it alternates between Fe^{2+} and Fe^{3+} as part of its normal function as an electron carrier.

Why use a chain of electron carriers instead of one reaction?

The oxidation of NADH leads to the pumping of protons at three sites across the membrane. When protons re-enter the matrix via ATP synthase, ATP is generated. Oxidation of NADH generates 2.5 molecules of ATP. If only a single reaction were employed, a lot of energy would be wasted, since there would be fewer proton pumping sites and thus less energy generation.

The oxidation of $FADH_2$ leads to the pumping of protons at only two sites across the membrane, bypassing the first site. This leads to only about 1.5 molecules of ATP being produced.

It is useful to note that until fairly recently it was thought that oxidation of NADH by the electron transport chain generated 3 ATP and oxidation of $FADH_2$ produced 2 ATP. However, recent studies on the ATP yield of oxidative phosphorylation have shown that the values are about 2.5 ATP for NADH and 1.5 for $FADH_2$. The reasons for the difference are complex, but basically the lower values compensate for additional protons used for phosphate transport into the mitochondrial matrix and the exchange of mitochondrial ATP for cytosolic ADP by ATP–ADP translocase.

The values 2.5 ATP for NADH and 1.5 for $FADH_2$ are used throughout this book.

Inhibitors of the respiratory chain

Inhibitors bind to a component of the chain and block the transfer of electrons at specific sites (Fig. 2.28). All the electron carriers of the chain before the block are reduced whereas those after the block remain oxidized.

Inhibitors of the electron transport chain	
Inhibitor	**Action**
rotenone and amytal	inhibits electron transfer within NADH dehydrogenase (complex I)
antimycin A	inhibits electron flow from reduced cytochrome b562 to cytochrome c_1 (complex III), therefore preventing proton pumping
cyanide, carbon monoxide, or azide	inhibits electron transfer in cytochrome oxidase (complex IV)
oligomycin and dicyclohexylcarbodiimide (DCCD)	blocks the proton channel part (Fo) of ATP synthase decreasing ATP synthesis

Fig. 2.28 Inhibitors of the electron transport chain.

As the electron transport chain and oxidative phosphorylation are tightly coupled, inhibition leads to a decrease in ATP synthesis.

Tetramethyl-*p*-phenyldiamine (TMPD) is an 'artificial electron donor': it transfers electrons directly to cytochrome c. Vitamin C (ascorbate) is required to reduce TMPD and they are both often used in combination to study the chain.

Generation of ATP via a proton gradient

The mechanism can be explained by the Chemiosmotic or Mitchell's hypothesis. The flow of electrons down the electron transport chain does not directly lead to ATP synthesis. Instead, electron transport is 'coupled' to pumping of protons across the inner mitochondrial membrane into the intermembrane space at complexes I, III, and IV. Proton translocation creates an electrochemical gradient across the membrane (both electrical and pH components). Energy stored in this proton gradient is used to make ATP by ATP synthase.

Structure of ATP synthase

ATP synthase consists of two subunits (see Fig. 2.26): Fo, a proton channel and F_1 the enzyme, ATP synthase. Protons re-enter the mitochondrial matrix normally only through the Fo proton channel. The movement of these protons activates ATP synthesis by the F_1 subunit. A flow of approximately 3 protons through ATP synthase are required to make each ATP. Therefore, electron transport and phosphorylation are 'coupled' by the proton gradient.

Uncoupling of the electron transport chain from phosphorylation

Any substance that increases the permeability of the inner mitochondrial membrane to protons, so that they can re-enter the mitochondrial matrix at sites other than ATP synthase causes uncoupling. As a result the re-entry of protons dissipates the proton gradient without ATP production.

Uncouplers

2,4-Dinitrophenol (DNP) is a lipophilic (lipid soluble) proton carrier that can diffuse freely across the inner mitochondrial membrane (see Fig. 2.29). It 'binds protons' and carries them across the membrane, dissipating the proton gradient. This results in a decreased flow of protons through ATP synthase and thus decreased ATP production (it 'short-circuits' ATP synthase). Therefore, electron transport occurs normally

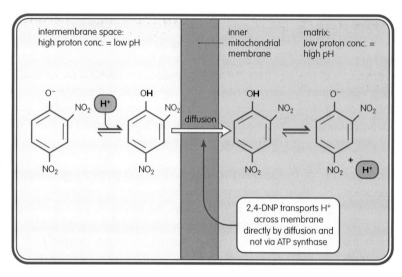

Fig. 2.29 The action of the uncoupler, 2,4-DNP is to transport protons across the mitochondrial membrane without the production of ATP, dissipating the proton gradient set up.

but with no consequent ATP production. The energy produced by electron transport is released as heat. Another uncoupling agent is FCCP (trifluoro-carbonylcyanide methoxyphenylhydrazone).

Uncoupling occurs physiologically in brown adipose tissue. Newborn babies and hibernating mammals contain brown fat, usually in their neck and upper back.

- What is the basic structure and function of ATP?
- Name the two processes of ATP production with examples.
- Define oxidative phosphorylation and know where it takes place within the cell.
- How does the electron transport chain produce ATP?
- What are the main components of the electron transport chain and which are the three proton-pumping sites?
- What is the action of inhibitors and of uncouplers on the chain?
- Describe the principle of respiratory control.

The mitochondria of brown fat contain the uncoupling protein thermogenin in their inner mitochondrial membrane. This acts as a proton channel and allows the dissipation of the proton gradient and thus the release of energy as heat, enabling them to keep warm.

Control of ATP generation: respiratory control

The principle of respiratory control is discussed on pp. 21–22 and it would be useful to recap on this now.

A supply of ADP (i.e. substrate) is necessary for ATP synthesis; a low concentration of ADP will result in decreased production of ATP. Since electron transport and ATP synthesis are tightly coupled, electron transport and thus oxidation of NADH and $FADH_2$ will also be inhibited.

GLYCOGEN METABOLISM

Role of glycogen

Excess dietary glucose is stored as glycogen. Glucose can be rapidly and easily mobilized from glycogen when the need arises, for example, between meals or during exercise. A constant supply of glucose is essential for life because it is the main fuel of the brain and the only energy source that can be used by cells lacking mitochondria or by active skeletal muscle (during anaerobic glycolysis). Glycogen is therefore an excellent short-term storage material that can provide energy immediately.

Comparison of the roles of liver and muscle glycogen		
	Liver glycogen	**Muscle glycogen**
Main function	**maintenance of blood glucose concentration**, particularly between meals and early stages of fasting	**fuel reserve for muscle contraction**
Other roles	**used as a fuel by any tissue** liver contains glucose-6-phosphatase, which removes the phosphate group from glucose-6-phosphate allowing glucose to leave the liver	none: **cannot leave muscle** muscle lacks glucose-6-phosphatase therefore glucose-6-phosphate cannot leave; enters glycolysis to generate energy instead
Size of stores	approximately 10% wet weight of liver; **stores last only about 12–24 h during a fast**	approximately 1–2% wet weight of muscle (however, humans have much more muscle than liver glycogen; and therefore about twice as much muscle glycogen as liver glycogen)
Hormonal control	glucagon and adrenaline promote glycogen breakdown insulin promotes synthesis	adrenaline promotes glycogen breakdown insulin promotes synthesis

Fig. 2.30 A comparison of the roles of liver and muscle glycogen.

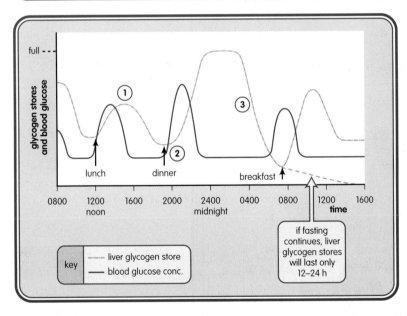

Fig. 2.31 A graph showing the approximate variation of liver glycogen stores and blood glucose against the time of day.
1. After a meal, glycogen stores rise; between meals glycogen stores fall as glucose is released from liver glycogen to help maintain the concentration of glucose in the blood.
2. After a meal there is an increase in blood glucose; between meals it stabilizes.
3. Overnight glycogen stores are mobilized to help maintain blood glucose concentration.

Glycogen stores

The main stores of glycogen are in muscle and in the liver where they have different functions (Fig. 2.30). Remember that muscle glycogen cannot leave muscle and therefore cannot contribute to the concentration of glucose in the blood. Fig. 2.31 is a graph showing the variation in liver glycogen stores and blood glucose plotted against the time of day.

Structure of glycogen

Glycogen is a large, highly branched polymer of glucose molecules. There are two types of linkages found between the glucose molecules (see Fig. 2.32a):
- Most are joined by an α-1,4 linkage to make straight chains.
- An α-1,6 linkage occurs every eight to 12 glucose residues to make branch points.

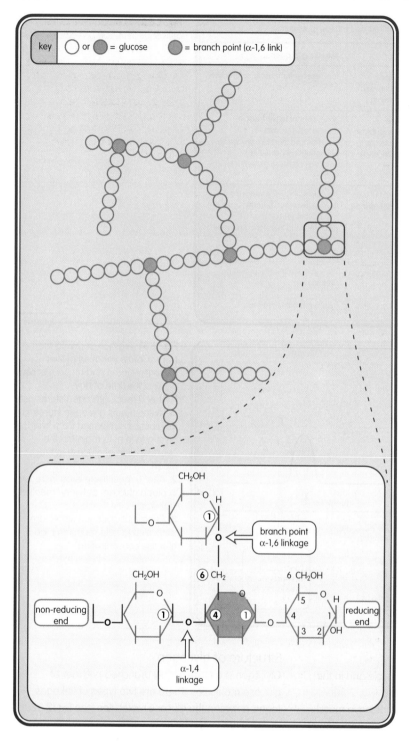

Fig. 2.32a The branched structure of glycogen showing the two types of linkages found between glucose molecules. Most glucose molecules are joined by α-1,4 linkages to make straight chains. α-1,6 linkages occur about every 8–12 glucose residues and enable branch points to be formed.

Glycogen is present in the cytosol as granules (the diameter varies between 100 and 400 Å). As well as glycogen, the granules contain the enzymes that catalyse glycogen synthesis and degradation and also some of the enzymes that regulate these processes.

Why is it an advantage to have a branched structure?
A branched structure creates a large number of exposed, terminal glucose molecules (i.e. many ends) that are easily accessible to the enzymes of glycogen breakdown. This enables rapid degradation and

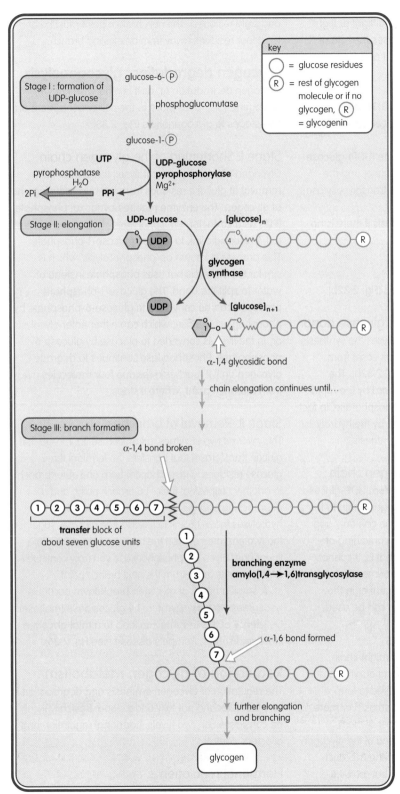

Fig. 2.32b Glycogen synthesis consists of three stages starting with the formation of UDP-glucose, which then takes part in the elongation of the glycogen molecule. When the growing glycogen chain is long enough a polysaccharide of between five and eight units is broken off and transferred to a neighbouring chain to form a branch chain.

glucose release when necessary (e.g. a 'fight or flight' response). Branching therefore increases the rate of glycogen synthesis and degradation. It also increases the solubility of glycogen.

Glycogen synthesis: glycogenesis
Glycogen synthesis takes place in the cell cytosol. The process requires:

- Three enzymes; Uridine diphosphate (UDP)-glucose pyrophosphorylase, glycogen synthase, and the branching enzyme, amylo(1,4→1,6)transglycosylase.
- The glucose donor, UDP-glucose.
- A primer to initiate glycogen synthesis if there is no pre-existing glycogen molecule.
- Energy.

There are three stages to glycogenesis (Fig. 2.32b).

Stage I: Initiation—formation of glucose donor
UDP-glucose pyrophosphorylase catalyses the synthesis of UDP-glucose (an activated form of glucose) from glucose-1-phosphate and UTP (see Fig. 2.32b). The reaction is reversible but is driven forward by the rapid hydrolysis of pyrophosphate by pyrophosphatase. In fact many biosynthetic reactions are driven by the hydrolysis of pyrophosphate—remember DNA synthesis.

Stage II: Elongation of the glycogen chain
Glycogen synthase transfers glucose from UDP-glucose to the C4 terminus of an existing glycogen chain to form an α-1,4 glycosidic linkage. The enzyme can only add glucose molecules to a chain already containing at least four or more glucose residues, that is, it cannot initiate chain synthesis but requires a primer. The primer can either be a glycogen fragment or in the absence of this the protein glycogenin can be used.

Stage III: Formation of branches
Glycogen synthase only forms linear, straight-chain glycogen molecules. A specific branching enzyme called amylo(1,4→1,6)transglycosylase is required to form branches. When the growing chain contains 11 or more residues, this enzyme transfers a number of them, usually seven, from the non-reducing end of the glycogen chain, to a neighbouring chain establishing a 'branch point'. Therefore an α-1,4 link is broken but an α-1,6 linkage is formed. The branching enzyme is very specific about the length of chain it transfers (usually between five

and eight residues). The new branch point must be at least four residues away from an existing branch.

Glycogen degradation: glycogenolysis
Glycogen degradation or, as it is otherwise known, glycogenolysis, takes place in the cell cytosol. There are two stages to glycogenolysis (Fig. 2.33).

Stage I: Shortening of the glycogen chain
Glycogen phosphorylase catalyses the sequential removal of glucose residues from the non-reducing end of glycogen. The enzyme requires pyridoxal phosphate (PLP) as a co-factor. Phosphorylase cleaves the terminal α-1,4 glycosidic link to release glucose-1-phosphate. This process is known as 'phosphorolysis' which is similar to hydrolysis but uses phosphate instead of water to split the bond. The glucose-1-phosphate produced can be converted to glucose-6-phosphate by phosphoglucomutase, which can either enter glycolysis or, in the liver, is converted to glucose by glucose-6-phosphatase. Phosphorylase continues to degrade glycogen until it reaches a residue four molecules away from a branch point, where it stops.

Stage II: Removal of branches
This involves two enzymes: a transferase ([α-1,4 →α-1,4] glucan transferase) that transfers the terminal three glucose residues (a trisaccharide) from one outer branch to another, 'exposing' the α-1,6 branch point; and a debranching enzyme, amylo-α-1,6 glucosidase, which hydrolyses the α-1,6 link to release free glucose. Together, the two enzymes convert the branched structure into a linear one. Glycogen phosphorylase can now continue until four units away from the next branch point.

A small amount of glycogen breakdown occurs in lysosomes via the enzyme α-1,4 glucosidase (maltase). Deficiency of this enzyme can lead to a fatal glycogen storage disorder, Pompe's disease (see Fig. 2.36).

Regulation of glycogen metabolism
The regulation of glycogen synthesis and degradation is very complex and not fully understood. Basically it can be considered on two levels: hormonal regulation and allosteric control.

Hormonal regulation
Glycogen synthase and phosphorylase are regulated by hormone-dependent reversible phosphorylation.

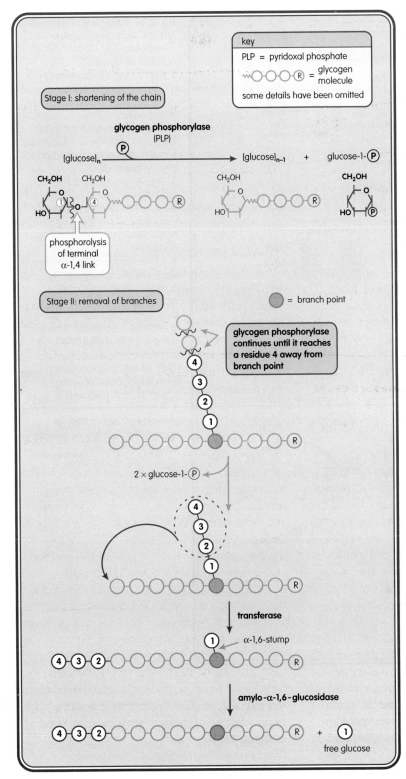

Fig. 2.33 Degradation of a glycogen showing the two stages necessary for its catabolism to monosaccharide units. Shortening of the glycogen chain releases glucose-1-phosphate while hydrolysis of a branch point releases free glucose.

33

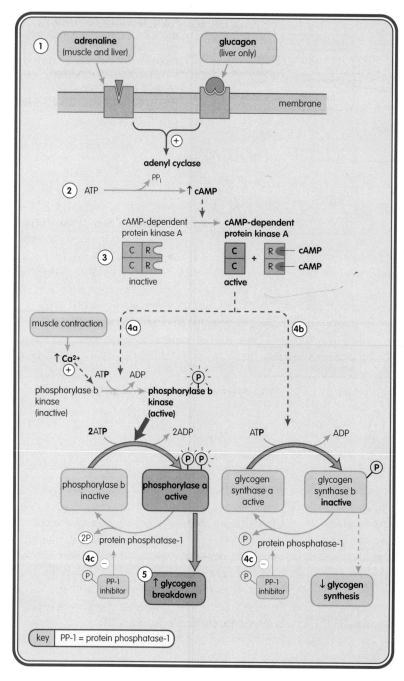

Fig. 2.34 The action of adrenaline and glucagon in glycogen metabolism. The mechanism of action is as follows:
1. The binding of adrenaline or glucagon activates adenyl cyclase via a G-protein coupled pathway (not shown).
2. Adenyl cyclase catalyses the formation of cAMP, which activates a cAMP-dependent protein kinase (protein kinase A).
3. This enzyme contains two regulatory (R) and two catalytic (C) subunits. cAMP binds to the regulatory subunits allowing the active catalytic subunits to dissociate.
4. cAMP-dependent protein kinase catalyses phosphorylation of:
a. phosphorylase b kinase, activating it;
b. glycogen synthase, inhibiting it;
c. protein phosphatase-inhibitor-I, activating it thus enabling it to inhibit protein phosphatase-I.
(Ca^{2+} released by contracting muscle also helps activate phosphorylase b kinase.)
5. Phosphorylation and activation of glycogen phosphorylase by phosphorylase b kinase activates glycogen breakdown.

Glycogen phosphorylase exists in two forms:
- Phosphorylase a, the active, phosphorylated form.
- Phosphorylase b, the inactive, dephosphorylated form.

Adrenaline (in muscle and liver) and glucagon (liver only) stimulate glycogen breakdown. They activate cAMP-dependent protein kinase A which, via the reaction cascade shown in Fig. 2.34, causes the phosphorylation of glycogen phosphorylase, thereby activating this enzyme.

Glycogen synthase also exists in two forms:
- Glycogen synthase a, the active, dephosphorylated form.
- Glycogen synthase b, the inactive phosphorylated form.

- ○ **Glucagon or adrenaline cause phosphorylation, which activates glycogen degradation.**
  - ○ **Dephosphorylation activates glycogen synthesis.**
- ⊙ **The most likely phosphorylation sites in enzymes are serine residues (they have a –CH₂OH side chain). With glycogen phosphorylase, phosphorylation occurs at two serine residues but with glycogen synthase, it occurs at nine serine residues.**

Adrenaline and glucagon are both catabolic hormones and therefore inhibit glycogen synthesis. Again they activate the cAMP-dependent protein kinase A, which phosphorylates glycogen synthase, inactivating it (remember, the opposite happens to glycogen phosphorylase (i.e. it is activated), which ensures that both pathways are not active at the same time). Therefore, glycogen synthase and phosphorylase are reciprocally regulated.

Phosphorylation of both glycogen synthase and phosphorylase is reversed by protein phosphatase-1, which removes the phosphate groups by hydrolysis. The actions of adrenaline and glucagon in glycogen metabolism are shown clearly in Fig. 2.34.

The action of insulin

The mechanism of action of insulin is unclear, however, it is an anabolic hormone and therefore stimulates

glycogen synthesis and inhibits breakdown. How does this occur? One possible explanation is that insulin activates the enzyme phosphodiesterase, which catalyses the breakdown of cAMP to AMP. A fall in cAMP levels leads to decreased activity of protein kinase A, (the enzyme that normally inactivates glycogen synthase). This results in dephosphorylation of both glycogen phosphorylase (inactivating it) and glycogen synthase (activating it). There are also other proposed mechanisms for the action of insulin but they are less well defined.

The mechanism of action of adrenaline and glucagon in glycogen metabolism shown in Fig. 2.34 is an example of an amplification pathway, in which the large number of steps involved amplify the hormonal signal, allowing the rapid release of glucose. Only one or two molecules of hormone bind to their receptors but they each cause the activation of a number of protein kinase molecules (100), which in turn activate many phosphorylase b kinase molecules (1000). This produces large numbers of active glycogen phosphorylase molecules (10 000) to degrade glycogen. If the binding of adrenaline directly activated glycogen phosphorylase it would require huge quantities of hormone for the same response.

Allosteric control
Liver glycogen phosphorylase

Glucose allosterically inhibits liver glycogen phosphorylase a. Phosphorylase a (phosphorylated, active form) contains two binding sites for glucose. The binding of glucose causes a conformational change; this exposes the phosphate groups, enabling their removal by protein phosphatase-I, thus converting it to phosphorylase b (the inactive form). Therefore, the product, glucose, inhibits glycogen breakdown. Glucose-6-phosphate also inhibits phosphorylase but activates glycogen synthase (Fig. 2.35).

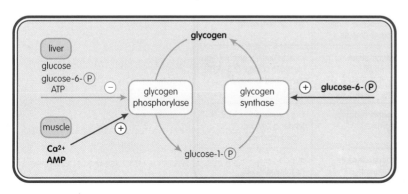

Fig. 2.35 Allosteric control of glycogen metabolism by glucose, glucose-6-phosphate, calcium ions, AMP, and ATP.

Muscle glycogen phosphorylase

The main allosteric control is effected by 5' AMP and Ca^{2+}. Calcium ions released during muscle contraction bind to calmodulin, a subunit of phosphorylase b kinase, activating it. For maximal activation, the enzyme also requires phosphorylation (Fig. 2.34).

AMP is an indicator of the energy status of the cell. High levels of AMP signal a low energy status (i.e. low ATP), for example, during intense exercise. Therefore AMP allosterically activates phosphorylase b; this increases glycogen breakdown in order to provide energy for muscle contraction.

Glycogen storage diseases

In this group of inherited diseases, each is caused by a defect in an enzyme required for either glycogen synthesis or degradation; they are very rare. They are all inherited as autosomal recessive disorders, except for type VIII which is sex-linked. The diseases either result in the production of an abnormal amount or an abnormal type of glycogen. The main glycogen storage diseases are summarized in Fig. 2.36.

Some of the more important ones are also discussed in Chapter 12.

- What are the different roles of liver and muscle glycogen in the body?
- What is the structure of glycogen?
- What is the basic outline of glycogen synthesis (name the site, the three main enzymes, and the three stages)?
- Describe glycogen breakdown (three enzymes and two stages).
- Explain the mechanism for the hormonal regulation of glycogen metabolism.
- Give two or three examples of glycogen storage disorders.

The main glycogen storage diseases			
Type	Enzyme deficiency	Glycogen structure and amount	Tissues affected
I von Gierke's disease	glucose-6-phosphatase	normal structure ↑ amount	liver and kidney are loaded with glycogen results in hypoglycaemia since glucose cannot leave the liver
II Pompe's disease	lysosomal α-1,4-glucosidase	normal structure ↑↑↑ amount	accumulation of glycogen in lysosomes in all organs usually fatal before the age of 2 years
III Cori's disease	amylo-1,6-glucosidase (debranching enzyme)	outer chains missing or very short ↑ amount	accumulation of branched polysaccharide in liver and muscle like type I but milder
IV Andersen's disease	branching enzyme	very long unbranched chains normal amount	liver failure causes death in the first year of life
V McArdle's disease	glycogen phosphorylase	normal structure ↑ amount	muscle has abnormally high glycogen content (2.5–4.1%) diminished exercise tolerance
VI Hers' disease	glycogen phosphorylase	normal structure ↑ amount	↑ liver glycogen tendency towards hypoglycaemia
VII Tarui's disease	phosphofructokinase	normal structure ↑ amount	muscle as for type V

Fig. 2.36 The main glycogen storage diseases. They either result in the production of an abnormal amount or an abnormal type of glycogen.

ROLE OF 2,3-BISPHOSPHOGLYCERATE

The Rapoport–Luebering shunt
Location
In red blood cells (RBCs), glycolysis is modified by the Rapoport–Luebering shunt, otherwise known as the 2,3-bisphosphoglycerate (2,3-BPG) shunt.

Pathway
There are two steps in the shunt (Fig. 2.37).
1. Bisphosphoglycerate mutase converts 1,3-BPG into 2,3-BPG.
2. 2,3-BPG is hydrolysed to 3-phosphoglycerate by 2,3-bisphosphoglycerate phosphatase.

ATP yield
Glycolysis is important to RBCs because it is their only energy source (they have no mitochondria and therefore must rely on anaerobic glycolysis). However, the shunt bypasses the energy-generating reaction, meaning therefore, there is effectively no net production of ATP.

Regulation of the shunt
Both reactions of the shunt are nearly irreversible. 3-phosphoglycerate stimulates bisphosphoglycerate mutase and therefore increases 2,3-BPG production. 2,3-BPG is a potent inhibitor of its own formation (i.e. negative feedback by the product).

Role of 2,3-BPG in haemoglobin function
Haemoglobin (Hb) is the oxygen-carrying protein found in RBCs. It has a high affinity for binding oxygen and therefore transports oxygen from the lungs to the tissues where it is needed. When Hb gets to the tissues, it has to release or 'unload' the oxygen. A low pH (acid) or an increased CO_2 concentration in the tissue favours unloading as both decrease the affinity of haemoglobin for oxygen; this is known as the Bohr effect.

2,3-BPG present in high concentrations in RBCs also helps unload oxygen from haemoglobin. Specifically, it is an allosteric effector that binds to and stabilizes deoxyhaemoglobin, reducing its affinity for oxygen therefore favouring the release of oxygen. 2,3-BPG fits in between the two β chains of haemoglobin in a

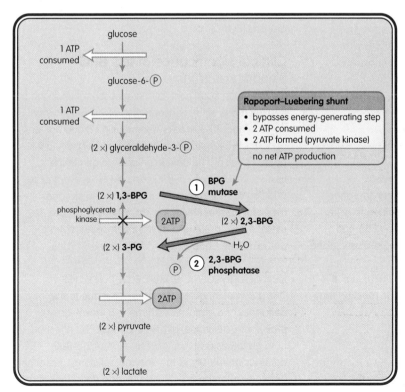

Fig. 2.37 The Rapoport–Luebering shunt in RBCs produces 2,3-BPG with no net energy production.

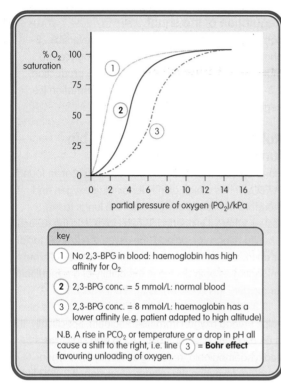

key

1 No 2,3-BPG in blood: haemoglobin has high affinity for O_2

2 2,3-BPG conc. = 5 mmol/L: normal blood

3 2,3-BPG conc. = 8 mmol/L: haemoglobin has a lower affinity (e.g. patient adapted to high altitude)

N.B. A rise in PCO_2 or temperature or a drop in pH all cause a shift to the right, i.e. line 3 = **Bohr effect** favouring unloading of oxygen.

Fig. 2.38 The effect of 2,3-BPG on haemoglobin is to decrease its affinity for oxygen causing a shift to the right in the oxygen saturation curve.

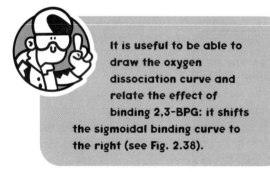

It is useful to be able to draw the oxygen dissociation curve and relate the effect of binding 2,3-BPG: it shifts the sigmoidal binding curve to the right (see Fig. 2.38).

'pocket' but only in the deoxygenated configuration. This pocket contains positively charged amino acids that form salt bridges with the negatively charged phosphate groups of 2,3-BPG, resulting in cross-linking of the β chains. 2,3-BPG cannot bind to oxyhaemoglobin as the gap between the β chains is too small in the presence of oxygen. The reaction may be written as follows:

$$HbO_2 + 2,3\text{-BPG} \rightarrow Hb\text{-}2,3\text{-BPG} + O_2$$
Deoxyhaemoglobin

The oxygen is therefore released for use by the tissues.

Main physiological effects of 2,3-BPG
Foetal haemoglobin
Foetal haemoglobin (HbF) contains two α chains and two γ chains $(\alpha_2\gamma_2)$ and is the major type of haemoglobin found in the foetus and in the newborn. HbF has a lower affinity for 2,3-BPG than normal adult haemoglobin (HbA) and therefore it has a higher affinity for oxygen (i.e. holds on to its oxygen). Why? HbF only binds 2,3-BPG weakly as its two γ chains lack some of the positively charged amino acids found in the β chains of HbA. As 2,3-BPG reduces the affinity of haemoglobin for oxygen, the weak interaction between HbF and 2,3-BPG means that HbF has a higher oxygen affinity than normal HbA. This enables placental oxygen exchange from the mother's circulation to the foetus.

Altitude acclimatization
The body responds to the chronic hypoxia observed at high altitude by increasing the concentration of 2,3-BPG in RBCs. This adaptation takes a few days. High levels of 2,3-BPG decrease the affinity of haemoglobin for oxygen, allowing greater unloading of oxygen to the tissues so that they receive enough oxygen despite its decreased availability. On return to low altitude, the concentration of 2,3-BPG returns to normal quite quickly. Similar, high concentrations of 2,3-BPG are observed in patients with chronic obstructive airways disease (COAD).

Clinical significance of 2,3 BPG
Blood transfusions
Storing blood in an acid–citrate–glucose medium leads to a decrease in the concentration of 2,3-BPG to low levels in about 1–2 weeks. The resulting blood has an abnormally high affinity for oxygen and if given to a patient it will not be able to unload oxygen to the tissues. The loss of 2,3-BPG can now be prevented by addition of substrates, e.g. inosine, to the storage medium. Inosine enters the RBC where it can be metabolized to 2,3-BPG by the pentose phosphate pathway (see Chapter 3).

Red cell glycolytic enzyme deficiencies
This group of inherited diseases occur due to the deficiency of a glycolytic enzyme (e.g. hexokinase, phosphofructokinase, pyruvate kinase). The effect on both glycolysis and the concentration of 2,3-BPG depends on the site of the enzyme deficiency, i.e. either before or after the 2,3-BPG shunt, or a deficiency of one

of the shunt enzymes. An abnormal concentration of 2,3-BPG affects the ability of the haemoglobin to transport and unload oxygen normally. Usually, this results in a haemolytic anaemia due to the decreased rate of glycolysis and thus ATP production, leading to increased haemolysis of red cells (see Chapter 12).

Causes of a raised concentration of 2,3-BPG
The main causes are:
- Long-term, smoking is known to cause an increase in the concentration of 2,3-BPG. This partly compensates for a decreased oxygen supply caused by the exposure to carbon monoxide.
- Chronic anaemia, which results in a decrease in the number of RBCs or the amount of haemoglobin, leading to decreased oxygen supply to the tissues. A compensatory increase in 2,3-BPG allows for greater unloading of oxygen to the tissues.
- Altitude acclimatization (see above).

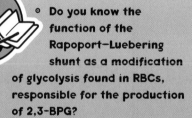

- Do you know the function of the Rapoport–Luebering shunt as a modification of glycolysis found in RBCs, responsible for the production of 2,3-BPG?
- What is the function of 2,3-BPG?
- Describe the effect of an increase or decrease in the concentration of 2,3-BPG. Be able to relate the changes to the oxygen dissociation curve.
- Describe the pathways for metabolism of fructose, galactose, and sorbitol and their site of entry into glycolysis (refer back to Fig. 2.12).

FRUCTOSE, GALACTOSE, ETHANOL, AND SORBITOL

Fructose metabolism
The main dietary source of fructose is the disaccharide sucrose, which is hydrolysed by sucrase in the small intestine to fructose and glucose; fructose is also found in fruit and honey. Unlike glucose, fructose can enter cells without the help of insulin. There are two pathways for fructose metabolism, one in muscle, the other in liver due to the presence of different enzymes in each tissue (see Fig. 2.39).
- In the liver, fructose is phosphorylated by the enzyme fructokinase to fructose-1-phosphate, which is then further metabolized to glyceraldehyde-3-phosphate to enter glycolysis or gluconeogenesis. Most dietary fructose is metabolized by the liver, such that little is left for metabolism by the muscle.
- In muscle, fructose is converted to fructose-6-phosphate by hexokinase to enter glycolysis after only one reaction.

Risks of excessive fructose ingestion
Fructose is metabolized rapidly compared with glucose. This is because it enters glycolysis as glyceraldehyde-3-phosphate, bypassing the rate-limiting step catalysed by phosphofructokinase, the key control point of glycolysis (see Fig. 2.2). Also, fructose entry into cells is independent of insulin.

As the rate-limiting step of glycolysis is bypassed, if fructose ingestion becomes too high it can result in an unregulated accumulation of glycolytic intermediates. For example, fructose-1-phosphate may accumulate, which will deplete the liver stores of phosphate and thus limit ATP production. A decrease in the concentration of ATP further activates glycolysis, leading to the increased production of lactic acid. If this continues it can lead to a potentially fatal lactic acidosis. For these reasons, intravenous fructose is no longer recommended for parenteral nutrition.

Inborn errors of fructose metabolism
These are genetic (autosomal recessive) diseases that are due to a deficiency in one of the key enzymes of fructose metabolism.
- Fructokinase deficiency is a congenital absence of fructokinase, meaning all fructose has to be metabolized by the hexokinase pathway (see Chapter 12).

- Hereditary fructose intolerance is a serious condition caused by a deficiency of fructose-1-phosphate aldolase (aldolase B), resulting in the accumulation of fructose-1-phosphate in the tissues (see Fig. 2.39). Phosphate is therefore sequestered in the cells and is not available to use. This leads to the inhibition of both glycogen phosphorylase (glycogenolysis) and aldolase A (enzyme of glycolysis and gluconeogenesis) since they are normally activated by phosphorylation. Glucose production is therefore inhibited which may lead to severe hypoglycaemia.

For a full discussion of these diseases see Chapter 12.

Galactose metabolism

The major dietary source of galactose is lactose in milk and milk products. Lactose is hydrolysed in the small intestine by lactase to galactose and glucose. The entry of galactose into cells is independent of insulin.

Metabolism of galactose

The metabolism of galactose has four steps (Fig. 2.40):
1. Phosphorylation to galactose-1-phosphate by galactokinase.
2. Galactose-1-phosphate uridyl transferase catalyses the transfer of the uridyl group of UDP-glucose to galactose-1-phosphate to make UDP-galactose and glucose-1-phosphate.
3. Glucose-1-phosphate can be converted to the glycolytic intermediate glucose-6-phosphate and enter glycolysis.
4. UDP-galactose is converted back to UDP-glucose by UDP-hexose-4-epimerase.

Inborn errors of galactose metabolism: Galactosaemia

This rare, autosomal recessive disorder is due to a deficiency of the enzyme galactose-1-phosphate uridyl transferase (see Chapter 12). It is occasionally caused by a deficiency of galactokinase or UDP-hexose-4-epimerase. The formation of UDP-galactose is

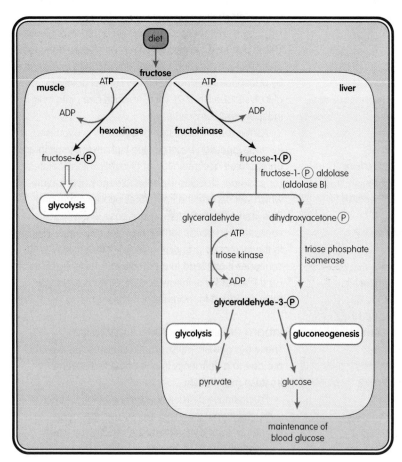

Fig. 2.39 The metabolism of fructose by liver and muscle cells leads to the production of intermediates that can then enter glycolysis.

prevented as is galactose metabolism, resulting in the accumulation of galactose in the blood and tissues. This can lead to an increase in galactose levels in the lens of the eye, where it is reduced by aldose reductase to galactitol, which is thought to contribute to cataract formation. The accumulation of galactitol also occurs in nerve tissue, liver, and kidneys.

Catabolism of ethanol

In the liver, three enzyme systems exist for the catabolism of ethanol (Fig. 2.41):

1. Cytosolic alcohol dehydrogenase pathway, probably the main route for the oxidation of ethanol. The activity of this enzyme is largely governed by the availability of NAD^+, which is required as a co-factor.

2. Microsomal ethanol oxidizing system (MEOS), which uses a cytochrome p450 enzyme system.

3. The peroxisome system, which uses the enzyme catalase.

The product of all three systems is acetaldehyde, which then enters mitochondria for further oxidation by aldehyde dehydrogenase to acetate. Certain races, in particular the Chinese, are genetically deficient in aldehyde dehydrogenase and consequently have a lower alcohol tolerance.

Metabolic effects of ethanol

The fate of acetate depends on the ratio of NADH to NAD^+. Both alcohol dehydrogenase and aldehyde dehydrogenase consume NAD^+, contributing to a high $NADH:NAD^+$, resulting in:

- Inhibition of the TCA cycle. A high $NADH:NAD^+$ ratio inhibits isocitrate dehydrogenase, α-ketoglutarate dehydrogenase, and citrate synthase (see Fig. 2.22).
- Inhibition of gluconeogenesis. A high $NADH:NAD^+$ ratio affects the dehydrogenase reactions, displacing the equilibrium in favour of the reduced compounds such that oxaloacetate is converted to malate and pyruvate to lactate (see Fig. 5.17). Therefore, less pyruvate and oxaloacetate (substrates) are available for gluconeogenesis by the liver. Acetate is therefore exported out of the liver for metabolism by other tissues.

Clinical significance of excessive ethanol ingestion

High levels of alcohol can lead to hyperlactataemia (i.e. favours conversion of pyruvate to lactate, see above). Since both lactate and urate share the same mechanism for renal tubular secretion, the more lactate produced the more urate will be retained. Urate may crystallize out in the joints especially in the toes, leading to gout.

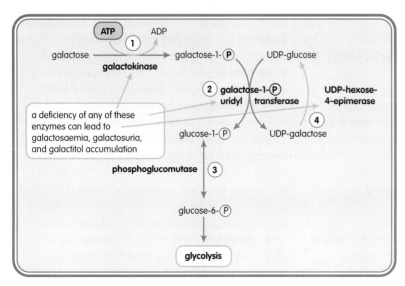

Fig. 2.40 The metabolism of galactose; a four-step pathway that converts galactose to glucose-6-phosphate, which can then enter glycolysis. (Numbers refer to text.)

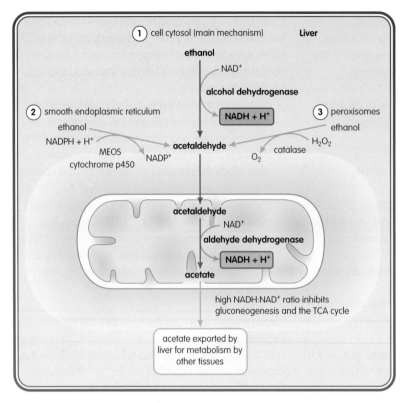

Fig. 2.41 Three enzyme systems are responsible for the metabolism of ethanol in the liver: cytosolic alcohol dehydrogenase (main mechanism), MEOS in smooth endoplasmic reticulum, and catalase in peroxisomes. The product, acetaldehyde, is then taken into the mitochondria for further metabolism to acetate. (Numbers refer to text on p. 41.)

Hypoglycaemia can develop in malnourished or fasting individuals after a heavy drinking session. The inhibition of gluconeogenesis leads to this hypo-glycaemia; medical students beware!

Alcohol can induce the cytochrome p450 enzymes that are responsible for the metabolism of many drugs, for example, barbiturates. Therefore, for an alcoholic patient on medication, the metabolism and effects of the drugs may be altered.

Sorbitol metabolism (polyol pathway)
Synthesis
Sorbitol is a sugar alcohol that can be synthesized endogenously from glucose by a number of tissues such as the lens and retina of the eye, the liver, kidney, and Schwann cells (the cells of the peripheral nervous system that make myelin).

Sorbitol synthesis requires the enzyme aldose reductase which reduces glucose to sorbitol.

Breakdown
Some tissues, especially the liver, also possess another enzyme, sorbitol dehydrogenase, which oxidizes sorbitol to fructose (Fig. 2.42).

In the liver, this provides a way for dietary sorbitol to enter glycolysis or gluconeogenesis and be metabolized further (see Fig. 2.39).

This is also a useful pathway in sperm and in the seminal vesicles where fructose is the preferred energy source.

Uses and complications of increased sorbitol
Sorbitol is used as a sweetener in many diabetic foods. It only has about one-half the sweetness of sucrose but, more importantly, it is safe because it is absorbed slowly from the intestine and also transported slowly across cell membranes. Therefore at normal levels there is little chance of it accumulating.

Problems arise when the endogenous production of sorbitol increases. Since sorbitol does not cross cell membranes easily it may remain 'trapped' in the cells. Aldose reductase has a high Km for glucose (about 60–70 mM). At normal blood glucose levels (3–5 mM), it is only slightly active, and the production of sorbitol is low. However, in poorly controlled diabetes, where blood glucose concentrations can reach as high as 15–20 mM on a daily basis, there is an increased production of sorbitol, which may accumulate within

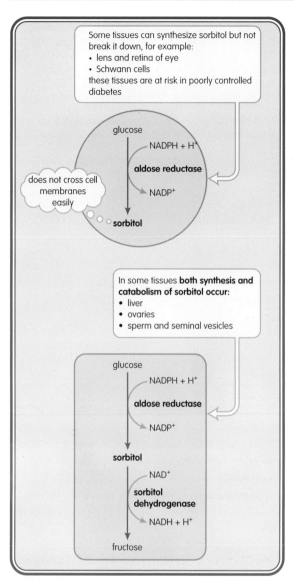

Some tissues can synthesize sorbitol but not break it down, for example:
• lens and retina of eye
• Schwann cells
these tissues are at risk in poorly controlled diabetes

does not cross cell membranes easily

glucose

NADPH + H⁺

aldose reductase

NADP⁺

sorbitol

In some tissues **both synthesis and catabolism of sorbitol occur:**
• liver
• ovaries
• sperm and seminal vesicles

glucose

NADPH + H⁺

aldose reductase

NADP⁺

sorbitol

NAD⁺

sorbitol dehydrogenase

NADH + H⁺

fructose

Fig. 2.42 The metabolism of sorbitol from glucose by aldose reductase. Some tissues contain the enzyme sorbitol dehydrogenase, which oxidizes sorbitol to fructose.

cells. This causes the greatest problems in tissues that lack sorbitol dehydrogenase to break down the sorbitol. For example:

• In the lens and retina of the eye the increased sorbitol exerts a strong osmotic effect, causing water retention; the lens swells and becomes opaque, leading to cataract formation.

• In Schwann cells, the increased levels of sorbitol disrupt cell structure and function, and demyelination of nerves and peripheral neuropathy ensues.

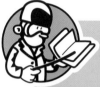

○ **Identify the tissues in which these pathways are particularly important.**

○ **Know briefly about enzyme deficiencies.**

○ **What is the significance of the sorbitol pathway in the development of complications of diabetes (see also Chapter 12)?**

○ **Describe the metabolism of ethanol and the clinical significance of excessive ethanol ingestion.**

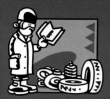

3. Production of NADPH

PENTOSE PHOSPHATE PATHWAY AND PYRUVATE–MALATE CYCLE

Pentose phosphate pathway

The pentose phosphate pathway (PPP), otherwise known as the hexosemonophosphate shunt or the phosphogluconate pathway, provides an alternative route for the metabolism of glucose. Most of the pathways that have already been discussed are concerned with the generation of ATP. However, in the pentose phosphate pathway no ATP is directly consumed or produced; instead, the pathway is concerned with the production of reducing power in the form of NADPH.

Like NADH, NADPH can be thought of as a high-energy molecule but instead of transferring its electrons to the electron transport chain to make ATP they are used for reductive synthetic reactions.

Location

Mainly the liver, lactating mammary glands, adipose tissue, adrenal cortex, and red blood cells (RBCs).

Site

Cell cytosol.

Main functions

The main functions of the pentose phosphate pathway are:
- Generation of NADPH necessary for reductive biosynthetic reactions, for example, fatty acid and cholesterol synthesis.
- Production of five-carbon, ribose sugar units for nucleotide and nucleic acid synthesis.
- In RBCs, NADPH is used to regenerate the reduced form of the anti-oxidant glutathione, which protects the cells against damage from reactive oxygen intermediates.

Pathway

The pathway has two stages:
- An irreversible oxidative phase (Fig. 3.1) that consists of three irreversible reactions results in the formation of ribulose-5-phosphate, CO_2, and two molecules of NADPH per molecule of glucose-6-phosphate oxidized.

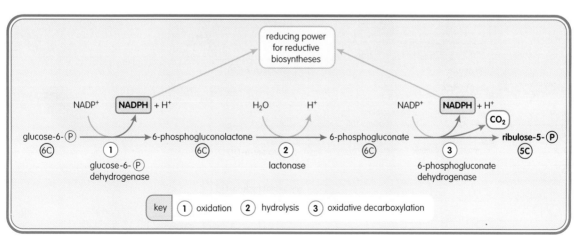

Fig. 3.1 The pentose phosphate pathway: phase I, the irreversible oxidative phase. Three irreversible reactions result in the production of two molecules of NADPH.

45

- A reversible non-oxidative phase (Fig. 3.2) that consists of a series of five, reversible sugar–phosphate interconversions whereby ribulose-5-phosphate is converted either to ribose-5-phosphate for nucleotide synthesis or to intermediates of glycolysis such as glyceraldehyde-3-phosphate or fructose-6-phosphate. The pathway is therefore linked with the needs of glycolysis.

It is not necessary to know the names of all the intermediates of the reversible phase; just be aware that it involves the interconversion of three, four, five, and seven carbon sugars as shown in steps 1 to 5 in Fig. 3.2. The sum of the reactions for the reversible phase is:
2 xylulose-5-phosphate + ribose-5-phosphate ↔
2 fructose-6-phosphate + glyceraldehyde-3-phosphate.

Fate of fructose-6-phosphate

The fate of fructose-6-phosphate formed in the pentose phosphate pathway depends on the specific needs of the tissue. For example, in liver, adipose tissue, and the adrenal cortex, fructose-6-phosphate promotes the synthesis of fatty acids.

How does this occur?

In the well-fed state, glucose is taken up by the liver and other tissues and phosphorylated to glucose-6-phosphate, which enters the pentose phosphate pathway to form fructose-6-phosphate. Accumulation of fructose-6-phosphate allosterically activates the rate-limiting enzyme of glycolysis, phosphofructokinase which, in turn, allows the formation of pyruvate. This is oxidatively

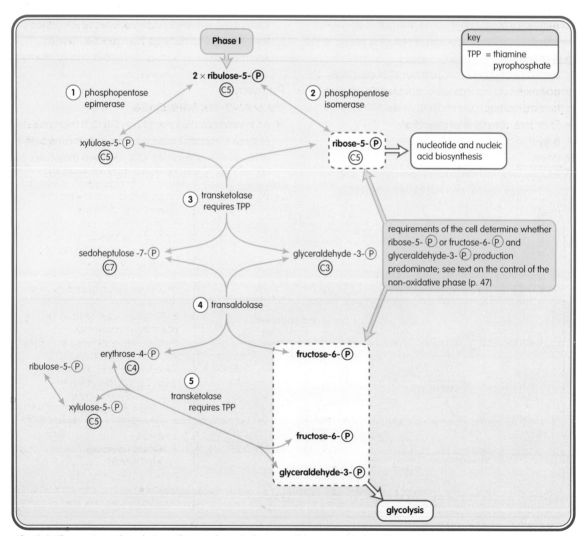

Fig. 3.2 The pentose phosphate pathway: phase II, the reversible non-oxidative phase.

decarboxylated to acetyl CoA, which can be used for fatty acid synthesis.

In RBCs, fructose-6-phosphate has a different fate. It is converted back to glucose-6-phosphate by the enzyme phosphoglucose isomerase to re-enter the pentose phosphate pathway therefore creating a cycle and thus a continual supply of substrate for the pentose phosphate pathway. This allows the continued production of NADPH required for the regeneration of reduced glutathione, the antioxidant which protects RBCs (see Fig. 3.4).

Control of the pentose phosphate pathway

The main control of the pathway is exerted at the first step, that is the glucose-6-phosphate dehydrogenase reaction.

Features are:
- This is an essentially irreversible reaction.
- The main controlling factor is the ratio of NADPH to $NADP^+$.
- As the cell uses up NADPH (e.g. during fatty acid synthesis) the concentration of $NADP^+$ increases. This activates the pathway increasing NADPH formation to compensate.
- Therefore, the pentose phosphate pathway is activated by a low NADPH:$NADP^+$.

Control of the non-oxidative phase is by the requirement for products, namely ribose-5-phosphate and NADPH (see Fig. 3.2). The individual needs of the cell for either of these determines whether production of ribose-5-phosphate, or fructose-6-phosphate and glyceraldehyde-3-phosphate predominates. For example:
- If the NADPH requirement is greater than the ribose-5-phosphate requirement, for example, in cells that take part in a lot of reductive synthetic reactions, all the ribose-5-phosphate formed is converted to fructose-6-phosphate and glyceraldehyde-3-phosphate. These are converted back to glucose-6-phosphate to re-enter the pentose phosphate pathway and therefore generate more NADPH.
- If the ribose-5-phosphate requirement is greater than the need for NADPH, for example, in cells with a high turnover and rate of nucleic acid formation, fructose-6-phosphate and glyceraldehyde-3-phosphate are converted to ribose-5-phosphate by further sugar interconversions.

Pyruvate–malate cycle

The pyruvate–malate cycle (Fig. 3.3) has two functions:
- The production of NADPH in the reaction catalysed

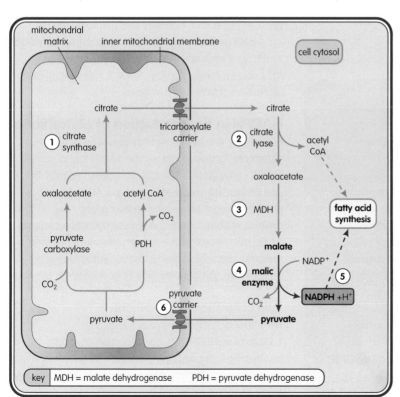

Fig. 3.3 The pyruvate–malate cycle operates between the cell cytosol and mitochondria. The reaction sequence is as follows:
1. Oxaloacetate and acetyl CoA condense to form citrate, which leaves the mitochondria via the tricarboxylate carrier.
2. Citrate is cleaved in the cytosol by citrate lyase back to oxaloacetate and acetyl CoA.
3. Acetyl CoA can be used for fatty acid synthesis whereas oxaloacetate is reduced to malate.
4. Malate is oxidatively decarboxylated by the malic enzyme, reforming pyruvate.
5. The reaction produces a significant amount of NADPH, which is used mainly for fatty acid synthesis.
6. Pyruvate is transported back into the mitochondria via a pyruvate carrier, where some of it is carboxylated to oxaloacetate and some converted to acetyl CoA.

47

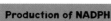
by the malic (malate dehydrogenase-decarboxylating) enzyme.

- The transport of acetyl CoA units from the mitochondria to the cytosol, the site of fatty acid synthesis by the citrate shuttle.

Glycolysis produces pyruvate, which enters the mitochondria where it is oxidatively decarboxylated to acetyl CoA, from which fatty acids can be synthesized. However, fatty acid synthesis takes place in the cell cytosol so that acetyl CoA requires a transport mechanism or 'carrier' to enable it to leave the mitochondria, namely, the citrate shuttle (discussed further in Chapter 4).

Sources of NADPH for fatty acid synthesis

The pentose phosphate pathway is the main source of NADPH: two molecules of NADPH are produced for each molecule of glucose entering the pathway. The pyruvate–malate cycle probably contributes between 25 and 40% of the total NADPH depending on the source of the acetyl units (i.e. glucose, amino acids, or lactate). For each acetyl CoA transferred from the mitochondria to the cytosol, one NADPH molecule is generated.

The pyruvate–malate cycle shows an inter-relationship between glucose metabolism and fatty acid synthesis. When the need for ATP is low, the oxidation of acetyl CoA by the TCA cycle is minimal thus providing acetyl CoA for fatty acid synthesis. Remember that these pathways are not all active at the same time.

THE ROLES OF NADPH

NADPH in lipid biosynthesis

NADPH like NADH is a high-energy molecule but its electrons, instead of being transferred to oxygen via the electron transport chain, are used for reductive biosyntheses, particularly for lipid synthesis. Each cycle of lipid synthesis in which the growing fatty acid chain is lengthened by two carbon atoms, employs two reductions, each requiring NADPH as co-factor. The pentose phosphate pathway and pyruvate–malate cycle both generate the NADPH necessary for fatty acid synthesis. Deficiency of NADPH leads to inhibition of fatty acid synthesis (see Chapter 4, for a more in-depth discussion of fatty acid synthesis).

NADPH in the production of glutathione

Glutathione is a tripeptide of three amino acids, glutamate, cysteine, and glycine, and is found in most cells. It can exist in two forms: an active, reduced form and an inactive, oxidized form (Fig. 3.4). Reduced glutathione contains a reactive thiol group (-SH) on the cysteine residue, which can reduce hydrogen peroxide (H_2O_2) and other reactive oxygen intermediates (free radicals), detoxifying them. That is, glutathione is an anti-oxidant and protects cells from damage.

Role of NADPH in glutathione metabolism (numbers refer to Fig. 3.4)

1. Glutathione (GSH) reduces hydrogen peroxide, inactivating it. The reaction catalysed by glutathione peroxidase (an enzyme containing selenium) produces oxidized, inactive glutathione.

- Locate and describe the main functions of the pentose phosphate pathway.
- Appreciate the two stages of the pathway (in which only phase I requires oxygen and generates NADPH).
- Describe the concept of reducing power and its importance to reductive biosynthetic reactions.
- Draw the pyruvate–malate cycle not forgetting its two parts: the malic enzyme and the citrate shuttle (see Chapter 4 also).
- What are the sources of NADPH for fatty acid synthesis?

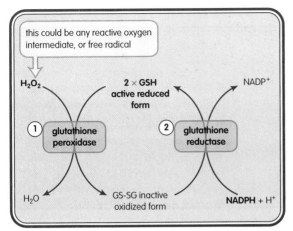

this could be any reactive oxygen intermediate, or free radical

H_2O_2

$2 \times GSH$ active reduced form

$NADP^+$

① glutathione peroxidase

② glutathione reductase

H_2O

GS-SG inactive oxidized form

$NADPH + H^+$

Fig. 3.4 The role of NADPH in glutathione metabolism. Glutathione is an antioxidant. It reduces hydrogen peroxide and other reactive oxygen intermediates, inactivating them. In doing so it undergoes oxidation to its inactive, oxidized form. NADPH is required for the regeneration of the active reduced form of glutathione by glutathione reductase, enabling it to continue its role as as antioxidant.

2.The active, reduced form of glutathione is regenerated by glutathione reductase, which requires NADPH as a reducing agent.

Therefore, NADPH indirectly provides the reducing power to inactivate hydrogen peroxide. This pathway is important in all cells of the body, but especially in RBCs.

Importance of NADPH in RBCs
RBCs do not contain mitochondria, therefore, they rely entirely on glycolysis and the pentose phosphate pathway. This means their only source of NADPH is the pentose phosphate pathway. Inhibition of the pathway would lead to a decrease in NADPH and therefore decreased activity of glutathione reductase. The amount of inactive, oxidized glutathione would increase, rendering the RBCs sensitive to oxidative damage by H_2O_2. This is seen in glucose-6-phosphate dehydrogenase deficiency, an X-linked condition in which oxidative damage leads to:
- The oxidation of haemoglobin to methaemoglobin, which cannot transport oxygen effectively (see below).
- The oxidation of membrane proteins and lipids, 'destabilizing' them, leading to an increased chance of cell lysis and thus haemolytic anaemia (see Chapter 12).

Action of free radicals
Reactive oxygen intermediates are formed from molecular oxygen in most cells, as either by-products of aerobic metabolism or from exogenous sources, for example, smoking, radiation, and the side effects of drugs and chemicals. They are highly reactive, and attack cell components such as proteins, DNA, and polyunsaturated fatty acids in cell membranes, resulting in disruption of membrane structure and cell integrity. Free radicals are thought to be partly responsible for the cell damage associated with inflammation, ageing, and certain cancers. They are detoxified by two main mechanisms, which are outlined below.

Enzyme inactivation
Several enzymes are responsible for the inactivation of free radicals:
- Glutathione peroxidase (a selenium-containing enzyme) removes hydrogen peroxide (Fig. 3.4).
- Catalase (an iron-containing enzyme) removes hydrogen peroxide according to the reaction:
$$H_2O_2 \rightarrow H_2O + \tfrac{1}{2}O_2$$
- Superoxide dismutase detoxifies the superoxide radical ($O_2^{\bullet-}$) as shown below:
$$2O_2^{\bullet-} + 2H^+ \rightarrow H_2O_2 + O_2$$
Superoxide dismutase exists in two forms: a copper- and zinc-containing cytoplasmic form and a manganese-containing mitochondrial form.

Deficiency of any of the trace elements contained in these enzymes can lead to their inhibition and thus an increase in cellular damage by free radicals (see Chapter 8).

Non-enzymatic inactivation: dietary anti-oxidants
Vitamins A, C, and E are anti-oxidants (see Chapter 8). An increased dietary intake of these vitamins is thought to decrease the incidence of heart disease (mainly vitamin E) and certain cancers (e.g. lung).

Prevention of oxidation of haemoglobin
The oxidation of the iron (Fe^{2+}; ferrous form) in haemoglobin by H_2O_2 or other free radicals, forms methaemoglobin (Fe^{3+}; ferric form), which cannot transport oxygen effectively. Methaemoglobin is usually only present at low concentrations because RBCs

49

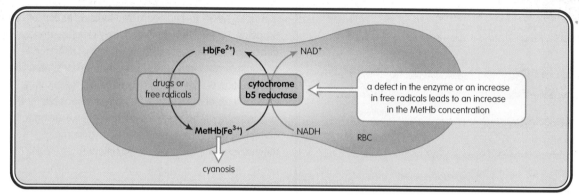

Fig. 3.5 The reduction of methaemoglobin. A defect in the enzyme cytochrome b5 reductase can lead to methaemoglobinaemia and cyanosis.

possess an efficient enzyme system, NADH-dependent cytochrome b5 reductase (methaemoglobin reductase), which catalyses the reduction of methaemoglobin to haemoglobin (Fig. 3.5).

The generation of excessive free radicals and the action of certain drugs or toxins can result in the increased formation of methaemoglobin. In this scenario, the cytochrome b5 reductase system cannot cope and the concentration of methaemoglobin in the blood rises, leading to methaemoglobinaemia. As methaemoglobin cannot carry oxygen, this results in poor perfusion of tissues and cyanosis (a dusky blue discoloration of skin). If adequate amounts of NADPH are present, the levels of glutathione in RBCs can cope with the excess free radicals and drugs and thus prevent oxidation of haemoglobin.

Newborn babies have only low concentrations of cytochrome b5 reductase and are therefore susceptible to methaemoglobinaemia.

Drug metabolism

A continual supply of reduced glutathione is required in the liver for the conjugation and detoxification of certain drugs and steroid hormones. This increases their excretion, thus preventing accumulation and toxicity. NADPH is necessary to maintain a continual supply of reduced glutathione as already described.

- Describe the origin of NADPH and its role in lipid synthesis.
- Describe the function of glutathione and the role of NADPH in its metabolism.
- What is the importance of NADPH to RBCs?
- Describe the role of NADPH in methaemoglobinaemia and drug metabolism.

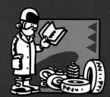

4. Lipid Metabolism

Overview of lipid biosynthesis

Fatty acids are an essential fuel and major energy source. The diet supplies a lot of the fat used by the body but a number of tissues can also synthesize fat *de novo* from acetyl CoA.

Working definition

Fatty acid synthesis, or lipogenesis as it is otherwise known, consists of a cyclical series of reactions in which a molecule of fatty acid is 'built up' by the sequential addition of two carbon units derived from acetyl CoA, to a growing fatty acid chain.

Fatty acid synthesis is not simply a reversal of the degradative pathway (i.e. β oxidation) but consists of its own set of reactions.

Location

Mainly in the liver, adipose tissue, and lactating mammary glands; there is a small amount in the kidney.

Site

Cell cytosol.

Fig. 4.1 shows an overview of lipid biosynthesis and the main steps involved in the formation of palmitate, a 16 carbon saturated fatty acid, beginning with the formation of acetyl CoA in the mitochondria, its transport into the cell cytosol where it is carboxylated to malonyl CoA, and then the characteristic sequence of reactions catalysed by fatty acid synthase. It would be a good idea to have a look at this diagram now, before you embark on the rest of this chapter.

The pentose phosphate pathway and the pyruvate–malate cycle generate the NADPH necessary for fatty acid synthesis (about 60% from the pentose phosphate pathway and 40% via the malic enzyme; see Chapter 3). The steps of fatty acid synthesis are now considered in more detail.

Production of acetyl CoA

Pyruvate dehydrogenase (PDH) catalyses the irreversible, oxidative decarboxylation of pyruvate to acetyl CoA in the mitochondrial matrix (Fig. 4.2). Details of this reaction are covered in Chapter 2. Acetyl CoA can also be produced by the degradation of fatty acids, ketone bodies, or amino acids.

Transport of acetyl CoA from mitochondria to the cytosol

The same pathway, namely the pyruvate–malate cycle, that produces NADPH for fatty acid synthesis also transports acetyl CoA from the mitochondria to the cell cytosol (see Fig. 4.2). The part of the cycle that transports acetyl CoA is called the citrate shuttle. Acetyl CoA is produced in the mitochondria but fatty acid synthesis occurs in the cytosol. The CoA portion of the molecule cannot cross the mitochondrial membrane. However, by condensing with oxaloacetate to form citrate, the acetyl group can be carried across by the tricarboxylate carrier. In the cytosol, citrate is cleaved by citrate lyase to release oxaloacetate for recycling and acetyl CoA for fatty acid synthesis.

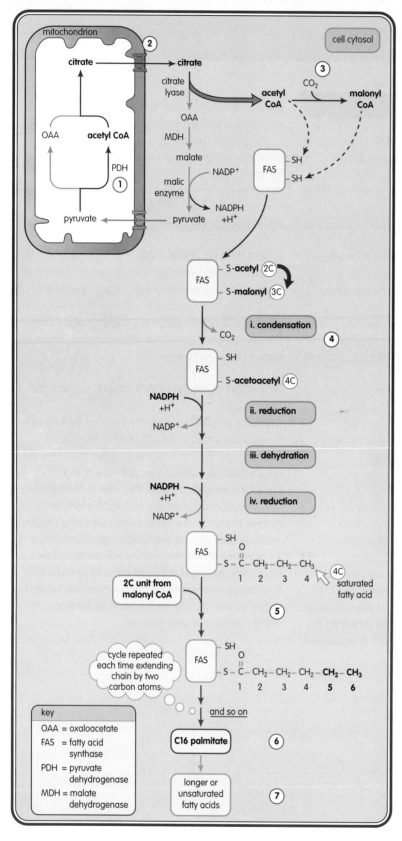

Fig. 4.1 An overview of lipid biosynthesis. The steps involved in the formation of palmitate:

1. Formation of the precursor, acetyl CoA from pyruvate in mitochondria.
2. Transport of acetyl CoA into the cytosol. Acetyl CoA combines with oxaloacetate to form citrate (citrate shuttle).
3. The carboxylation of acetyl CoA to malonyl CoA by acetyl CoA carboxylase.
4. The initiation of the synthesis of a new fatty acid molecule requires both acetyl CoA and malonyl CoA. They attach to the enzyme, fatty acid synthase and condense to form acetoacetyl ACP. This then undergoes a characteristic sequence of reactions catalysed by fatty acid synthase to make a four-carbon saturated fatty acid.
5. Fatty acid synthase also catalyses the sequential addition of further two carbon units from malonyl CoA to the growing fatty acid chain.
6. Elongation by fatty acid synthase stops on formation of palmitate (C16).
7. Further elongation and insertion of double bonds is carried out by other enzymes.

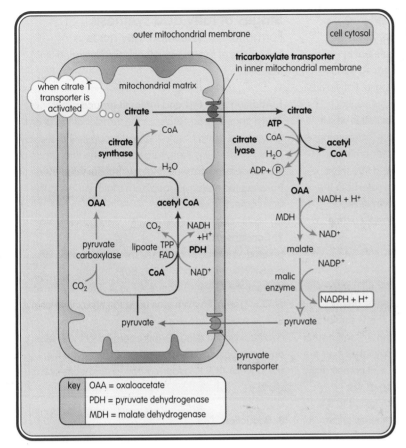

Fig. 4.2 Production and transport of acetyl CoA by the citrate shuttle.

Fate of acetyl CoA: the TCA cycle vs fatty acid synthesis

Normally in mitochondria, any citrate formed enters the TCA cycle for oxidation and the generation of ATP. However, when the concentration of ATP is high, enzymes of the TCA cycle, especially isocitrate dehydrogenase, are inhibited because there is no need to generate further energy. The concentration of citrate rises, which activates the tricarboxylate transporter and thus citrate is transported into the cytosol. As ATP is also needed for fatty acid synthesis, the high levels of both ATP and citrate favour lipogenesis.

Production of malonyl CoA from acetyl CoA

This is the irreversible, rate-limiting step of fatty acid synthesis (Fig. 4.3). The carboxylation of acetyl CoA is catalysed by acetyl CoA carboxylase, which requires the vitamin biotin as a co-factor. Biotin is covalently attached to a lysine residue of the enzyme and takes part in the reaction. The carboxylation is a two-stage process:

- The biotin group of the enzyme is first carboxylated.
- This activates CO_2 and enables its transfer to acetyl CoA.

Biotin is therefore a 'carrier of activated CO_2' and is in fact the co-factor for other carboxylases, including pyruvate carboxylase (see Chapter 5).

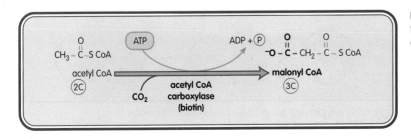

Fig. 4.3 Carboxylation of acetyl CoA to malonyl CoA by acetyl CoA carboxylase.

Fatty acid synthase

Fatty acid synthesis requires several enzymes. In bacteria, these enzymes are all separate but in eukaryotes they are joined together forming a multi-enzyme complex called fatty acid synthase. Fatty acid synthase is a dimer of two identical subunits, each containing seven different enzymatic activities which each catalyse a different reaction of fatty acid synthesis. Each subunit also contains an acyl carrier protein. Subunits of fatty acid synthase are folded into three domains joined by flexible regions (Fig. 4.4). Both the acyl carrier protein and one of the enzymes, the condensing enzyme (β-ketoacyl synthase), contain important thiol (sulphydryl) groups.

Function of the acyl carrier protein

The acyl carrier protein contains the vitamin pantothenic acid as a 4-phosphopantetheine prosthetic group, which contains a terminal thiol group. This is similar to the pantothenic acid group of coenzyme A (see Chapter 2). In fact, the acyl carrier protein actually takes over the role of CoA in fatty acid synthesis, that is, it carries acyl groups on its thiol group. Consequently, all the intermediates of fatty acid synthesis are joined to the acyl carrier protein. The phosphopantetheinyl group forms a long flexible arm that carries the growing fatty acyl chain from one active site to the next in fatty acid synthase, enhancing the efficiency of the overall synthetic process and minimizing any side reactions.

Stages of fatty acid synthesis
Formation of saturated fatty acids

The stages of fatty acid synthesis are illustrated in Fig. 4.5.

1. Addition of acetyl and malonyl groups

Acetyl transacylase catalyses the transfer of the acetyl group from acetyl CoA to the thiol group (SH) of the acyl carrier protein. It is then transferred to the thiol group of the condensing enzyme. Malonyl transacylase then transfers the malonyl group from malonyl CoA to the acyl carrier protein.

2. Condensation

β-ketoacyl synthase catalyses the condensation of acetyl (2C) and malonyl (3C) groups to form acetoacetyl-ACP (4C). The reaction is driven by the loss of CO_2. (The ATP which was used to carboxylate acetyl CoA to malonyl CoA (Fig. 4.3) is stored in malonyl CoA; decarboxylation releases this energy and thus helps to drive elongation). The next three steps convert the acetoacetyl-ACP to a four-carbon, saturated fatty acyl chain.

3. Reduction

The keto group at C3 (the β carbon) is reduced to an alcohol group by β-ketoacyl reductase. The reducing agent for this reaction is NADPH.

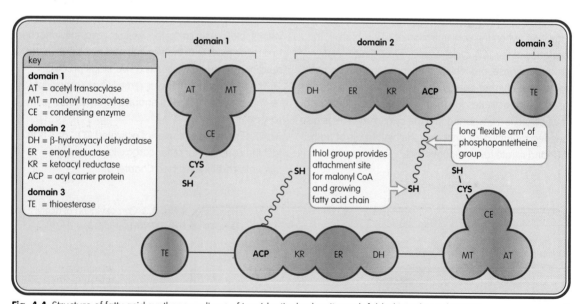

Fig. 4.4 Structure of fatty acid synthase: a dimer of two identical subunits each folded into three domains.

4. Dehydration

The removal of water by β-hydroxyacyl dehydratase introduces a double bond.

5. Reduction

Enoyl reductase catalyses the second reduction producing a saturated four-carbon fatty acyl chain. This completes the first elongation cycle.

6. Site-to-site transfer

The four-carbon chain is transferred to the thiol group of the cysteine residue of the condensing enzyme.

7. Addition of a second malonyl CoA to the acyl carrier protein.

The four-carbon chain condenses with malonyl CoA and steps 2–6 are repeated to form a saturated six-carbon fatty acyl chain.

The cycle is in fact repeated a further five times until a 16-carbon chain, palmitate, is made, i.e. seven cycles altogether (Fig. 4.5). The enzyme thioesterase then catalyses the release of palmitate. Therefore, the synthesis of one molecule of palmitate uses one molecule of acetyl CoA and seven of malonyl CoA. The overall reaction for the synthesis of palmitate is:

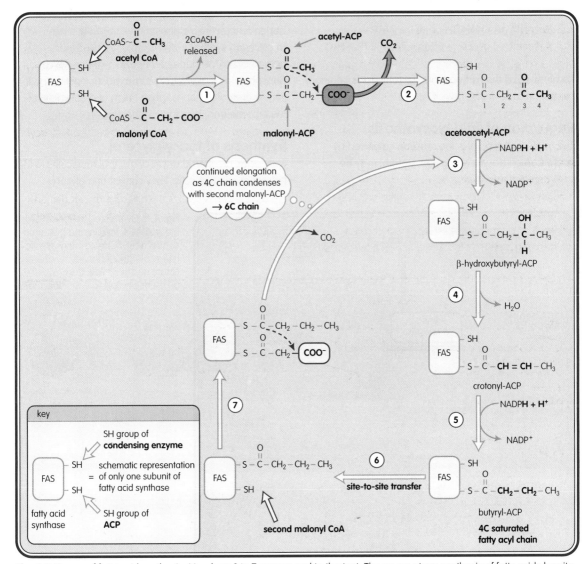

Fig. 4.5 Stages of fatty acid synthesis. Numbers 1 to 7 correspond to the text. The seven-stage synthesis of fatty acids has its cyclical part in steps 3–7 which add two carbons to the growing fatty acid chain for each cycle of the pathway.

It is worth remembering the characteristic set of reactions, namely the reduction, dehydration, reduction motif of fatty acid synthesis. The opposite of these reactions is the oxidation, hydration, and oxidation that occurs in the TCA cycle (Chapter 2) and fatty acid breakdown.

$$8\,\text{acetyl CoA} + 14\text{NADPH} + 14\text{H}^+ + 7\text{ATP} \rightarrow$$
$$\text{palmitate} + 14\text{NADP}^+ + 8\text{CoA} + 7\text{ADP} + 7\text{Pi} + \text{H}_2\text{O}$$

Remember, all the carbon atoms of fatty acids originally come from acetyl CoA.

Regulation of lipid biosynthesis

The main control point is the reaction catalysed by acetyl CoA carboxylase (Fig. 4.6). Control may be considered at two levels:

Allosteric regulation

Acetyl CoA carboxylase can exist in two forms: an inactive protomer or subunit form and an active polymer or filamentous form. Citrate activates acetyl CoA carboxylase by promoting the polymerization of protomers to active filaments. How? A rise in citrate concentration indicates that the substrate acetyl CoA and ATP are available for fatty acid synthesis (since an increase in ATP inhibits enzymes of the TCA cycle leading to a build-up of citrate).

Acetyl CoA carboxylase is inhibited by the product, palmitoyl CoA, which causes the depolymerization of filaments.

Reversible phosphorylation

Acetyl CoA carboxylase is also controlled by hormone-dependent reversible phosphorylation in a similar way to glycogen synthase (see Chapter 2). Glucagon activates a cAMP-dependent protein kinase which phosphorylates acetyl CoA carboxylase, inactivating it. Insulin promotes dephosphorylation and activation of the enzyme and thus lipid synthesis.

Synthesis of triacylglycerol

Fatty acids are stored as triacylglycerol molecules in the cytosol of adipose cells. They consist of a glycerol

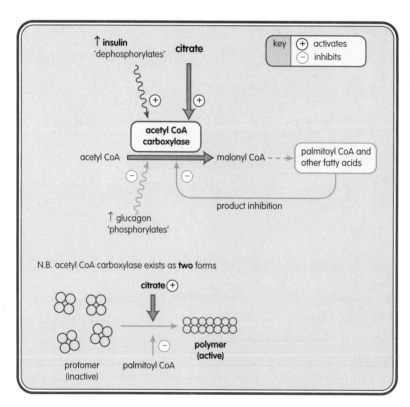

Fig. 4.6 Overall regulation of lipid biosynthesis. Insulin and glucagon control acetyl CoA carboxylase via reversible phosphorylation whereas citrate and palmitoyl CoA allosterically regulate the enzyme.

backbone esterified with three fatty acids.
Triacylglycerol formation can be thought of in three
main stages (the numbers correspond to Fig. 4.7).

1. Formation of glycerol-3-phosphate
This occurs either directly by the phosphorylation of
glycerol by glycerol kinase or by the reduction of the
glycolytic intermediate, dihydroxyacetonephosphate by
glycerol-3-phosphate dehydrogenase.

2. Activation of fatty acids
Fatty acyl CoA synthetase activates the fatty acids by
attaching them to CoA. The reaction requires ATP.

3. Esterification of glycerol-3-phosphate
Acyl transferase 'adds' the activated fatty acids to
glycerol-3-phosphate in stages.

During the synthesis of triacylglycerol, the
intermediate phosphatidate formed can also be used

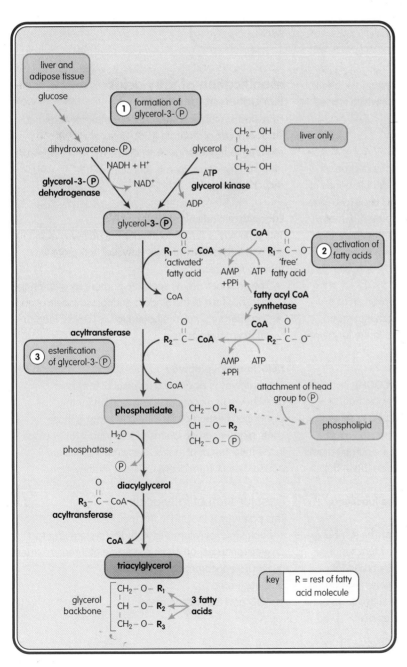

Fig. 4.7 Triacylglycerol synthesis
consists of three distinct stages as
described in the text.

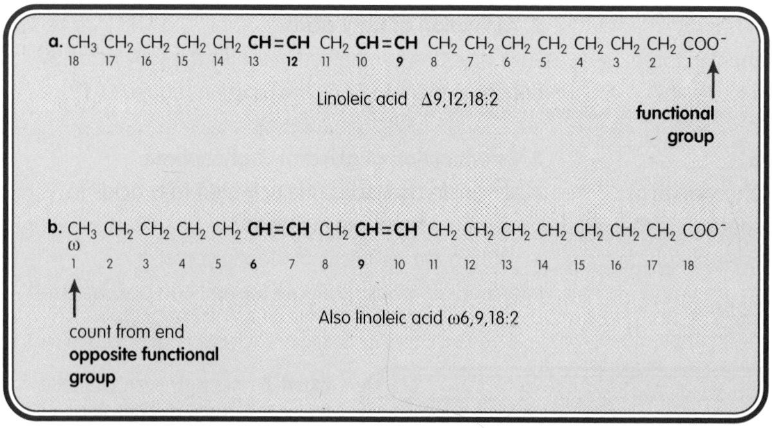

a. CH_3 CH_2 CH_2 CH_2 CH_2 **CH=CH** CH_2 **CH=CH** CH_2 CH_2 CH_2 CH_2 CH_2 CH_2 CH_2 COO^-
   18   17   16   15   14   **13 12**   11 **10   9**   8   7   6   5   4   3   2   1

Linoleic acid $\Delta 9,12,18:2$

functional group

b. CH_3 CH_2 CH_2 CH_2 CH_2 **CH=CH** CH_2 **CH=CH** CH_2 CH_2 CH_2 CH_2 CH_2 CH_2 CH_2 COO^-
   ω
   1   2   3   4   5   **6   7**   8   **9   10**   11   12   13   14   15   16   17   18

count from end opposite functional group

Also linoleic acid $\omega 6,9,18:2$

Fig. 4.8 The two ways of defining the position of a double bond:
a. By counting from the functional group.
b. By counting from the end opposite (ω) the functional group.

for the synthesis of phospholipids, for example, addition of choline to form phosphatidyl choline, which is used for membrane biosynthesis.

Nomenclature of fatty acids

Fatty acids vary in chain length and in the degree of unsaturation. The configuration of the double bonds in most unsaturated fatty acids in animals is *cis* (*cis* refers to the orientation of the substituent groups, i.e. methyl groups to the double bond. *Cis* means that the methyl groups are on the same side of the double bond compared with *trans*, where they are on opposite sides—remember 'A' level Chemistry!)

There are two ways of defining the position of a double bond: by counting from the functional group and by counting from the end opposite to the functional group (Fig. 4.8a and b).

Counting from the functional group (COOH)

Used by chemists; the position of the double bond is represented by the symbol Δ, followed by a number. For example, $\Delta 9,12, 18:2$, means an 18-carbon fatty acid containing two double bonds between the carbon atoms 9 and 10 and 12 and 13, that is linoleic acid (Fig. 4.8a).

Counting from the end opposite to the functional group

Used by biologists and more confusing! The symbol ω is used to depict the end opposite to the functional group. For example, $\omega 6,9, 18:2$ is an 18-carbon fatty acid containing two double bonds between the carbon atoms 6 and 7 and 9 and 10. From Fig. 4.8b, it can be seen however, that this is also linoleic acid.

Modification of fatty acids
Elongation of fatty acids

Fatty acid synthase only produces palmitate (C16) and a small amount of stearate (C18). Other enzymes are required to make longer fatty acids. These enzymes are found on the endoplasmic reticulum and in mitochondria.

Endoplasmic reticulum pathway

This pathway is similar to the normal pathway and steps of fatty acid synthesis. However, there are two main differences:

- The enzymes are all separate and are located on the cytosolic face of the smooth endoplasmic reticulum.
- The intermediates are bound to CoA rather than to an acyl carrier protein.

Mitochondrial pathway

This pathway is basically a reversal of fatty acid breakdown (β oxidation). It is important for the elongation of short chain fatty acids, that is those containing 14 carbon atoms or less, and it takes place in the mitochondrial matrix. Two carbon units are added directly from acetyl CoA, not malonyl CoA.

Desaturation of fatty acids

This pathway is located in the membrane of the smooth endoplasmic reticulum (Fig. 4.9). The system is in fact an electron transport chain consisting of three enzymes:

- NADH-cytochrome b_5 reductase.
- Cytochrome b_5.
- Fatty acyl CoA desaturase.

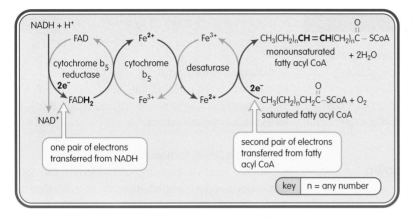

Fig. 4.9 The desaturation pathway located in the smooth endoplasmic reticulum, is responsible for the introduction of double bonds at positions Δ4, Δ5, Δ6, and Δ9.

Two pairs of electrons are passed down the chain: one pair comes from the single bond of the fatty acid and one pair from NADH. Mammalian systems have four different desaturase enzymes capable of producing double bonds at positions Δ4, Δ5, Δ6, and Δ9. Unsaturated fatty acids are necessary for the synthesis of important membrane phospholipids and intracellular messengers such as prostaglandins.

Essential fatty acids

Mammals can only form double bonds at the positions Δ4, Δ5, Δ6, and Δ9, but lack the enzymes needed to create double bonds beyond the ninth carbon atom. Therefore, certain polyunsaturated fatty acids (PUFAs) that are vital for health, cannot be synthesized endogenously and must be taken in from the diet. The

principal essential fatty acids are linoleic (C18:2) and α-linolenic (C18:3) acids, of the ω6 and ω3 series, respectively (see Fig. 4.10). From these, other important unsaturated fatty acids can be made. For example, arachidonic acid (C20:4) is synthesized from linolenic acid and is the precursor molecule for prostaglandin, leukotriene, and thromboxane molecules. Fish oils are a particularly good source of the ω3 series.

- Describe the overall process of lipid biosynthesis — remembering to mention its location, site, and use of the citrate shuttle.
- Describe the basic structure of fatty acid synthase and the function of the acyl carrier protein.
- Summarize the control of fatty acid synthesis.
- How are fatty acids stored?
- Briefly describe the pathways for long chain and unsaturated fatty acid production, that is, where they occur and what they do.
- What are the main essential fatty acids and why are they essential?

Essential fatty acids (EFAs)				
ω series	No. of C atoms	No. of double bonds	Position of double bonds	Name
ω3 series ω3,6,9	18	3	*cis* Δ9,12,15	α-linolenic acid (EFA)
ω6 series ω6,9	18	2	*cis* Δ9,12	**linoleic acid** (EFA)
ω6,9,12	18	3	*cis* Δ6,9,12	γ-linolenic acid (made from linolenic acid)
ω6,9,12,15	20	4	*cis* Δ5,8,11,14	arachidonic acid

Fig. 4.10 Essential fatty acids.

LIPID BREAKDOWN

Triacylglycerol stores in adipose tissue serve as the body's major fuel reserve. Fatty acids are easily mobilized to provide energy during prolonged exercise or starvation. The oxidation of fat yields about 9 kcal/g (38.6 kJ) of energy compared with only 4 kcal/g (16.8 kJ) for protein and carbohydrate.

An overview of lipid breakdown

Working definition
Lipid breakdown is the process by which a molecule of fatty acid is degraded by the sequential removal of two carbon units, producing acetyl CoA which can then be oxidized to CO_2 and H_2O by the TCA cycle.

Location
Many tissues, especially liver and muscle. Certain tissues are unable to oxidize fatty acids, namely the brain, RBCs, and adrenal medulla, because they lack the necessary enzymes.

The four stages of lipid breakdown
Lipid breakdown can be conveniently divided into four main stages.

1. Hydrolysis of triacylglycerol by lipase: lipolysis
Lipolysis occurs in the cell cytosol of adipose cells. The hydrolysis of triacylglycerol produces glycerol and free fatty acids. The free fatty acids travel in the blood bound to albumin and are taken up by muscle or liver cells for oxidation.

2. Activation of fatty acids
Before they can be oxidized, fatty acids are activated by attachment to CoA to form acyl CoA molecules; this takes place in the cell cytosol.

3. Transport into mitochondria
β Oxidation occurs in the mitochondrial matrix. The acyl CoA molecules are transported into the mitochondria by the carnitine shuttle.

4. β Oxidation
Fatty acids are degraded by a cyclical sequence of four reactions: oxidation, hydration, oxidation, thiolysis. This results in the shortening of the fatty acid chain by two carbon atoms per sequence. The two carbons are removed as acetyl CoA. For even-numbered saturated fatty acids this is straightforward, but other enzymes are necessary for the oxidation of unsaturated and odd-numbered fatty acids (see later).

These steps are now considered in more detail.

Lipolysis
The initial event in the breakdown of fat is the hydrolysis of triacylglycerol stores in adipose tissue. Triacylglycerol is converted into glycerol and three, free fatty acids in two steps (Fig. 4.11):

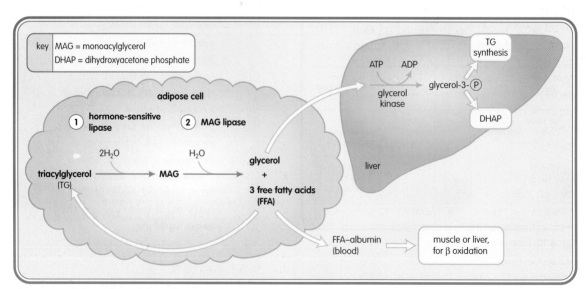

Fig. 4.11 Hydrolysis of triacylglycerol to glycerol and free fatty acids (numbers refer to the text).

1. A hormone-sensitive lipase hydrolyses triacylglycerol at the C1 and C3 positions to form monoacylglycerol.
2. A monoacylglycerol specific lipase removes the remaining fatty acid.

The glycerol produced cannot be metabolized by adipose tissue because adipose tissue does not contain glycerol kinase. Glycerol is transported to the liver where it is phosphorylated, either to be used again to make triacylglycerol or to be converted to dihydroxyacetone phosphate (DHAP), a glycolytic intermediate. The free fatty acids produced are either re-esterified to triacylglycerol in the adipose tissue or travel in the blood to be taken up by the cells for oxidation.

Activation of fatty acids to fatty acyl CoA
Fatty acyl CoA synthetase (thiokinase) activates fatty acids by attaching them to CoA. The reaction occurs on the cytosolic face of the outer mitochondrial membrane and requires ATP, which is hydrolysed to AMP and pyrophosphate (PPi), breaking a high-energy phosphate bond. The reaction is made irreversible by the rapid hydrolysis of the pyrophosphate to two free inorganic phosphates by pyrophosphatase, consuming a second high-energy phosphate bond (Fig. 4.12). Therefore the activation of a fatty acid consumes 2ATP equivalents. Fatty acids are non-polar molecules and can easily diffuse out of cells but the attachment to a polar molecule such as CoA, 'traps' the fatty acid inside.

Transport of fatty acyl CoA molecules into mitochondria
The activation of fatty acids occurs in the cytosol but the enzymes for β oxidation are in the mitochondrial matrix. The inner mitochondrial membrane is relatively impermeable to long-chain acyl CoA molecules, so a special transporter system is required to 'carry' the fatty acid across. The carnitine shuttle consists of three enzymes: a translocase and two carnitine acyltransferases, CAT I and II as shown in Fig. 4.12.

β Oxidation
Acyl CoA molecules inside the mitochondrial matrix undergo β oxidation, a cyclical sequence of four reactions (numbers refer to Fig. 4.13).

1. Oxidation
The oxidation of acyl CoA introduces a double bond between the C2 and C3 atoms. The $FADH_2$ formed

enters the electron transport chain to produce 1.5ATP (see Chapter 2). In mitochondria there are three types of acyl CoA dehydrogenase, which act on long, medium, and short chain fatty acids, respectively. A deficiency in medium chain acyl CoA dehydrogenase has been recognized (this is discussed further in Chapter 12).

2. Hydration
Hydration is the addition of water across the double bond between C2 and C3 by enoyl CoA hydratase.

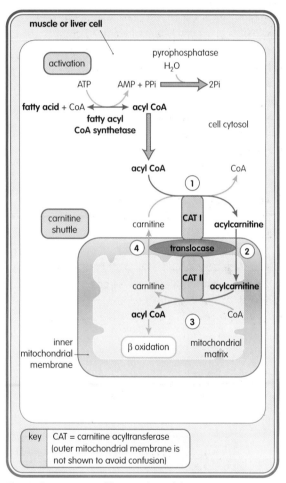

Fig. 4.12 Activation of fatty acids and their transport into mitochondria by the carnitine shuttle.
1. The acyl group is transferred from CoA to carnitine by carnitine acyltransferase I, an enzyme found on the cytosolic side of the inner mitochondrial membrane.
2. Acylcarnitine is transported across the membrane by the translocase to the mitochondrial matrix.
3. The acyl group is transferred back to CoA by carnitine acyltransferase II, located on the inner surface of the inner mitochondrial membrane.
4. Carnitine is returned to the cytosolic side in exchange for another acylcarnitine.

61

Lipid Metabolism

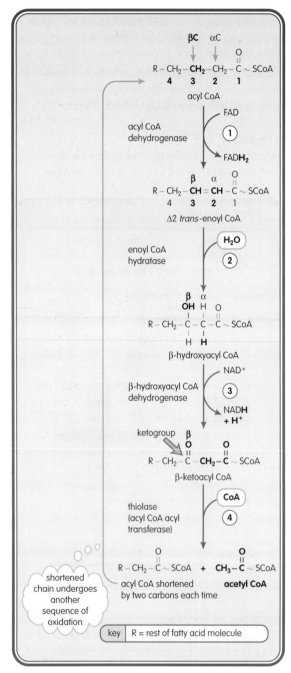

For even-numbered, saturated fatty acids, $(n \div 2) - 1$ cycles are required for complete oxidation, where n = the number of carbons of the fatty acid.
e.g. C16 palmitate requires $(16 \div 2) - 1 = 7$ cycles.

3. Oxidation by NAD⁺

β-hydroxyacyl CoA dehydrogenase converts the OH group at C3 (the β carbon) to a keto group. The NADH produced enters the electron transport chain to make 2.5 ATP molecules. These three reactions of oxidation, hydration, and oxidation resemble the last three reactions of the TCA cycle which convert succinate to oxaloacetate (see Chapter 2).

4. Thiolytic cleavage by CoA

Thiolase cleaves the molecule to release acetyl CoA and acyl CoA is shortened by two carbon atoms. The shortened acyl CoA is ready to undergo another sequence of β oxidation. The four steps are repeated until the fatty acid is oxidized completely to acetyl CoA. The last round of oxidation produces two molecules of acetyl CoA.

ATP yield from the oxidation of the fatty acid palmitate

Each round of β oxidation produces one molecule each of FADH₂, NADH, and acetyl CoA. The β oxidation of palmitate requires seven cycles, producing 7 FADH₂, 7 NADH, and 8 acetyl CoA in total (see Fig. 2.21).

ATP yield

The activation of palmitate to palmitoyl CoA consumes 2 molecules of ATP. β oxidation generates:

- 7 FADH₂, which are oxidized by the electron transport chain to generate 10.5 ATP.
- 7 NADH, which are oxidized by the chain to generate 17.5 ATP.
- 8 acetyl CoA, which are oxidized by the TCA cycle to generate 80 ATP (remember, oxidation of each acetyl CoA by the TCA cycle yields 10 ATP).

Fig. 4.13 β Oxidation pathway. The cyclical sequence of four reactions; oxidation, hydration, oxidation, and thiolysis, shortens the fatty acid chain by two carbons each cycle. This continues until the fatty acid is completely oxidized to acetyl CoA.

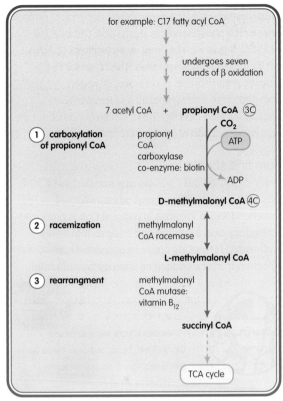

Fig. 4.14 Oxidation of odd-numbered fatty acids produces propionyl CoA, which is metabolized to succinyl CoA in three steps to enter the TCA cycle.

Therefore the total energy generated from the oxidation of a molecule of palmitate is 106 ATP.

Oxidation of odd-numbered fatty acids

The oxidation of odd-numbered fatty acids (Fig. 4.14) is essentially the same as for even-numbered fatty acids except that the last round of β oxidation produces one molecule of acetyl CoA and one of propionyl CoA (3C), instead of two molecules of acetyl CoA. Propionyl CoA is metabolized to succinyl CoA, which can then enter the TCA cycle.

Oxidation of unsaturated fatty acids

In the oxidation of unsaturated fatty acids, most of the reactions are the same as for saturated fatty acids except two additional enzymes are involved, enoyl CoA isomerase and 2,4-dienoyl reductase. Naturally occurring unsaturated fatty acids contain *cis* double bonds. These are not easily metabolized by the enzymes of β oxidation, particularly enoyl CoA hydratase which is specific for the *trans* configuration of double bonds.

However, enoyl CoA isomerase converts a *cis* to a *trans* double bond thus enabling β oxidation to proceed.

During the oxidation of some unsaturated fatty acids, for example, linoleic acid (*cis* Δ9,12, 18:2), the intermediate 2,4-dienoyl CoA is produced. This, again, is not a substrate for enoyl CoA hydratase, however NADPH-dependent 2,4-dienoyl reductase reduces it to *trans* enoyl CoA, thus enabling β oxidation to continue. This 2,4-dienoyl CoA reductase enzyme has only recently been described.

It was previously thought an epimerase enzyme was required for oxidation of unsaturated fatty acids but it is now known that this enzyme is only present in peroxisomes and not in mitochondria.

Peroxisomal β oxidation

Oxidation of fatty acids can also occur in peroxisomes, in the kidney and in the liver. Approximately 5–10% of the total oxidation of fatty acids occurs in peroxisomes, with the rest in mitochondria. The pathway of β oxidation in mitochondria and peroxisomes is identical; it is the enzymes that are different. The enzymes of peroxisomes are more versatile and can oxidize a wider range of substrates, including prostaglandins. The main function of peroxisomal oxidation is the shortening of long chain fatty acids, for example those greater than 22–24 carbon atoms, preparing them for β oxidation by the mitochondrial system.

Different enzymes of peroxisomal and mitochondrial β oxidation
Oxidation
The FAD-containing enzyme acyl CoA oxidase, passes its electrons directly to oxygen, so no ATP is formed. Energy is dissipated as heat instead.

Hydration and oxidation
These are performed by the bifunctional enzyme which has both enoyl CoA hydratase and 3-hydroxyacyl CoA dehydrogenase activity.

Thiolysis
Thiolase cleaves acyl CoA, releasing acetyl CoA and a shortened acyl chain.

Oxidation continues until acyl CoA molecules are fewer than 22 carbons in length, at which point they diffuse out of the peroxisomes, via a pore-forming protein in the peroxisomal membrane, for further oxidation in mitochondria.

Regulation of lipid breakdown

The control of lipid breakdown is exerted at three levels (Fig. 4.15): lipolysis, carnitine shuttle, and β oxidation.

Control of lipolysis

Hormone-sensitive lipase (see Fig. 4.11) is regulated by reversible phosphorylation. Adrenaline during exercise, and glucagon and adrenocorticotrophic hormone (ACTH) during starvation, activate adenylate cyclase, which increases the levels of cAMP. This activates a cAMP-dependent protein kinase, which phosphorylates

lipase, activating it. The same cAMP-dependent protein kinase also phosphorylates acetyl CoA carboxylase, inhibiting it (see Fig. 4.6); that is, it stimulates lipolysis but inhibits fatty acid synthesis. This is similar to the reciprocal mechanism of control of glycogen phosphorylase and synthase by reversible phosphorylation (see Fig. 2.34). Insulin brings about the dephosphorylation of lipase, inhibiting lipolysis.

Carnitine shuttle

Malonyl CoA inhibits carnitine acyl transferase I (CAT I), thus inhibiting the entry of acyl groups into mitochondria. An increase in malonyl CoA is produced during fatty acid synthesis and ensures that newly synthesized fatty acids are not transported into mitochondria for oxidation as soon as they are made.

In exams you will often be asked to compare the processes of fatty acid synthesis and degradation. Fig. 4.16 should give you an idea of the main points to include.

○ Describe the four main stages of lipid breakdown and name the site of each.
○ **Summarize the function and mechanism of the carnitine shuttle.**
○ Describe the four steps of β oxidation.
○ **Work out the approximate ATP yield from the oxidation of a fatty acid such as palmitate.**
○ **Which enzymes are required for the oxidation of odd-numbered and unsaturated fatty acids?**
○ Describe the three main control sites of lipid breakdown.

Fig. 4.15 Regulation of lipid breakdown. Control is exerted at three levels. **1.** lipolysis, **2.** the carnitine shuttle, **3.** β oxidation.

Comparison of fatty acid synthesis and degradation		
	Synthesis	**Degradation**
Active	after meals: fed state	fasting and prolonged exercise
Main tissues involved	liver and adipose tissue	muscle and liver
Site	cytosol	mitochondria
2C donor/product	acetyl CoA	acetyl CoA
Active fatty acid carrier	attached to ACP	attached to CoA
Enzymes	FAS: enzymes all part of multi-enzyme complex	probably not associated
Oxidant/reductant	NADPH	NAD^+ and FAD
Allosteric control	citrate activates acetyl CoA carboxylase; palmitoyl CoA inhibits it	malonyl CoA inhibits CAT I
Hormonal control	insulin activates acetyl CoA carboxylase; adrenaline and glucagon inhibit it	adrenaline and glucagon activate lipase; insulin inhibits it
Product	palmitate	acetyl CoA

Fig. 4.16 Comparison of fatty acid synthesis and degradation.

Inhibition of β oxidation by NADH and $FADH_2$

The oxidation reactions require a supply of FAD and NAD^+, which are regenerated via the electron transport chain. The enzymes of β oxidation have to compete with the dehydrogenase enzymes of the TCA cycle for NAD^+ and FAD because both pathways are usually active at the same time.

CHOLESTEROL METABOLISM

Role of cholesterol in the body

Cholesterol has many functions in the body, including being:
- An essential component of cell membranes.
- A precursor of the five major classes of steroid hormones: progestogens, oestrogens, androgens, glucocorticoids, and mineralocorticoids.
- A precursor of bile acids and vitamin D.

The body therefore requires a continuous supply of cholesterol.

Sources of cholesterol

Cholesterol can either be obtained from the diet or be synthesized endogenously by the body. Regulatory mechanisms exist which try to balance the amount of cholesterol made by the body daily with both the dietary intake and the amount excreted, either in bile or as bile salts to enable control of the plasma cholesterol level. Failure of this control may lead to high plasma cholesterol levels and an increased risk of cardiovascular disease in particular, coronary heart disease, stroke, and peripheral vascular disease.

Cholesterol synthesis

Cholesterol is a 27-carbon steroid molecule. All 27 carbon atoms of cholesterol come from acetyl CoA. It is one of a large group of compounds derived from the five-carbon isoprene group (others include ubiquinone and the vitamins A, E, and K). The easiest way to view cholesterol synthesis is to divide it into two stages (Fig. 4.17):
- Stage I: The formation of the isoprene unit, isopentenyl pyrophosphate (IPP). This is formed by the condensation of three molecules of acetyl CoA to 3-hydroxy-3-methylglutaryl CoA (HMG-CoA), followed by the loss of CO_2.
- Stage II: The progressive condensation of isoprene units to form cholesterol. Six, five-carbon isoprene units link up to form squalene (30 C atoms) which cyclizes to lanosterol, from which cholesterol arises.

Location

Cholesterol is made by most tissues (except RBCs) but the main site of synthesis is the liver.

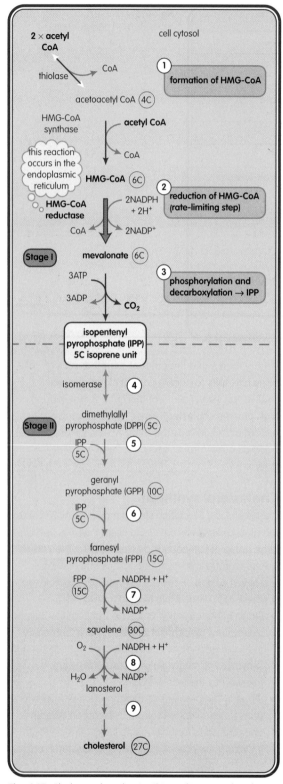

Fig. 4.17 Cholesterol synthesis. This multi-stepped pathway is divided into two stages. The final steps in stage II are still not fully understood (numbers refer to the text).

Site

Cell cytosol, although some of the enzymes are found in the endoplasmic reticulum.

These stages are now considered in more detail and are clearly illustrated in Fig. 4.17.

Stage I: Formation of IPP

1. Formation of HMG-CoA from acetyl CoA

This occurs in two steps:

- Two molecules of acetyl CoA condense to form acetoacetyl CoA (4C).
- HMG-CoA synthase catalyses the addition of a third molecule of acetyl CoA to form HMG-CoA (6C).

HMG-CoA is also an intermediate in the synthesis of ketone bodies. However, ketone body formation occurs in the mitochondria whereas the reactions of cholesterol synthesis occur in the cell cytosol. The liver therefore contains two isoenzymes of HMG-CoA synthase: a cytosolic enzyme for cholesterol synthesis and a mitochondrial enzyme for ketone body formation.

2. Reduction of HMG-CoA to mevalonic acid (mevalonate)

This is the irreversible, rate-limiting step of cholesterol synthesis and thus the most important control site. The enzyme HMG-CoA reductase is found in the endoplasmic reticulum and requires NADPH as a reducing agent.

3. Phosphorylation and decarboxylation of mevalonate to IPP

Mevalonate is converted to IPP in three reactions requiring three molecules of ATP. The first two reactions are phosphorylations forming a 5-pyrophosphome-valonate intermediate (not shown in Fig. 4.17) which is then decarboxylated to form isopentenyl pyrophosphate (IPP).

Stage II: Progressive condensation of isoprene units to cholesterol

4. Isomerization of IPP to dimethylallyl pyrophosphate

The five-carbon isoprene units then link up in a stepwise fashion as shown in Fig. 4.17.

5. IPP and dimethylallyl pyrophosphate condense to form the 10-carbon, geranyl pyrophosphate

6. Another IPP condenses with geranyl pyrophosphate to form the 15-carbon, farnesyl pyrophosphate

7. Squalene synthase catalyses the reductive condensation of two molecules of farnesyl pyrophosphate, forming the 30-carbon molecule, squalene

All three condensation reactions (5, 6, and 7) release pyrophosphate (which 'drives' the reactions), making them favourable.

8. Cyclization of squalene to lanosterol (30C) by squalene monoxygenase

9. Conversion of lanosterol to cholesterol

The exact pathway is not known but it is thought to consist of about 20 steps! Basically, three methyl groups are removed to produce a 27-carbon molecule followed by the migration of the double bond to the Δ5 position to produce cholesterol (Fig. 4.18).

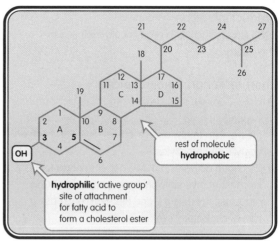

Fig. 4.18 Structure of cholesterol.

Regulation of cholesterol synthesis

Regulation is necessary in order to prevent high plasma cholesterol levels which may lead to cholesterol deposition in arterial walls and the formation of atherosclerotic plaques. Indeed the primary control site is the rate-limiting enzyme HMG-CoA reductase (Fig. 4.19).

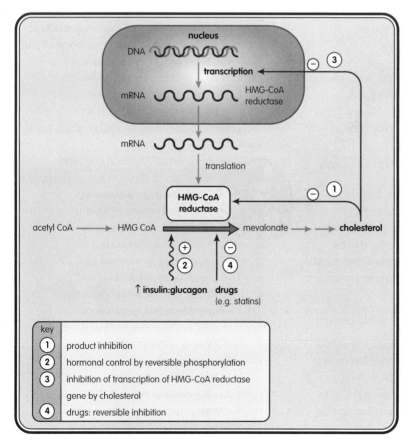

Fig. 4.19 Control of HMG-CoA reductase. This enzyme is not only affected by cholesterol as its product in an allosteric fashion but also because cholesterol actually down-regulates the transcription of HMG-CoA reductase which catalyses the rate-limiting step of cholesterol synthesis.

Product inhibition

HMG-CoA reductase is allosterically inhibited by cholesterol.

Short-term hormonal regulation

- HMG-CoA reductase is also regulated by hormone-dependent reversible phosphorylation by a similar mechanism to glycogen synthase (see Fig. 2.34) and acetyl CoA carboxylase.
- Glucagon activates a cAMP-dependent protein kinase that reversibly phosphorylates HMG-CoA reductase, inhibiting it and therefore decreasing the rate of cholesterol synthesis.
- Insulin dephosphorylates the enzyme leading to its activation and an increase in cholesterol synthesis.

Long-term regulation of HMG-CoA reductase

- This is probably the most important control mechanism.
- The amount of cholesterol, both dietary and endogenous, taken up by cells affects the amount of HMG-CoA reductase synthesized.
- A high cholesterol level in cells causes a decrease in the rate of transcription of the HMG-CoA reductase gene inhibiting it, leading to a reduction in cholesterol synthesis.

High intracellular levels of cholesterol also suppress the synthesis of cholesterol receptors, resulting in a decrease in the uptake of cholesterol by the cell. A low intracellular cholesterol concentration stimulates receptor synthesis.

Packaging of cholesterol

Most of the cholesterol in the blood is in the form of cholesterol esters, formed by the addition of a fatty acid to the C3-OH group (see Fig. 4.18). Esterification makes the cholesterol more hydrophobic enabling it to be packaged and stored easily. Two enzyme systems are responsible for the esterification of cholesterol (numbers refer to Fig. 4.20):

1. In cells:
- If the cholesterol taken up or synthesized by cells is not immediately required then it is esterified by acyl CoA:cholesterol acyl transferase (ACAT).
- ACAT transfers a fatty acid from a fatty acyl CoA to cholesterol, forming a cholesterol ester that can be stored in the cell.

2. In high density lipoprotein:
- A similar enzyme known as lecithin:cholesterol acyl transferase (LCAT) is found associated with high density lipoprotein (HDL).
- HDL is responsible for picking up free cholesterol from peripheral tissues and transporting it to the liver, that is, it acts as a cholesterol scavenger.
- LCAT catalyses the transfer of a fatty acid from the phospholipid, phosphatidylcholine to cholesterol.
- HDL then carries cholesterol esters to the liver either to be reused or excreted.

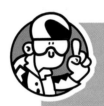

For patients with a high plasma cholesterol (hypercholesterolaemia), treatment includes drugs that reversibly inhibit HMG–CoA reductase. Therefore these drugs, known as statins, decrease the rate of cholesterol synthesis by cells. Cells compensate for lower cholesterol levels by increasing the synthesis and thus the number of cholesterol receptors on the cell surface. This increases cholesterol uptake by the cells and therefore reduces plasma cholesterol.

- What are the main functions of cholesterol?
- What are the sources of cholesterol and why is it important to control the plasma cholesterol level?
- Name the location and the site of cholesterol synthesis and outline the pathway.
- How is cholesterol synthesis regulated?
- Name the enzymes responsible for the esterification of cholesterol.

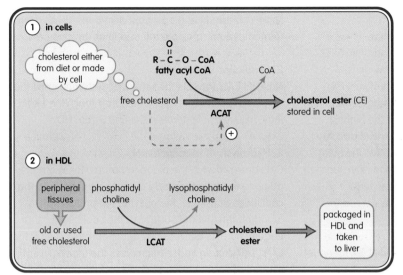

Fig. 4.20 Two enzyme systems are responsible for the esterification of cholesterol; acyl CoA:cholesterol acyl transferase in cells and lecithin: cholesterol acyl transferase in HDL (refer to text on p. 68).

TRANSPORT OF LIPIDS

Lipoproteins

Lipids are insoluble in aqueous solution and therefore are transported in the plasma in association with proteins to form lipoproteins (Fig. 4.21). Lipoproteins function both to solubilize the lipids and to provide an efficient transport system for them. If the system fails, the plasma lipid concentration will increase. Long term, a high plasma cholesterol level is associated with an increased risk of coronary heart disease.

Apolipoproteins are only weakly associated with lipoprotein complexes and can therefore be transferred easily between them. They have a number of functions including acting:

• In a structural role.
• As recognition sites or ligands for receptors.
• As activators or co-enzymes for enzymes involved in lipid metabolism.

The functions of the major apolipoproteins are summarized in Fig. 4.22.

Fig. 4.21 The basic structure of a lipoprotein particle consists of a non-polar lipid core containing triacylglycerol (TG) and cholesterol esters surrounded by a polar outer coat of phospholipids, free cholesterol, and proteins known as apolipoproteins.

Functions of the major apolipoproteins	
Apolipoprotein	**Function**
A-I	activates lecithin:cholesterol acyl transferase
A-II	activates hepatic lipase
B-48	structural (CM); recognized by remnant receptor increases cholesterol uptake
B-100	structural; binds to LDL receptor increases cholesterol uptake
C-I	co-factor for lecithin:cholesterol acyl transferase
C-II	activates lipoprotein lipase
C-III	inhibits lipoprotein lipase?
E	binds to apo. B/E receptor and increases cholesterol uptake

Fig. 4.22 Functions of major apolipoproteins.

Classes of lipoprotein

There are five main classes of lipoproteins: chylomicrons (CM), very low density lipoprotein (VLDL), intermediate density lipoprotein (IDL), low density lipoprotein (LDL), and high density lipoprotein (HDL). They are classified according to increasing density, with CM having the lowest density and HDL the highest. Remember, protein is more dense than lipid and so HDL, with the highest density, must contain the most protein. Lipoproteins differ in composition, size, function, and the apolipoproteins present on their surface. These properties are summarized in Fig. 4.23.

Pathways of lipid transport

Lipids can either be obtained from the diet (exogenous lipid) or synthesized by the body (endogenous lipid). There are two different pathways for lipid transport in the body; HDL takes part in both of these pathways:

- Exogenous pathway: chylomicrons (CMs) transport dietary lipid absorbed from the intestine to the tissues (Fig. 4.24).
- Endogenous pathway: VLDL, IDL, and LDL transport endogenously synthesized triacylglycerol and cholesterol from the liver to the tissues (Fig. 4.25).

These pathways can now be considered in more detail.

Exogenous pathway (numbers refer to Fig. 4.24)

1. CM formation

CMs are assembled in intestinal mucosal cells from dietary fat. They contain mainly triacylglycerol with some cholesterol and apolipoprotein B-48. These newly formed chylomicrons are referred to as nascent CMs.

2. Circulation of CMs

Nascent CMs travel in the lymphatic system to enter the blood via the thoracic duct. When they reach the blood they acquire apolipoprotein C-II and E from HDL.

3. Hydrolysis of triacylglycerol

CMs are carried in the blood to tissues, for example, adipose tissue and muscle. As they pass through the capillaries of tissues, the enzyme lipoprotein lipase, found on the luminal surface of the capillary endothelium, is activated by apolipoprotein C-II on the CMs. Lipoprotein lipase hydrolyses the triacylglycerol content of CMs to glycerol and free fatty acids. The fatty acids are taken up by cells either for oxidation or storage as triacylglycerol.

4. Formation of CM remnants

The removal of triacylglycerol leaves behind a much smaller CM remnant particle. Apolipoprotein C-II is returned to HDL. Apolipoproteins B-48 and E are recognized by remnant receptors on liver cells and the CM remnants are taken up by the liver and degraded. Cholesterol released from the remnants inhibits HMG-CoA reductase and thus the endogenous synthesis of cholesterol by the liver (see Fig. 4.19).

Classification and properties of lipoproteins				
Class	Main composition	Diameter (nm)	Source and function	Major apolipo-proteins
CM	90% triacylglycerol	500	transport of **dietary** triacylglycerol	A-I, II, B-48, C-I, II, III, E
VLDL	65% triacylglycerol	43	transport of **endogenously** synthesized triacylglycerol from the liver to peripheral tissues	B-100, C-I, II, III, E
IDL	35% phospholipid 25% cholesterol	27	formed by partial breakdown of VLDL, precursor of LDL	B-100,C-III, E
LDL	50% cholesterol 25% protein	22	formed by breakdown of IDL; carries cholesterol to peripheral tissues	B-100
HDL	55% protein 25% phospholipid	8	formed in the liver; 2 main functions: • reverse cholesterol transport removes 'used' cholesterol from tissues and takes it to liver; 'cholesterol scavenger' • provides apolipoproteins C-II and E for chylomicrons and VLDL	A-I, II, C-I, II, III, D, E

Fig. 4.23 Classification and properties of lipoproteins.

Endogenous pathway (numbers refer to Fig. 4.25)
The liver is the main site of lipid synthesis.

1. Assembly of VLDL
VLDL is synthesized in the liver mostly from triacylglycerol and is released as nascent VLDL particles containing surface apolipoprotein B-100. Like CMs, VLDL acquires apolipoprotein C-II and E from HDL. VLDL transports endogenous triacylglycerol to peripheral tissues.

2. Hydrolysis by lipoprotein lipase (LPL) in tissues
Lipoprotein lipase removes triacylglycerol in the same way as for CMs. VLDL becomes smaller in size and more dense (VLDL remnant).

3. Formation of IDL and LDL
Some triacylglycerol, phospholipids, and apolipoprotein C-II are transferred to HDL, converting VLDL to the denser lipoprotein, IDL. Cholesterol esters are transferred from HDL to IDL in exchange for triacylglycerol and phospholipid by cholesterol ester transfer protein. Some of the IDL is taken up by the liver

via receptors that recognize both apolipoprotein B and apolipoprotein E on the surface of IDL (not shown in Fig. 4.25); but the rest forms LDL. Therefore, the sequence is VLDL → IDL → LDL.

4. LDL provides cholesterol for peripheral tissues
LDL binds to LDL receptors on cell membranes and is internalized by receptor-mediated endocytosis. The LDL receptor recognizes apolipoprotein B-100 on the LDL. Lysosomal enzymes hydrolyse LDL releasing free cholesterol into the cell.

5. HDL metabolism
HDL is made in the liver and has two main functions:
- It accepts 'used' free cholesterol from peripheral tissues and lipoproteins and esterifies it by the action of LCAT (see Fig. 4.20). The cholesterol esters formed are either transferred to VLDL or IDL to form LDL or are carried back to the liver by 'reverse cholesterol transport'.
- HDL also provides apolipoproteins for other lipoproteins (CMs and VLDL) as already described.

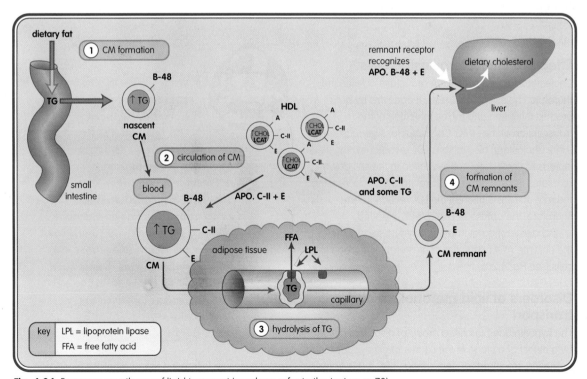

Fig. 4.24 Exogenous pathway of lipid transport (numbers refer to the text on p. 70).

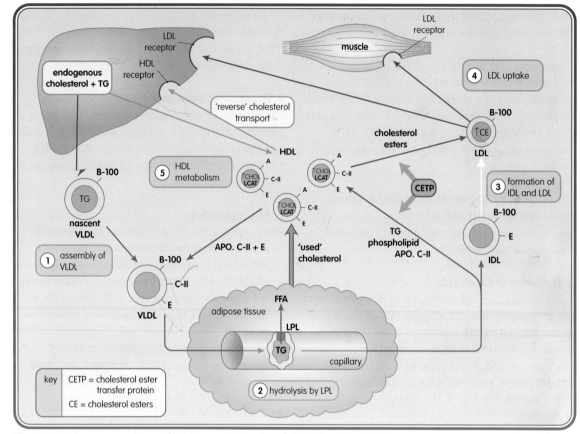

Fig. 4.25 Endogenous pathway of lipid transport (numbers refer to the text on p. 71).

Effects of cholesterol inside cells

Cholesterol inhibits HMG-CoA reductase activity and therefore cholesterol synthesis. It does this by both product inhibition and by the inhibition of the transcription of the HMG-CoA reductase gene (see Fig. 4.19). Cholesterol also inhibits LDL receptor synthesis. An increased cholesterol concentration in the cell down-regulates the synthesis of LDL receptors by decreasing the rate of transcription of the LDL receptor gene. Therefore, the uptake of cholesterol is limited.

If cholesterol is not immediately required by the cell, the enzyme ACAT esterifies cholesterol for storage in cells (see Fig. 4.20).

Disorders of lipid metabolism and transport

The hyperlipidaemias are a group of disorders caused by a defect at a stage in the course of either lipoprotein formation, transport, or degradation (Fig. 4.26). They result in the accumulation of lipids in the blood and in

Whereas an increase in LDL-cholesterol is harmful, an increase in HDL-cholesterol has a protective effect because it removes old cholesterol and takes it to the liver for degradation and excretion. It is known that one or two glasses of red wine each day increases the levels of HDL. Unfortunately, this is only seen with one or two glasses, so most people will not notice this beneficial effect!

most cases an increased risk of atherosclerosis and coronary heart disease. The clinical aspects of these

Fig. 4.26 Disorders of lipid metabolism: hyperlipidaemias.

Type	Name	Cause	Effect on lipoproteins
I	**familial LPL deficiency or apo C-II deficiency** autosomal recessive	decreased or absent LPL activity	increased CMs cause a milky serum increased triacylglycerol may cause acute pancreatitis
IIa	**familial hypercholesterolaemia** autosomal dominant (1:500)	deficiency or total absence of LDL receptors (occasionally caused by a defect in apolipoprotein B-100)	decreased uptake of LDL by tissues and increased plasma cholesterol concentration homozygotes have no receptors and die of coronary heart disease in childhood
IIb	**familial combined hyperlipidaemia** autosomal dominant	overproduction of apolipoprotein B by liver	increased VLDL secretion leads to increased LDL (increased plasma cholesterol and triacylglycerol)
III	**remnant hyperlipidaemia** (familial dys-β-lipoproteinaemia)	abnormal apolipoprotein E decrease in remnant clearance by liver	increased IDL; increased risk of peripheral vascular disease and coronary heart disease
IV	**familial hypertriglyceridaemia**: mild form	overproduction of VLDL by the liver	increased VLDL
V	**familial hypertriglyceridaemia**: severe form	overproduction of VLDL by the liver	increased VLDL and increased CMs

Title: Disorders of lipid metabolism: hyperlipidaemias

disorders are covered in Chapter 12. Commonly the disorders occur as a result of a deficiency in either:
- An enzyme, for example, LPL deficiency.
- An apolipoprotein, for example, apolipoprotein C-II deficiency.
- A receptor, for example, LDL receptor.

Drugs used to control lipid metabolism
There are two main approaches to the treatment of hyperlipidaemias: diet and/or drugs. This is discussed fully in Chapter 12. The main drugs used to control lipid metabolism are illustrated in Fig. 4.27.

- Describe the basic structure and functions of lipoproteins.
- Name the five main types of lipoproteins and their properties.
- Outline the two pathways for lipid transport in the body.
- Describe the main apolipoproteins and their role.
- Give two or three examples of hyperlipidaemias (I, IIa, and IIb are the most common).
- Give two or three examples of drugs used to control lipid metabolism and their action.

Drug	Mechanism of action
statins: simvastatin, lovastatin	inhibit **HMG-CoA reductase**, decreasing cholesterol synthesis; cell compensates for lower cholesterol by increasing LDL receptor synthesis, resulting in increased cholesterol uptake thus leading to decreased plasma cholesterol
fibrates: bezafibrate, gemfibrozil	activate LPL (main effect), thus lowering plasma TG; suppress HMG-CoA reductase, leading to increased uptake of LDL by liver
anion exchange resins: cholestyramine, colestipol	bind bile acids in gastrointestinal tract preventing their reabsorption and therefore decrease plasma LDL levels
nicotinic acid	decreases VLDL production by liver and thus LDL; increases LPL activity, leading to decreased triacylglycerol
fish oils	increase the concentration of polyunsaturated fatty acids; reduce triacylglycerol synthesis in the liver

Title: Main drugs used to control lipid metabolism

Fig. 4.27 Main drugs used to control lipid metabolism.

KETONE BODIES

The roles of the ketone bodies

Ketone bodies, namely acetoacetic acid, 3-hydroxybutyric acid, and acetone, provide an alternative fuel for cells and are produced at low levels all the time. However, they are only produced in significant quantities during adverse states such as starvation, prolonged severe exercise, or uncontrolled diabetes, that is, they are produced when the glucose concentration is limiting.

Starvation

In the fed state, the brain uses only glucose as its energy source since fatty acids cannot cross the blood–brain barrier. During starvation, the brain adapts to using ketone bodies as its major fuel because they are soluble and can therefore cross the blood–brain barrier. This reduces the need for glucose which, during starvation, when glycogen reserves are depleted, comes from the breakdown of muscle protein into amino acids, which are then oxidized to glucose by gluconeogenesis. Therefore, the use of ketone bodies as a fuel spares glucose and preserves muscle protein. In starvation the production of ketone bodies is usually controlled so that their rate of formation is equal to their rate of use. This prevents the accumulation of acidic ketone bodies so the pH of the blood remains buffered within normal limits.

Metabolic adaptation to starvation, exercise, and diabetic states are very common topics for exam questions. The use of ketone bodies is just one adaptation; see Chapters 5 and 7 for others. You must know which fuels are used and why.

Diabetes

In well-controlled diabetes, tissues receive an adequate glucose supply and ketone body production is minimal. Severe, uncontrolled diabetes leads to the massive production of acidic ketone bodies, to the point where the rate of formation is far greater than the rate of use. This can lead to life-threatening, severe ketoacidosis as the accumulation of hydrogen ions exceeds the buffering capacity of the blood.

Synthesis of ketone bodies

Ketone bodies are formed from acetyl CoA arising mainly from the β oxidation of fatty acids (Fig. 4.28).

Location

Liver mitochondria.

Pathway

The synthesis of ketone bodies (ketogenesis) is a five-step pathway and is illustrated in Fig. 4.28. Three molecules of acetyl CoA condense to form HMG-CoA, which is then cleaved to acetoacetate. The first two reactions are the same as for cholesterol synthesis but ketone bodies are formed in the mitochondria, whereas cholesterol is synthesized in the cytosol (see Fig. 4.17).

3-Hydroxybutyrate is formed by the reduction of acetoacetate. The ratio of 3-hydroxybutyrate to acetoacetate formed depends on the availability of NADH.

The spontaneous decarboxylation of acetoacetate forms acetone but usually only a small amount is made. Acetone can be smelt on the breath when the concentration of ketone bodies is high, especially in people with poorly controlled diabetes.

Control of the pathway

Acetyl CoA formed by β oxidation of fatty acids usually enters the TCA cycle. During starvation or diabetes, the oxaloacetate necessary for acetyl CoA to combine with, to form citrate, is directed to gluconeogenesis to help maintain the blood glucose. Therefore, acetyl CoA is used to form ketone bodies instead.

Use of ketone bodies

Ketone bodies are carried in the blood to various tissues, mainly the heart, muscle, and the brain, where they are oxidized in mitochondria to acetyl CoA which can enter the TCA cycle (Fig. 4.29). Ketone bodies are important sources of energy for these tissues. In fact, the heart uses ketone bodies as a fuel in preference to glucose. The liver, although the site of synthesis, cannot use ketone bodies because it lacks 3-ketoacyl CoA transferase. RBCs also cannot metabolize ketone bodies because they have no mitochondria.

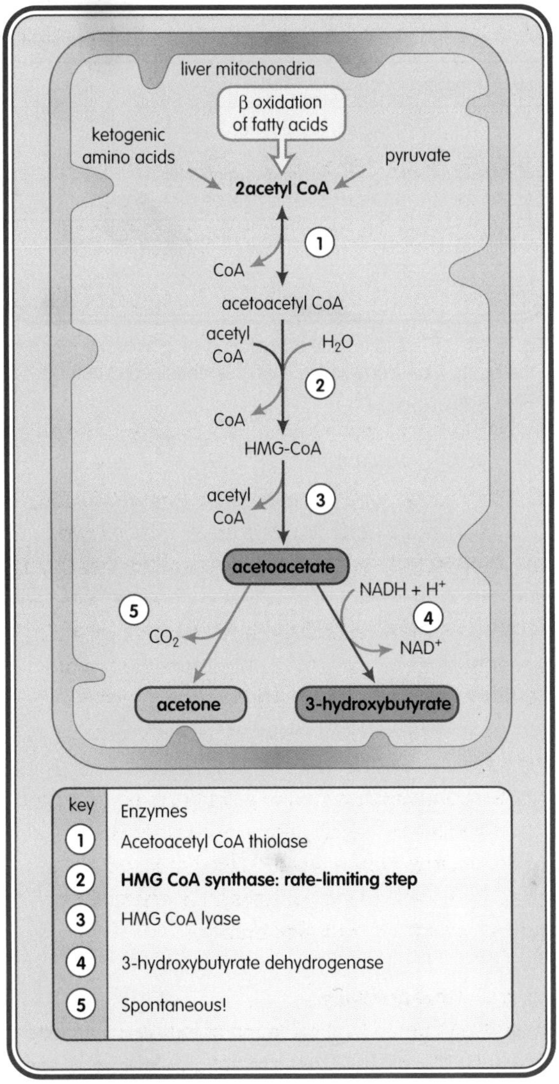

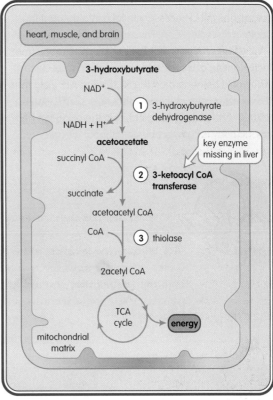

Fig. 4.29 Oxidation and use of ketone bodies. The pathway has three reactions:
1. The oxidation of 3-hydroxybutyrate back to acetoacetate.
2. The activation of acetoacetate, which involves the transfer of CoA from succinyl CoA, catalysed by 3-ketoacyl CoA transferase. Therefore, only tissues with this enzyme can oxidize ketone bodies (i.e. not the liver).
3. Thiolase cleaves acetoacetyl CoA to produce two molecules of acetyl CoA, which enter the TCA cycle for oxidation and ATP production.

Fig. 4.28 Synthesis of ketone bodies. The five-step pathway to synthesize ketone bodies takes place in liver mitochondria; the first two steps are the same as for cholesterol synthesis.

ATP yield from the oxidation of ketone bodies

The oxidation of 3-hydroxybutyrate produces two molecules of acetyl CoA. The oxidation of each acetyl CoA by the TCA cycle yields 10 molecules of ATP. There is no net formation of NADH (the NADH formed in the breakdown of 3-hydroxybutyrate is used in its synthesis). Thus, the oxidation of 3-hydroxybutyrate produces 20 molecules of ATP. However, in order to calculate the true, total ATP yield from the oxidation of a ketone body, it is necessary to take into account the origin of the acetyl CoA. For example, if the acetyl CoA used in the synthesis of 3-hydroxybutyrate arose from the oxidation of a fatty acid, a total of 26 molecules of ATP would be generated (Fig. 4.30). The ATP yield from the oxidation of a glucose molecule is 32 ATP (see Fig. 2.20). Therefore, the ATP yield from the oxidation of a ketone body is comparable with that of glucose,

showing that ketone bodies are an excellent energy source and substitute for glucose during adverse states such as starvation.

ATP yield if acetyl CoA arose from a fatty acid	
	ATP yield
two ATP required to activate fatty acid → acyl CoA	−2

to form two acetyl CoA, fatty acid undergoes two rounds of β oxidation
    releases two NADH → electron transport chain
    releases two FADH$_2$ → electron transport chain
	5
	3

oxidation of two molecules acetyl CoA by TCA cycle	20
total	26 ATP

Fig. 4.30 ATP yield from the oxidation of 3-hydroxybutyrate if the acetyl CoA from which it was synthesized arose from a fatty acid.

- **What are the main roles of ketone bodies in the body and when are they produced?**
- **What is the location of ketone body synthesis?**
- **Describe the pathways for the synthesis and breakdown of ketone bodies.**
- **Name the tissues that can use ketone bodies and the tissues that cannot.**
- **Discuss the ATP yield from the oxidation of a ketone body compared with that of glucose.**

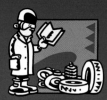

5. Protein Metabolism

BIOSYNTHESIS OF NON-ESSENTIAL AMINO ACIDS

Essential amino acids

In the body there are 20 amino acids, nine of which are essential; the other 11 are non-essential. The essential amino acids are those which cannot be synthesized by the body and therefore have to be obtained from the diet.

These nine essential amino acids are:

- Histidine (His) (infants only).
- Valine (Val).
- Leucine (Leu).
- Isoleucine (Ile).
- Lysine (Lys).
- Methionine (Met).
- Threonine (Thr).
- Phenylalanine (Phe).
- Tryptophan (Trp).

Histidine and also arginine are only regarded as essential during periods of rapid cell growth such as infancy, childhood, or illness. At other times arginine is synthesized in sufficient quantities by the body.

Non-essential amino acids

These 11 amino acids can be synthesized by the body from intermediates of the TCA cycle and other metabolic pathways. They are:

- Tyrosine (Tyr).
- Glycine (Gly).
- Alanine (Ala).
- Cysteine (Cys).
- Serine (Ser).
- Aspartate (Asp).
- Asparagine (Asn).
- Glutamate (Glu).
- Glutamine (Gln).
- Arginine (Arg).
- Proline (Pro).

The pathways for the synthesis of these non-essential amino acids will be considered in this chapter.

Key reactions of amino acid metabolism

There are two main reactions essential to amino acid metabolism: transamination and oxidative deamination. You must know about them.

Transamination converts one amino acid into another

Working definition

Aminotransferases (or transaminases) catalyse the transfer of the α-amino group (NH_3^+) from an amino acid to an α-keto acid (either pyruvate, oxaloacetate, or most often α-ketoglutarate) (Fig. 5.1). A new amino acid and a new keto-acid are formed. If the acceptor is

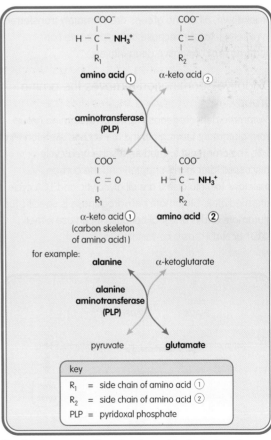

Fig. 5.1 Transamination of amino acids. Aminotransferases (or transaminases) catalyse the transfer of the α-amino group (NH_3^+), from an amino acid to an α-keto acid (either pyruvate, oxaloacetate, or most often α-ketoglutarate).

α-ketoglutarate then glutamate is produced. All transamination reactions are fully reversible. Remember, the amino group is not released.

Site
Aminotransferases are found in both the cytosol and the mitochondria.

Mechanism
Aminotransferases all require pyridoxal phosphate (PLP), a vitamin B_6 derivative as a co-factor. The pyridoxal phosphate is covalently linked to a lysine residue in the active site of the enzyme and therefore takes part in the reaction. The two most common aminotransferases are alanine aminotransferase (ALT) and aspartate aminotransferase (AST).

Aminotransferases are central to amino acid metabolism. They are used both for the synthesis of amino acids and for their breakdown. During breakdown, all amino groups are ultimately transferred to α-ketoglutarate because only glutamate can undergo rapid oxidative deamination.

Oxidative deamination removes the amino group
Glutamate dehydrogenase removes the amino group from glutamate leaving behind the carbon skeleton (Fig. 5.2). The ammonia formed enters the urea cycle (discussed later in this chapter) and the carbon skeletons (α-keto acids) are all glycolytic and TCA cycle intermediates. Glutamate dehydrogenase is specific for glutamate and is unusual because it can use either NAD^+ or $NADP^+$ as a co-factor.

Site
Mitochondria.

Control
The reaction is reversible. ATP and GTP allosterically inhibit the enzyme; GDP and ADP activate it. Therefore, when energy levels are low, amino acids are deaminated to provide α-ketoglutarate for the TCA cycle to generate energy. Deamination can also be achieved by other minor enzymes (see p. 86).

Biosynthetic pathways of non-essential amino acids
Tyrosine
Tyrosine is formed by the hydroxylation of the essential amino acid phenylalanine by phenylalanine hydroxylase (Fig. 5.3). This is an irreversible reaction; phenylalanine therefore cannot be made from tyrosine. The enzyme requires the co-factor tetrahydrobiopterin, which takes part in the hydroxylation. The genetic deficiency of phenylalanine hydroxylase leads to phenylketonuria, a disease characterized by an accumulation of phenylalanine (this is discussed fully in Chapter 12). Tyrosine is the precursor of the catecholamines, namely dopamine, adrenaline, and noradrenaline, as well as melanin and the hormone thyroxine. Its synthesis is regulated by the demand for these molecules.

Serine, glycine, and cysteine
These three amino acids are all formed from glycolytic intermediates. Both glycine and cysteine can be formed from serine.

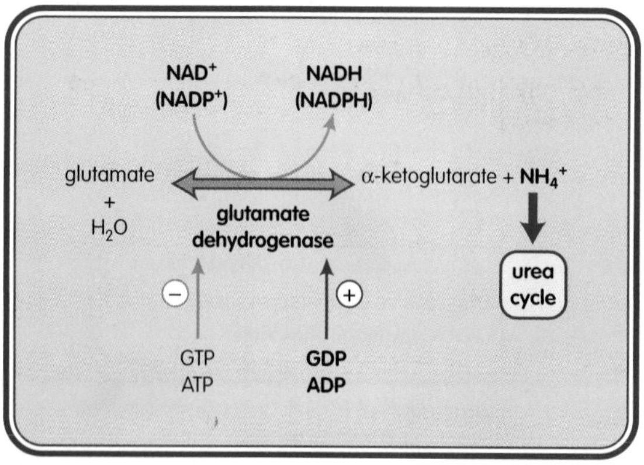

Fig. 5.2 Oxidative deamination of glutamate. Glutamate dehydrogenase removes the amino group from glutamate leaving behind the carbon skeleton, α-ketoglutarate.

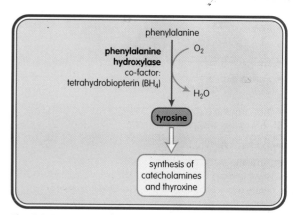

Fig. 5.3 Tyrosine synthesis. Tyrosine is formed by the hydroxylation of the essential amino acid phenylalanine by phenylalanine hydroxylase.

Serine synthesis

There are a number of possible pathways available for the synthesis of serine (letters refer to Fig. 5.4).

a. The phosphorylated pathway (the main pathway) takes place in the cell cytosol. Serine is formed from the glycolytic intermediate 3-phosphoglycerate in three steps: oxidation, transamination to 3-phosphoserine, and hydrolysis to serine.

b. Serine can also be synthesized from glycine in mitochondria. Serine hydroxymethyl transferase transfers a hydroxymethyl group to glycine. The reaction is reversible; glycine and serine are thus interconvertible. The enzyme requires pyridoxal phosphate as a co-factor.

Glycine synthesis

c. Glycine synthesis takes place via two main pathways both of which occur in mitochondria (see Fig. 5.4):

- From serine by serine hydroxymethyl transferase (this is merely a reversal of serine synthesis).
- Glycine can also be formed from CO_2, NH_4^+, and N^5N^{10}- methylene tetrahydrofolate (THF) (a donor of one-carbon units, see Chapter 6) in a reaction catalysed by glycine synthase (glycine cleavage enzyme).

Glycine has many functions in the body, for example:

- Protein synthesis, especially of collagen, glutathione, creatine, and porphyrins, and purine synthesis.
- The metabolism and excretion of drugs.
- Acts as an inhibitory neurotransmitter in the brain.

Cysteine synthesis

Cysteine is formed from serine and the essential amino acid methionine in the cell cytosol (Fig. 5.5). Cysteine synthesis is dependent on an adequate supply of methionine in the diet. A large number of steps are involved but only the main ones are shown (numbers refer to Fig. 5.5):

1. Activation of methionine and the formation of homocysteine (details of this reaction are in Fig. 6.2).

2. Condensation of serine with homocysteine to form cystathionine.

3. Hydrolysis by cystathionase to form cysteine and homoserine.

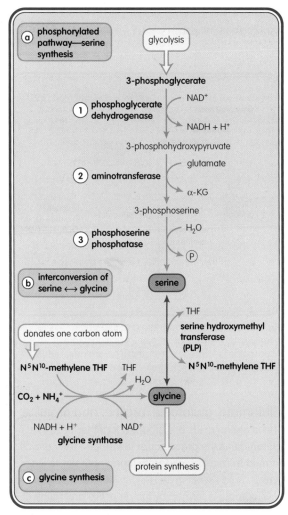

Fig. 5.4 Serine and glycine synthesis. A number of pathways are available to synthesize serine:
a. The phosphorylated pathway is the main pathway and occurs in the cell cytosol.
b. Serine is also synthesized from glycine in mitochondria by serine hydroxymethyl transferase. This is a reversible reaction and therefore is also a pathway for glycine synthesis.
c. lycine can also be formed from CO2, NH4+, and N5 N10methylene-THF in mitochondria.

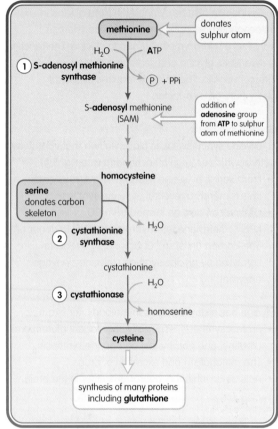

Fig. 5.5 Synthesis of cysteine. Cysteine is formed from serine and the essential amino acid methionine in the cell cytosol. Some of the steps have been omitted (numbers refer to text on p. 79).

Alanine

Alanine is formed by a simple one-step transamination of pyruvate (Fig. 5.6). The formation depends on the demand for glycolysis and thus the energy status of the cell.

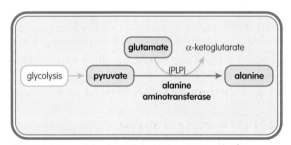

Fig. 5.6 Transamination of pyruvate to form alanine. Alanine is formed by a simple one-step transamination of pyruvate. The formation depends on the demand for glycolysis and thus the energy status of the cell.

Aspartate and asparagine synthesis

Asparagine is the amide derivative of the acid aspartate (Fig. 5.7).

1. Aspartate is formed by the transamination of oxaloacetate (a TCA cycle intermediate). Aspartate is an important amino acid in metabolism because of its role as an amino group donor in the urea cycle and in purine and pyrimidine synthesis.

2. Asparagine is formed by the transfer of an amide group from glutamine to aspartate. The reaction requires ATP and the equilibrium lies in favour of asparagine synthesis.

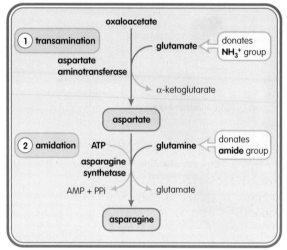

Fig. 5.7 Synthesis of aspartate and asparagine. Aspartate is formed by the transamination of oxaloacetate (1). Asparagine is formed by transfer of an amide group from glutamine to aspartate (2) (refer to text above).

Glutamate, glutamine, proline, and arginine

These amino acids are grouped together because glutamate is the precursor of the others. They are all formed from a-ketoglutarate (numbers refer to Fig. 5.8).

1. Glutamate is formed by the reductive amination of a-ketoglutarate by glutamate dehydrogenase. Glutamate has a key role in amino acid metabolism since it is the only amino acid that can undergo rapid oxidative deamination (see Fig. 5.2). Glutamate is also formed by transamination of most other amino acids.

2. Glutamine is formed by the amidation of glutamate by glutamine synthetase (like asparagine). Glutamine is used for purine and pyrimidine synthesis. As well as

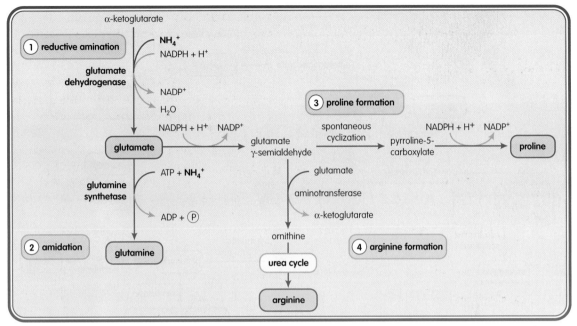

Fig. 5.8 Synthesis of glutamate, glutamine, proline, and arginine. Glutamate is the precursor of the other amino acids in this group. They are all formed from α-ketoglutarate (numbers refer to text).

producing glutamine for protein synthesis, the reaction serves as a pathway for the removal of ammonia in the liver and the kidney.

3. Proline is synthesized from glutamate in three steps: reduction of glutamate to glutamate-g-semialdehyde, a spontaneous cyclization, and then reduction to proline.

4. Arginine is formed by the reduction of glutamate to glutamate-g-semialdehyde, which is transaminated to ornithine. Ornithine is metabolized by the urea cycle to form arginine (discussed later in this chapter).

It is not necessary to learn these pathways in detail; a basic outline is all you need. Fig. 5.9 is an overview of amino acid synthesis. If all fails just learn that!

- ○ Define essential and non-essential amino acids, and be able to list the essential ones.
- ○ What are transamination reactions. What are their uses in amino acid metabolism?
- ○ Describe the oxidative deamination of glutamate and its significance for the breakdown of all amino acids.
- ○ Outline the synthesis of essential amino acids: know the major substrates involved, any important enzymes and intermediates formed along the pathway, and the types of reactions.

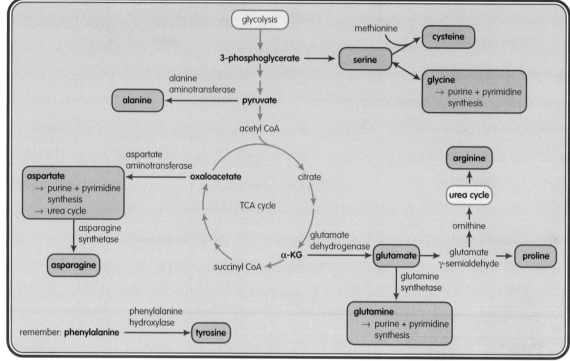

Fig. 5.9 Overview of the biosynthesis of non-essential amino acids. If all else fails, just learn this!

PROTEIN BREAKDOWN AND THE DISPOSAL OF NITROGEN

Protein turnover

Most proteins in the body are constantly being synthesized from amino acids and degraded back to them. Therefore, there is a continual turnover of protein.

Amino acid pool

This is a 'pool' of amino acids present in the body in dynamic equilibrium with tissue protein (Fig. 5.10). Amino acids are continually taken from the pool for protein synthesis and replaced by the hydrolysis of dietary and tissue protein. Any amino acids not immediately used are lost since protein cannot be stored. In a healthy adult, the total amount of protein in the body is constant so that the rate of protein synthesis is equal to the rate of protein breakdown. In an average 70 kg person, about 300 g of protein is synthesized each day and 300 g is degraded. Fig. 5.11 shows how this protein is used.

Nitrogen balance

The breakdown of protein leads to a net daily loss of nitrogen (as urea) from the body, which corresponds usually to about 35–55 g protein lost each day.

The amino acid pool can be thought of in terms of a sink without a plug therefore requiring a continual daily input to keep it topped up, because protein is not stored.

Therefore, a normal diet must provide at least 35–55 g of protein every day. Under these conditions the body is said to be in nitrogen balance because the dietary intake is equal to the loss from the body.

Positive nitrogen balance

This occurs when nitrogen intake is greater than nitrogen loss from the body. Three conditions are associated with this:

- Growth.
- Pregnancy.
- Convalescence.

Negative nitrogen balance

This occurs when nitrogen intake is less than nitrogen loss from the body. Conditions associated with this are:

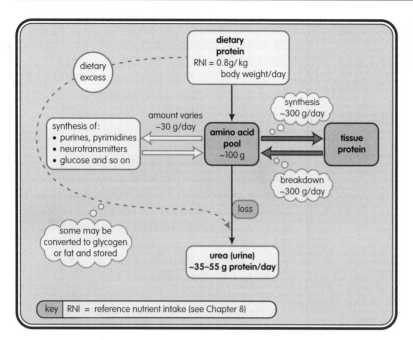

Fig. 5.10 Amino acid pool. This is a 'pool' of amino acids present in the body in dynamic equilibrium with tissue protein.

Daily turnover of tissue protein	
Amount	**Use**
70 g	turnover of digestive enzymes and gut cells
20 g	synthesis of plasma proteins
8 g	synthesis of haemoglobin
20 g	white blood cell turnover
75–100 g	turnover of muscle cells
80–100 g	varies
	N.B. under certain conditions (e.g. stress, infection, or pregnancy) the synthesis of certain proteins may increase

Fig. 5.11 Daily turnover of tissue protein. In an average 70 kg person the daily turnover of protein is about 300 g/day.

- Malnutrition.
- Starvation.
- Cachexia (seen in advanced stages of cancer).
- Post-trauma (surgery, severe burns, or sepsis).
- Lack of an essential amino acid (remember, all 20 are needed for protein synthesis).

This is discussed further in Chapter 8.

Rate of protein turnover

Between 1 and 2% of the total body protein is turned over daily. The rate of protein turnover varies for individual proteins and depends to a certain extent on the function of the protein:
- Regulatory proteins, for example, digestive enzymes, lactate dehydrogenase, or RNA polymerase have short half-lives (minutes to hours).
- Structural proteins, for example, collagen, have long half-lives and last for years.
- Haemoglobin has an intermediate half-life of about 120 days.

Protein degradation
There are two possible pathways for protein degradation; the end result of each is the breakdown of proteins to their constituent amino acids by proteases.

Ubiquitin pathway
The ubiquitin pathway degrades abnormal proteins and short-lived cytosolic proteins; it is ATP-dependent and is located in the cell cytosol (Fig. 5.12).

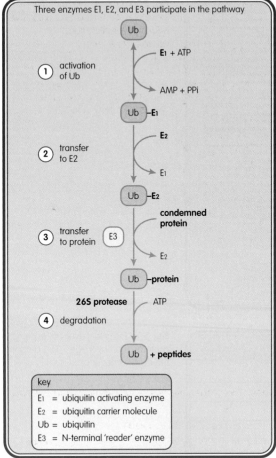

Three enzymes E1, E2, and E3 participate in the pathway

① activation of Ub

Ub → E1 + ATP

→ AMP + PPi

Ub —E1

② transfer to E2

E2

E1

Ub —E2

③ transfer to protein

condemned protein

E3

E2

Ub —protein

26S protease — ATP

④ degradation

Ub + peptides

key

E1 = ubiquitin activating enzyme
E2 = ubiquitin carrier molecule
Ub = ubiquitin
E3 = N-terminal 'reader' enzyme

Fig. 5.12 Ubiquitin pathway degrades abnormal proteins and short-lived cytosolic proteins; it is ATP-dependent and is located in the cytosol (numbers refer to text).

Structure of ubiquitin

Ubiquitin is a small, basic protein that attaches to proteins to be destroyed. The attachment of ubiquitin targets the protein for degradation—it is a 'tagging' system. At the carboxyl-terminal of ubiquitin is a glycine residue that attaches to lysine residues on target proteins to form: ubiquitin-C-glycine—lysine-target protein.

Mechanics of the pathway

The ubiquitin pathway consists of four stages (steps below refer to Fig. 5.12): The enzymes E1, E2, and E3 participate in the pathway.

1. The activation of ubiquitin by attachment to E1, the ubiquitin activating enzyme. The reaction is driven by the hydrolysis of ATP.

2. The transfer of activated ubiquitin to E2, the ubiquitin carrier molecule.

3. E3 catalyses the transfer of ubiquitin to the target

protein. The E3 enzyme actually 'reads' the N-terminal amino acid on proteins to determine whether a protein may be easily tagged with ubiquitin (see below).

4. The degradation of the labelled protein by 26S protease complex (also called megapain or endopeptidase) to peptides.

Lysosomal pathway

The lysosomal pathway degrades long-lived, membrane or extracellular proteins and organelles, for example, mitochondria. It is ATP-independent and is located in lysosomes (Fig. 5.13). Initially, the proteins must enter lysosomes and there are two possible processes by which proteins can do this:

- Endocytosis, by which extracellular proteins enter cells for degradation in lysosomes.
- Autophagy for intracellular proteins or organelles; these are engulfed by the plasma membrane or endoplasmic reticulum to form autophagosomes.

The end result of both is the degradation of proteins by lysosomal proteases (cathepsins).

Lysosomal activity and therefore protein degradation is increased in starvation (an increase in protein breakdown provides substrates for gluconeogenesis) and many disease states including diabetes, hyperthyroidism, and chronic inflammatory diseases.

Signals for degradation

Protein degradation (ubiquitinylation) is not random but is influenced by some structural aspect of the protein.

N-end rule

This divides proteins into short- and long-lived by the nature of their N (amino)-terminal amino acid:

- Examples of stabilizing N-terminal residues are methionine, glycine, alanine, and serine. These are not easily tagged by ubiquitin and proteins containing these have long half-lives.
- Examples of destabilizing N-terminal residues are phenylalanine, tryptophan, aspartate, arginine, and lysine. These are signals for rapid ubiquitin tagging.

It is the E3 enzyme that actually reads the N-terminal residues.

PEST region

Proteins containing PEST regions [-Pro-Glu-Ser-Thr] (named according to the one-letter nomenclature for

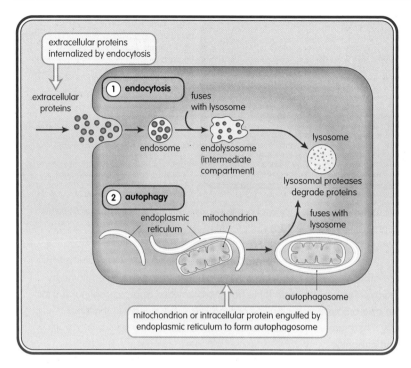

Fig. 5.13 Lysosomal pathway degrades long-lived, membrane or extracellular proteins and organelles, for example, mitochondria. Extracellular proteins enter cells by endocytosis where, as intracellular proteins, they are engulfed by the endoplasmic reticulum to form autophagosomes.

amino acids) are rapidly degraded and have short half-lives. For example, cAMP-dependent protein kinase.

Conformational changes
The binding of ligands to receptors often causes a conformational change that may expose a PEST region or a region susceptible to the action of proteases.

Disposal of protein nitrogen and the urea cycle
An overview
Any amino acids surplus to the body's requirements are degraded. The amino group is removed, forming ammonia, which is extremely toxic. Ammonia is therefore converted to a non-toxic compound, namely urea, by the urea cycle for excretion in the urine. A small amount of ammonia can also be incorporated into glutamine (see Fig. 5.8). The removal of the amino group from amino acids leaves behind the carbon skeletons (α-keto acids). Their metabolism is discussed later in this chapter.

The major site of amino acid degradation is the liver. Nitrogen disposal can be divided into two main stages:
- The removal of the amino group from amino acids.
- The formation of urea via the ornithine cycle.

These two stages are now considered in more detail.

Removal of amino group
There are two possible routes for the removal of the amino group.

Transdeamination
Transdeamination is transamination linked to oxidative deamination (see Figs 5.1 and 5.2):
- Transamination is the transfer of amino groups from amino acids to form glutamate in the cytosol.
- Oxidative deamination catalysed by glutamate dehydrogenase, removes the amino group from glutamate. The reaction occurs in mitochondria and the amino group released then enters the urea cycle.

Transamination
This involves two transamination reactions (numbers refer to Fig. 5.14):
1. The first transfers the amino group to a-ketoglutarate, forming glutamate.
2. In the second, aspartate aminotransferase transfers the amino group from glutamate to oxaloacetate, forming aspartate.

85

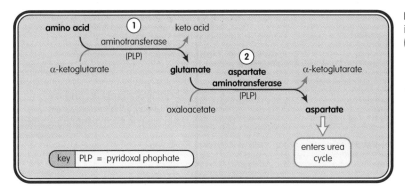

Fig. 5.14 Transamination route involves two transamination reactions (for details, see text on p. 85).

Aspartate then enters the urea cycle by condensing with citrulline. In this way, a second amino group enters the urea cycle providing a second nitrogen atom to form urea.

Deamination can also be achieved by other enzymes but these are only minor pathways. For example, there is a non-specific l-amino acid oxidase but it is not very important physiologically. There are also specific enzymes such as serine and threonine dehydratases, which deaminate serine and threonine respectively, by removal of H_2O and NH_4^+, and cysteine desulphydrase, which deaminates cysteine and produces hydrogen sulphide as a by-product.

Formation of urea by the ornithine cycle

The urea cycle consists of five reactions (described below) that synthesize the organic compound urea from two inorganic compounds, CO_2 and NH_4^+ (Fig. 5.15). Urea, NH_2–CO–NH_2, contains two nitrogen atoms: one nitrogen is supplied by ammonia formed by the transdeamination of amino acids; the other derives from aspartate. The cycle uses a carrier molecule, ornithine, which is regenerated (this is similar to the way the TCA cycle uses oxaloacetate).

Location
Liver hepatocytes, mainly in the periportal cells.

Site
The first two reactions occur in mitochondria, the last three in the cytosol.

Urea cycle (numbers refer to Fig. 5.15)
1. Formation of carbamoyl phosphate
This is the irreversible, rate-limiting step of the pathway, catalysed by carbamoyl phosphate synthase I (CPSI). The reaction consumes two molecules of ATP. (There is also a carbamoyl phosphate synthase II enzyme in the cytosol but this is only involved in pyrimidine synthesis [see Chapter 6].)

2. Formation of citrulline
The carbamoyl group is transferred to ornithine by ornithine transcarbamylase. Specific transporters for citrulline and ornithine are present in the inner mitochondrial membrane.

3. Synthesis of argininosuccinate
Argininosuccinate synthase catalyses the condensation of citrulline with aspartate. The reaction is driven by the cleavage of ATP to AMP and pyrophosphate, which is rapidly hydrolysed to two inorganic phosphates. Therefore the reaction consumes two ATP equivalents.

4. Cleavage of argininosuccinate to fumarate and arginine by argininosuccinate lyase

5. Cleavage of arginine to ornithine and urea by arginase
Arginase is specific to the liver, meaning that only the liver can produce urea. The urea formed is transported in the blood to the kidneys for excretion in urine.

Fate of fumarate
The fumarate formed is converted to malate by fumarase. Malate either can be converted to oxaloacetate and then aspartate in the cytosol as shown in Fig. 5.15, or it can be transported into mitochondria and enter the TCA cycle first. There is evidence to suggest that both are possible and it is a matter of debate as to what actually happens. Either way, the NADH formed can be oxidized by the electron transport chain to produce 2.5 molecules of ATP.

$$CO_2 + NH_4^+ + 3ATP + aspartate + 2H_2O \rightarrow$$
$$urea + fumarate + 2ADP + AMP + 4Pi$$

The ATP yield
The overall reaction can be written as:
- Four ATP equivalents are consumed for every molecule of urea formed (reactions **1** and **3**).
- The conversion of fumarate to oxaloacetate produces NADH, which is oxidized by the electron transport chain to generate 2.5 ATP.

Therefore, overall 1.5 ATP are consumed for every molecule of urea formed by the cycle (i.e. energy is required, not generated).

Control of the urea cycle
Control can be considered at two levels:

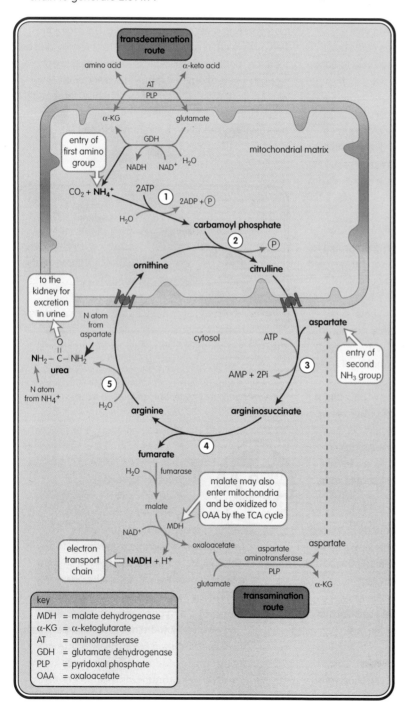

Fig. 5.15 The urea cycle consists of five reactions that synthesize the organic compound urea from two inorganic compounds: CO_2 and NH_4^+ (numbers refer to text on p. 86).

Short-term allosteric control

The main control of the urea cycle is by N-acetyl glutamate (formed from acetyl CoA and glutamate), which allosterically activates carbamoyl phosphate synthase I, the enzyme which catalyses the rate-limiting step of the urea cycle. How does this work? Following a protein-rich meal, the excess amino acids are deaminated resulting in an increased concentration of glutamate and thus N-acetyl glutamate. N-acetyl glutamate activates carbamoyl phosphate synthase I and thus the urea cycle to cope with the extra nitrogen load.

Long-term regulation

Changes in the diet are thought to induce or repress transcription of the urea cycle enzymes. For example, in starvation, the increased breakdown of tissue protein induces the synthesis of enzymes to cope with the extra load of ammonia.

Why is it beneficial to form urea?

Ammonia is extremely toxic. By converting ammonia to urea, a non-toxic, organic compound it can be excreted easily by the kidneys. Urea possesses a number of properties which favour its formation:

- It is a small, uncharged, and water-soluble molecule. It can therefore diffuse across membranes easily and be excreted in the urine.
- Nearly 50% of its weight is nitrogen, making it a very efficient nitrogen carrier and excretory product.
- Little energy is used up in its synthesis—only about 1.5 ATP are required for every mole of urea formed.

A normal diet produces 35–55 g of urea each day. In birds, ammonia is converted to uric acid for excretion, which is very insoluble, as I am sure most people know.

Ammonia toxicity

Ammonia is one of the most toxic compounds produced by the body. Elevated levels (hyperammonaemia) can cause symptoms of ammonia intoxication: tremors, slurred speech, and blurred vision. At very high concentrations, ammonia causes irreversible brain damage, coma, and death. It is therefore essential that ammonia is detoxified rapidly to urea by the liver.

Proposed mechanisms of ammonia toxicity

Ammonia toxicity targets the brain and central nervous system. Whilst the effects of ammonia toxicity are well-known, its mechanism of action is still unclear. An increase in the concentration of ammonia causes a shift in the equilibrium of the glutamate dehydrogenase reaction towards glutamate formation (Fig. 5.16). This leads to a depletion of α-ketoglutarate, which results in a decrease in TCA cycle activity and therefore ATP production. Shifting the equilibrium of the reaction also leads to an increase in the ratio of NAD$^+$ to NADH, which also results in a decrease in ATP levels. The brain and nervous system require large amounts of energy and are therefore particularly susceptible to ammonia toxicity.

High levels of ammonia may also react with glutamate, forming glutamine, which may damage the brain directly. Decreasing the level of glutamate (a neurotransmitter) in the brain may also cause

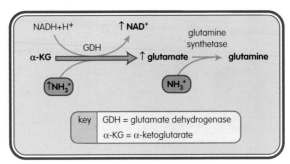

Fig. 5.16 Mechanisms of ammonia toxicity. An increase in the concentration of ammonia causes a shift in the equilibrium of the glutamate dehydrogenase reaction towards glutamate formation, which leads to the depletion of α-ketoglutarate, a substrate of the TCA cycle.

A genetic deficiency in each of the urea cycle enzymes has been identified; all are rare, the most common being ornithine transcarbamylase deficiency. These deficiencies each result in a failure to make urea, leading to hyperammonaemia and irreversible mental retardation from ammonia toxicity. Ammonia toxicity is also seen in patients with liver damage due to cirrhosis.

problems. Remember, these are only proposed mechanisms—the true mechanism is not yet known.

> ◦ **Describe the concepts of protein turnover, the amino acid pool, and nitrogen balance.**
> ◦ **Outline the two pathways of protein degradation; know the types of proteins degraded by each.**
> ◦ **Give two examples of signals for protein degradation.**
> ◦ **Describe transdeamination and transamination reactions and their significance to the urea cycle.**
> ◦ **Give the location, site, and basic outline of the five main reactions of the urea cycle.**
> ◦ **Name one inherited cause and one acquired cause of hyperammonaemia, and a possible mechanism for ammonia toxicity.**

GLUCONEOGENESIS AND THE METABOLISM OF AMINO ACIDS TO GLUCOSE AND FAT

Role of protein as an energy source
Fed state
In the fed state, protein undergoes digestion in the stomach and small intestine to release amino acids, which are taken up by cells and used for the synthesis of proteins and other molecules. However, if amino acids are present in excess of the body's requirements, they can either be used directly as a fuel to produce ATP or converted to glycogen or fat and stored for later use, that is, they provide an energy store. Amino acids are never stored as protein.

Starvation
Following prolonged exercise or during starvation, the body has to rely on its energy stores for fuel. Glycogen reserves last only between 12 and 24 h and are quickly depleted. The main concern is how to maintain the blood glucose concentration and provide fuel for the brain and RBCs. Fat, as has already been shown, cannot be converted to glucose (see Fig. 2.15). The brain adapts to using ketone bodies as its main fuel although it still requires some glucose, but RBCs cannot metabolize ketone bodies at all because they have no mitochondria (see Chapter 4). Therefore, alternative substrates for glucose production via gluconeogenesis are required. Lactate and glycerol can provide some glucose but the majority is obtained by the breakdown of muscle protein to release amino acids. Many of these amino acids produced from muscle protein are transaminated to alanine and glutamine, which are released into the blood. Alanine is taken up by the liver for gluconeogenesis. Glutamine is taken up by the small intestine to be used as a fuel and by the kidney to form glucose via gluconeogenesis.

Gluconeogenesis
Gluconeogenesis is defined as 'the production of glucose from non-carbohydrate sources'. For a period of starvation of longer than about 12 h or during prolonged exercise, glucose has to be formed from alternative substrates to maintain the blood glucose concentration. Gluconeogenesis is the process in which glucose is produced from:

- Glycerol (released by triacylglycerol hydrolysis (see Fig. 4.11).
- Lactate (from anaerobic glycolysis in RBCs and active skeletal muscle).
- Amino acids (breakdown of muscle protein).

Location
Liver (in prolonged starvation it can also occur in the cortex of the kidney).

Site
Cell cytosol—except for the first step, the carboxylation of pyruvate, which occurs in mitochondria.

Pathway
Gluconeogenesis is not simply a reversal of glycolysis. Some of the reactions of glycolysis are reversible and are common to both glycolytic and gluconeogenic pathways. However, the three essentially irreversible reactions of glycolysis, namely those catalysed by hexokinase, phosphofructokinase (PFK)-1 , and

pyruvate kinase, have to be bypassed. How this is achieved is shown in Fig. 5.17, and explained in stages 1–3 below.

1. Conversion of pyruvate to phosphoenol pyruvate

The conversion of pyruvate to phosphoenolpyruvate (PEP) occurs via two reactions:

a. The carboxylation of pyruvate to oxaloacetate. Pyruvate carboxylase is found in the mitochondria but PEP-carboxykinase and the other enzymes involved are in the cytosol. The oxaloacetate formed is unable to cross the inner mitochondrial membrane; therefore it is reduced to malate, which is transported into the cytosol where it is re-oxidized. Pyruvate carboxylase requires the vitamin biotin as a co-factor and has a similar mechanism to acetyl CoA carboxylase (see Chapter 4).

b. The decarboxylation and phosphorylation of oxaloacetate by PEP-carboxykinase.

2. Hydrolysis of fructose-1,6-bisphosphate

The hydrolysis of fructose-1,6-bisphosphate by fructose-1, 6-bisphosphatase bypasses the PFK reaction, (rate-limiting step of glycolysis).

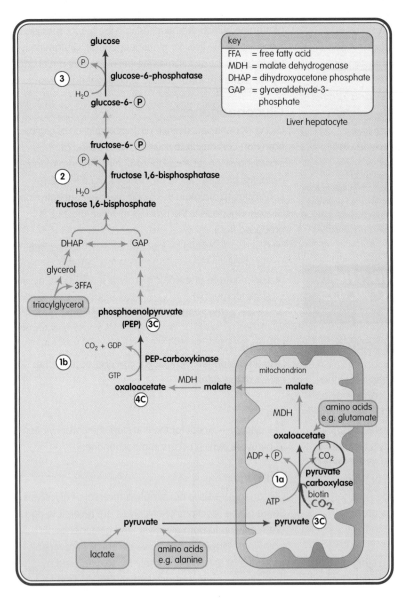

Fig. 5.17 Gluconeogenesis is not simply a reversal of glycolysis. The three essentially irreversible reactions of glycolysis have to be bypassed. The first reaction, the carboxylation of pyruvate to oxaloacetate, occurs in the mitochondrial matrix. The rest of the reactions occur in the cell cytosol. Details of the individual reactions 1 to 3 are found in the text.

3. Hydrolysis of glucose-6-phosphate

The hydrolysis of glucose-6-phosphate by glucose-6-phosphatase bypasses the irreversible hexokinase reaction to form free glucose. This enzyme is unique to the liver.

Amino acid breakdown

Amino acid breakdown involves two stages:
- The removal of amino groups by transamination and oxidative deamination (see Figs 5.1 and 5.2).
- The catabolism of the carbon skeletons.

The carbon skeletons of amino acids can be metabolized to intermediates of the TCA cycle and glycolytic pathway. In fact, the breakdown of all 20 amino acids converges to produce seven products: pyruvate, acetyl CoA, acetoacetyl CoA, α-ketoglutarate, succinyl CoA, fumarate, and oxaloacetate (Fig. 5.18). Depending on the energy status of the cell, these products can either be oxidized to generate energy or used to synthesize glycogen or fat.

Concepts of amino acid catabolism

Metabolically, amino acids can be classified into two types: ketogenic and gluconeogenic.

Ketogenic amino acids

These are amino acids that are broken down to either acetyl CoA or acetoacetyl CoA and are therefore able to form ketone bodies, hence ketogenic meaning 'ketone forming'. Only leucine and lysine are purely ketogenic (see Fig. 5.18). Isoleucine, phenylalanine, tryptophan, and tyrosine are both ketogenic and glucogenic, that is, their breakdown yields some acetyl CoA and acetoacetyl CoA and some precursors of glucose.

Glucogenic amino acids

These are amino acids that can be broken down to either pyruvate or one of the intermediates of the TCA cycle. They can be channelled into gluconeogenesis for glucose synthesis, hence the term glucogenic ('glucose forming').

Pathways of amino acid catabolism

Amino acids can be divided into seven groups based on their breakdown product. Several breakdown pathways are possible for each amino acid, but only the main ones are discussed here:
- Five amino acids form pyruvate, that is alanine, serine, glycine, cysteine, and threonine (Fig. 5.19).

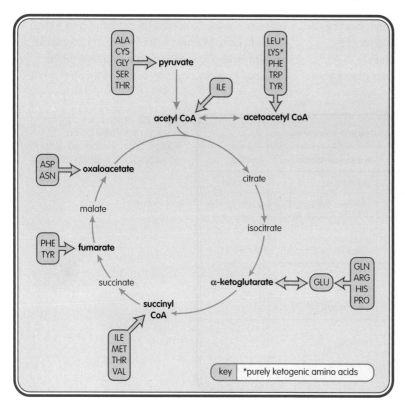

Fig. 5.18 Entry points of amino acid carbon skeletons into the TCA cycle and glycolytic pathways. The breakdown of all 20 amino acids converges to produce only seven products: pyruvate, acetyl CoA, acetoacetyl CoA, α-ketoglutarate, succinyl CoA, fumarate, and oxaloacetate. These products, depending on the energy status of the cell, can either be oxidized to generate energy or used to synthesize glycogen or fat.

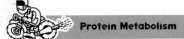

Breakdown of amino acids to pyruvate			
Amino acid	**Important reactions**	**Enzymes involved**	**Product**
alanine	transamination	alanine aminotransferase	pyruvate
serine	deamination and dehydration	serine dehydratase	pyruvate
glycine	methylation to serine followed by dehydration	serine hydroxymethyl transferase serine dehydratase	pyruvate
cysteine	two main steps: • oxidation to cysteine sulphinate • transamination	cysteine dioxygenase cysteine aminotransferase	pyruvate
threonine	aminoacetone pathway	threonine dehydrogenase	pyruvate

Fig. 5.19 Breakdown of amino acids to pyruvate. Five amino acids form pyruvate.

- Two amino acids form oxaloacetate:
  - Aspartate: transamination of aspartate by aspartate aminotransferase produces oxaloacetate.
  - Asparagine: hydrolysis of asparagine by asparaginase releases ammonia and forms aspartate, which can undergo transamination to oxaloacetate.
- Five amino acids form glutamate and α-ketoglutarate (Fig. 5.20).
- Four amino acids form succinyl CoA (Fig. 5.21).
- Phenylalanine and tyrosine form fumarate. The hydroxylation of phenylalanine by phenylalanine hydroxylase produces tyrosine (a reversal of its synthesis [see Fig. 5.3]). Tyrosine is then transaminated and undergoes a series of reactions to form fumarate. Some acetoacetyl CoA is also produced, therefore it is both a ketogenic and glucogenic amino acid.
- Isoleucine forms acetyl CoA: its breakdown actually produces both acetyl CoA and succinyl CoA (see Fig. 5.21).
- Leucine, lysine, and tryptophan form acetoacetyl CoA. (Phenylalanine and tyrosine can also produce some acetoacetyl CoA). Leucine is a branched chain amino acid and its breakdown is discussed below.

Lysine undergoes a number of reactions: a reduction to saccharopine, two oxidations to form aminoadipate, transamination to α-ketoadipate, and then further reactions to eventually form acetoacetyl CoA (it is not

Breakdown of amino acids to glutamate and α-ketoglutarate			
Amino acid	**Important reactions**	**Enzymes involved**	**Product**
glutamine	hydrolysis	glutaminase	glutamate
glutamate	oxidative deamination	glutamate dehydrogenase	α-ketoglutarate
proline	two main steps: • oxidation → pyrroline-5-carboxylate • oxidation → glutamate	proline oxygenase dehydrogenase	glutamate
arginine	two steps: • cleaved to ornithine (part of urea cycle) • transamination	arginase aminotransferase	glutamate
histidine	two main steps: • deamination and hydrolysis to N-formiminoglutamate (FIGlu) • transfer of formimino group to THF	histidase glutamate formiminotransferase	glutamate

Fig. 5.20 Breakdown of amino acids to glutamate and α-ketoglutarate. five amino acids form glutamate and α-ketoglutarate.

Breakdown of amino acids to succinyl CoA			
Amino acid	Important reactions	Enzymes involved	Product
isoleucine (BCAA)	three reactions: • transamination • oxidative decarboxylation • dehydrogenation	BCAA aminotransferase BCAA α-ketoacid dehydrogenase	succinyl CoA and acetyl CoA
valine (BCAA)	all BCAAs have a similar breakdown pathway	as above	succinyl CoA
methionine	condensation with ATP to form SAM hydrolysis to homocysteine	SAM synthase	succinyl CoA
threonine	dehydration to α-ketobutyrate	threonine dehydratase	succinyl CoA

Fig. 5.21 Breakdown of amino acids to succinyl CoA. Four amino acids form succinyl CoA. (Only the important reactions are shown.) (SAM, S-adenosylmethionine; BCAA, branched chain amino acids.)

You are not going to be asked to discuss the different degradation pathways of the amino acids. Know about transamination and deamination reactions and where the amino acid carbon skeletons feed into the TCA cycle: learn Fig. 5.18.

necessary to know this in detail). The breakdown of tryptophan is even more complicated!

Branched chain amino acids (BCAA)
The branched chain amino acids are isoleucine, leucine, and valine, and these are degraded by a common pathway of three reactions:
- Transamination: a single enzyme, branched chain amino acid aminotransferase, transaminates all three amino acids.
- Oxidative decarboxylation: again by one enzyme, the branched chain amino acid, α-ketoacid dehydrogenase, which requires thiamine pyrophosphate as a co-factor. A deficiency of this enzyme causes an accumulation of the keto acids of branched chain amino acids in the urine; this is called maple syrup urine disease (see Chapter 12).
- Dehydrogenation.

Not all tissues can oxidize branched chain amino acids: the liver has limited ability because it lacks the branched chain amino acid aminotransferase. Branched chains amino acids are mainly oxidized by peripheral tissues, in particular, muscle.

Regulation of amino acid catabolism
During fasting and starvation, gluconeogenesis is active (Fig. 5.22).

Hormonal control
In starvation, the levels of glucagon, cortisol, and adrenocorticotrophic hormone are high, which activates gluconeogenesis and inhibits glycolysis. The actions of glucagon are:
- It activates a cAMP-dependent protein kinase which causes phosphorylation and inactivation of pyruvate kinase in the glycolytic pathway (see Fig. 2.10).
- It decreases the formation of fructose-2,6-bisphosphate, the allosteric activator of phosphofructokinase-1 (glycolyic enzyme) but inhibitor of fructose-1,6-bisphosphatase (gluconeogenic enzyme, see Fig. 2.8).
- It increases the rate of transcription and thus the rate of synthesis of PEP carboxykinase. Glucagon inhibits the rate of transcription of pyruvate kinase.

Allosteric activation by acetyl CoA
During starvation, the rate of lipolysis and β oxidation is high, leading to a large increase in the amount of acetyl CoA. Acetyl CoA allosterically activates pyruvate carboxylase, stimulating gluconeogenesis. It has an opposite inhibitory effect on pyruvate dehydrogenase.

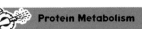
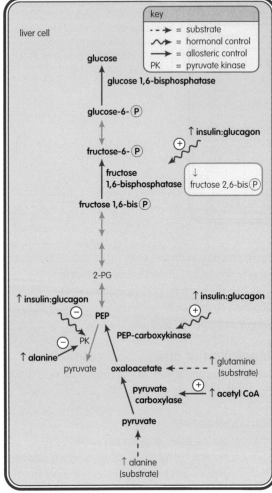

Fig. 5.22 Regulation of gluconeogenesis: fasting and starved state. Control is at two levels. Hormonal control: glucagon activates gluconeogenesis. Allosteric control: acetyl CoA activates pyruvate carboxylase. An increased supply of amino acids, alanine and glutamine activate gluconeogenesis.

Therefore, the pyruvate formed will be channelled into gluconeogenesis, rather than into the TCA cycle. An increased supply of substrates, particularly of the amino acids alanine, and glutamine, favours gluconeogenesis. A high concentration of cortisol favours mobilization of amino acids from muscle.

Disorders of amino acid metabolism
These arise due to inherited deficiencies of enzymes involved in amino acid metabolism. They are very rare and include phenylketonuria, albinism, alkaptonuria, maple syrup urine disease, and histidinaemia; you may see some of them when you do paediatrics. They are covered in detail in Chapter 12.

- Describe the role of protein as an energy source in both the fed and the fasted state.
- Outline gluconeogenesis, including its definition, location, site, and three unique reactions.
- Give examples of glucogenic and ketogenic amino acids.
- Name the ultimate breakdown product for each amino acid (see Fig. 5.18).
- Describe the control of gluconeogenesis.

AMINO ACID METABOLISM IN INDIVIDUAL TISSUES

Amino acid transport
Several transporters exist for 'carrying' amino acids across the cell membrane. The concentration of free amino acids outside the cell is much lower than the concentration of free amino acids inside. Therefore most amino acid transporters function as active transport systems in which the movement of amino acids into cells, against their concentration gradient, is driven by the hydrolysis of ATP.

Five main transport systems exist based on the specificity of the transporter for the side chain of the amino acid (Fig. 5.23), that is there is one for basic amino acids, another for acidic amino acids and so on.

The γ-glutamyl cycle
Unlike the specific transport systems described in Fig. 5.23, the γ-glutamyl cycle transports a wide range of amino acids into cells, being particularly active for neutral amino acids.

Function
The γ-glutamyl cycle is responsible for the active transport of amino acids into cells via the synthesis and breakdown of a glutathione carrier (Fig. 5.24). Three molecules of ATP are required for the transport of each amino acid molecule into the cell.

Location/site
Kidney renal tubular cells and the endoplasmic reticulum of hepatocytes and brain cells.

Amino acid Metabolism
Amino acids are taken up into tissues by active transport and used for protein synthesis. Excess amino acids are not stored by the body; those not immediately required are degraded. The role of protein as an energy source has already been outlined; here we consider amino acid metabolism in individual tissues during the absorptive (fed) state and post-absorptive state.

Absorptive (fed) state
A summary of amino acid metabolism in tissues during the absorptive state is given in Fig. 5.25.

Small intestine
After a protein-rich meal, protein digestion takes place in the small intestine. The amino acids released are absorbed by intestinal epithelial cells. A large proportion of amino acids are transaminated to alanine, which is released into the hepatic portal vein and taken to the liver. Therefore, alanine is the major amino acid secreted by the gut and the principal carrier of nitrogen in the plasma.

Liver
Alanine and other diet-derived amino acids received from the small intestine have a number of possible fates:
- Protein synthesis.
- Transamination to glutamate, which may be oxidatively deaminated to produce NH_4^+, which in turn enters the urea cycle. (Some NH_4^+ comes from the hydrolysis of glutamine in the small intestine.) The urea formed is taken to the kidneys for excretion. Some of the glutamate formed may also be used for protein synthesis.

Specific transport systems for amino acids		
Amino acid specificity	Amino acids transported	Diseases resulting from a defect of the carrier system
small, neutral amino acids	alanine, serine, threonine	non-specific
large, neutral and aromatic amino acids	isoleucine, leucine, valine, tyrosine, tryptophan, phenylalanine	Hartnup's disease: a defect in the intestinal and renal transporter for neutral amino acids
basic amino acids	arginine, lysine, cysteine, ornithine	cystinuria: a defect in kidney tubular reabsorption of all four basic amino acids
proline and glycine	proline, glycine	glycinuria
acidic amino acids	glutamate, aspartate	non-specific

Fig. 5.23 Specific transport systems for amino acids.

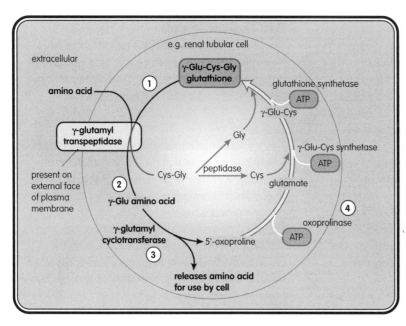

Fig. 5.24 γ-Glutamyl cycle for amino acid transport.
1. Glutathione is formed in the cell and transported to the external surface of the plasma membrane.
2. The enzyme, γ-glutamyl transpeptidase, catalyses the transfer of a γ-glutamyl group from glutathione to the amino acid. This enables uptake of the γ-glutamyl amino acid by the cell (or the cells of other organs if it travels in the blood first).
3. γ-glutamyl cyclotransferase releases the amino acid for use by the cell.
4. The glutathione is reformed by the action of oxoprolinase, γ-glutamyl-cysteinyl synthetase, and glutathione synthetase, in three ATP-dependent reactions.

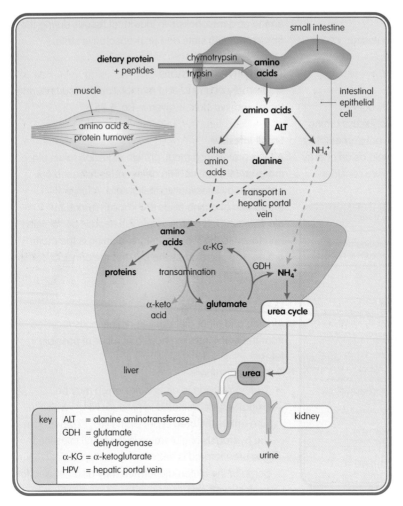

Fig. 5.25 Summary of amino acid metabolism in tissues during the absorptive state. (refer to text for explanation).

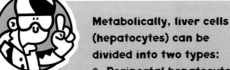
Metabolically, liver cells (hepatocytes) can be divided into two types:
- Periportal hepatocytes, which receive blood from the hepatic portal vein and are mainly involved in amino acid degradation reactions such as glutamine hydrolysis and urea synthesis.
- Perivenous hepatocytes, which drain into the hepatic vein and are mainly involved with amino acid synthesis, for example, glutamine synthesis.

Post-absorptive state

The post-absorptive state is the period four to eight hours after a meal when there is no dietary supply of amino acids. A summary of amino acid metabolism in tissues in the post-absorptive state is given in Fig. 5.26.

Muscle

The breakdown of muscle protein releases amino acids, which are transaminated to alanine and glutamine. Glutamine is formed in two steps: transamination to glutamate and amidation to glutamine. Nucleic acid turnover provides the NH_4^+ for this reaction. The glutamine released is taken up by the intestine and the kidney. The alanine formed goes to the liver. The breakdown of muscle protein also releases branched chain amino acids, which are taken up primarily by the brain (especially valine).

Gut

Glutamine has two main fates; respective degrees depend on the energy status of the cell:

- Firstly, it can be used for nucleotide synthesis to compensate for the very high turnover rate of intestinal cells (see Chapter 6).
- Secondly, it undergoes hydrolysis to glutamate to release NH_4^+, which travels to the liver to enter the urea cycle.

The glutamate formed is transaminated either to alanine or citrulline (a urea cycle intermediate), both of which are taken to the liver.

Liver

In the liver alanine is either:

- Converted to pyruvate and then to glucose by gluconeogenesis, providing an energy source for the muscle. The reactions form the glucose–alanine cycle (Fig. 5.27).
- Or transaminated to glutamate. The extent of each depends on the energy state of the cell.

Glutamate can be deaminated to form NH_4^+, which enters the urea cycle. During starvation or acidosis, glutaminase activity is reduced resulting in a decrease in glutamine hydrolysis and NH_4^+ production. This leads

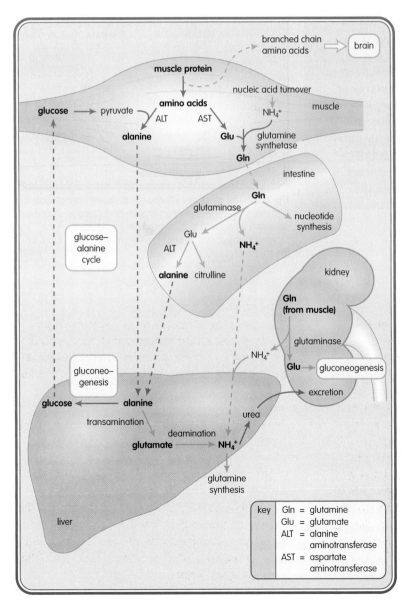

Fig. 5.26 Summary of amino acid metabolism in tissues in the post-absorptive state (refer to text for explanation).

to a decrease in the urea cycle and amino acid breakdown. A reciprocal increase is seen in the activity of glutamine synthetase and amino acid synthesis.

Kidney

Glutamine released from muscle is taken up by kidney cells. It is hydrolysed by glutaminase to release ammonia for excretion. In starvation, glutamate serves as a substrate for gluconeogenesis (see Fig. 5.17).

The glucose–alanine cycle

The glucose–alanine cycle (see Fig. 5.27) shows how carbon skeletons alternate between protein and glucose. Alanine from muscle is converted back to glucose in the liver for use by muscle. This is very similar to the Cori cycle in which lactate formed by active skeletal muscle is taken to the liver to be converted back to pyruvate and then to glucose by gluconeogenesis (see Chapter 7). The glucose formed is then taken back to muscle.

○ **Describe the principles involved in amino acid transport, and give two examples of transporters.**

○ **What are the main features of amino acid metabolism in tissues in the absorptive and post-absorptive state (be able to draw Figs 5.25 and 5.26)?**

○ **Describe the glucose–alanine cycle and its role in muscle.**

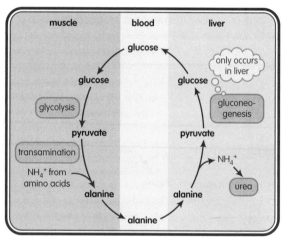

Fig. 5.27 The glucose–alanine cycle shows how carbon skeletons alternate between protein and glucose. Alanine released by muscle is converted back to glucose in the liver by gluconeogenesis. The glucose formed is taken back to the muscle for use.

6. Purines, Pyrimidines, and Haem

ONE-CARBON POOL

Concepts

Single carbon units can exist in a number of oxidation states, for example, methane, formaldehyde, and methanol. They are used in the synthesis and elongation of many organic compounds. In order to do this, carbon units require a carrier to 'activate' them and to enable their transfer to the molecule being synthesized. The main carriers used are folate and S-adenosyl methionine. The one-carbon pool refers to single carbon units attached to these carriers.

S-adenosyl methionine

S-adenosyl methionine (SAM) is a high-energy compound formed by the condensation of the amino acid methionine with ATP. It contains an activated methyl group, which can be transferred easily to a variety of molecules. SAM is the main methyl group donor used in biosynthetic reactions, for example, the methylation of noradrenaline to adrenaline.

Folate

The active form of folate is **5,6,7,8-tetrahydrofolate** (**THF**). THF is a carrier of a number of one-carbon units which bind to its nitrogen atoms at positions N^5, N^{10}, or both to form the compounds shown below. THF receives these one-carbon fragments from donors such as serine, glycine, or histidine and transfers them to intermediates in the synthesis of other amino acids, purines, and thymidine.

THF compound	one-carbon unit
N^{10}-formyl THF	$-CHO$
N^5-formimino THF	$-CH=NH$
N^5,N^{10}-methenyl THF	$=CH-$
N^5,N^{10}-methyleneTHF	$-CH_2$
N^5-methyl	$-CH_3$

These THF compounds are all interconvertible except the N^5-methyl group; along with SAM they comprise the one-carbon pool.

Students always tend to find the concept of the one-carbon pool confusing. All you need to realize is that THF and SAM are just carriers of one-carbon groups which are used in the synthesis of a range of molecules, mainly, amino acids, purines, and pyrimidines.

Folate metabolism
Formation of THF

THF is formed by the two-step reduction of folate by dihydrofolate reductase (Fig. 6.1). Dihydrofolate reductase is competitively inhibited by methotrexate, a folic acid analogue used in the treatment of certain cancers. By

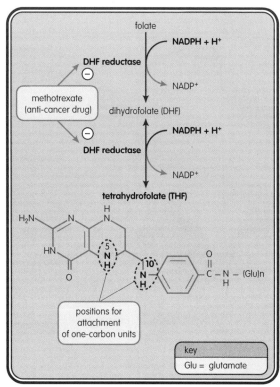

Fig. 6.1 Formation of THF. THF is formed by the two-step reduction of folate by dihydrofolate reductase.

inhibiting folate synthesis, methotexate can decrease the amount of THF available for purine and pyrimidine formation, thus decreasing DNA and RNA synthesis in cells.

Methyl-folate trap (Fig. 6.2)

Reactions involving the transfer of methyl groups result in the formation of N^5-methyl THF. Unlike the other THF compounds, it is not interconvertible, therefore the THF cannot be released and is trapped. Normally, however, the methionine salvage pathway is present. Methionine is formed by methylation of homocysteine using N^5-methyl THF as the methyl group donor, releasing the THF. Homocysteine methyltransferase catalyses the reaction and requires vitamin B_{12} as an essential co-factor (methylcobalamin). In vitamin B_{12} deficiency, this pathway is inhibited and THF remains as N^5-methyl THF. Eventually, all of the body's folate can become trapped resulting in folate deficiency secondary to B_{12} deficiency (see Chapter 8 also). This results in decreased nucleotide synthesis, and DNA and RNA formation. As blood cells require high levels of nucleotides for their turnover, they are particularly sensitive to folate deficiency, which can lead to megaloblastic anaemia.

Amino acids and the one-carbon pool

The synthesis and breakdown of certain amino acids produces THF carriers that can then be used in the synthesis of other amino acids and nucleotides. The following reactions demonstrate the use of the one-carbon pool.

Formation of SAM from methionine (numbers refer to Fig. 6.2)

1. Condensation of ATP and methionine to form SAM.
2. SAM contains an activated methyl group that can be donated to a number of acceptor molecules, forming S-adenosyl homocysteine.
3. The hydrolysis of S-adenosyl homocysteine releases adenosine to form homocysteine.
4. Homocysteine can be used either for the synthesis of the amino acid cysteine (see Chapter 5), or for
5. the regeneration of methionine in the methionine salvage pathway.

Serine to glycine conversion

The reaction sequence for the conversion of serine to glycine is shown in Fig. 6.3.

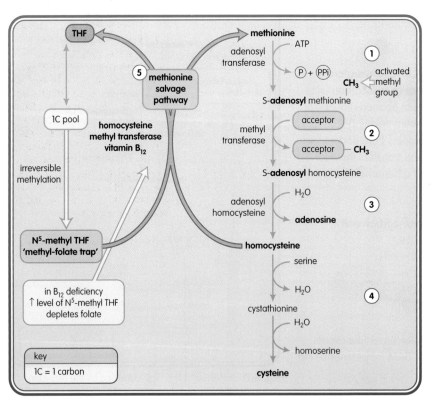

Fig. 6.2 Formation of S-adenosyl methionine and the **methionine salvage pathway**. SAM is formed by condensation of ATP and methionine. It contains an activated CH_3 group that can be transferred to a number of acceptor molecules. Homocysteine released from hydrolysis of S-adenosyl homocysteine can either be used for synthesis of the amino acid cysteine or for the methionine salvage pathway. The methionine salvage pathway reverses the methyl-folate trap. (Numbers refer to text above.)

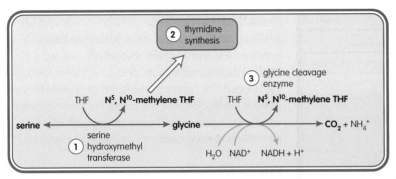

Fig. 6.3 Serine to glycine conversion.
1. Serine hydroxymethyl transferase transfers a methyl group from serine to tetrahydrofolate (THF) forming N^5,N^{10}-methylene THF and glycine.
2. This methyl group can then be used for the synthesis of thymidine (discussed later in this chapter).
3. The glycine cleavage enzyme (glycine synthase) oxidatively decarboxylates glycine generating N^5,N^{10}-methylene THF and CO_2.

- **What is the one-carbon pool?**
- **Describe the formation of THF.**
- **What is the significance of the methyl–folate trap to both folate and vitamin B$_{12}$ metabolism (see also Chapter 8)?**
- **Describe the use of one-carbon units in the synthesis of amino acids.**

PURINE METABOLISM

Structure and function of purines

The purines are the nitrogenous bases adenine, guanine, and hypoxanthine. Purines have a double-ring structure consisting of a six-carbon ring and a five-carbon ring. They are nearly always found with a pentose sugar (5C) attached to the nitrogen atom at N9 to form a nucleoside, for example, adenosine. The sugar is usually ribose or deoxyribose. Phosphorylation of the sugar at the C5 position leads to the formation of mono-, di-, and tri-nucleotides as shown in Fig. 6.4.

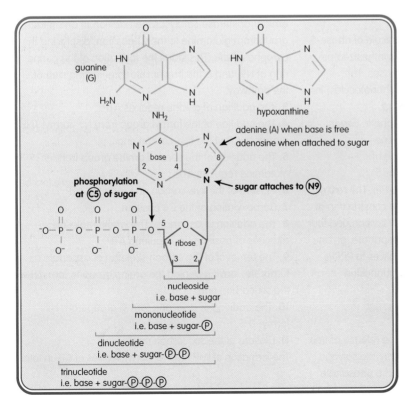

Fig. 6.4 Structure of purines, nucleosides and nucleotides. Purines are the nitrogenous bases adenine, guanine and hypoxanthine. They can either exist as free bases or with a pentose sugar, usually ribose or deoxyribose attached at the N9 position to form a nucleoside. For example, adenine is the free base, adenosine is the nucleoside; or guanine is the free base, guanosine is the nucleoside. The nucleoside of hypoxanthine is called inosine. Phosphorylation of the sugar at the C5 position leads to the formation of mono-, di- and tri-nucleotides as shown.

Main functions of purines	
Functions	**Examples**
building blocks of DNA and RNA	adenine and guanine
components of co-factors, particularly adenine	NAD+, FAD, CoA
energy currency in cell	ATP, GTP, AMP, etc.
regulatory compounds for enzymes of metabolic pathways	ATP, ADP, NAD+, etc.
cell-signalling molecules	cAMP, cGMP, GTP, G–proteins
neurotransmitters and smooth muscle effectors	cGMP

Fig. 6.5 Main functions of purines.

The phosphate groups cause these molecules to be negatively charged. The main functions of purines are listed in Fig. 6.5.

An overview of purine metabolism

The diet provides negligible amounts of purines because they are broken down in the gut to form uric acid. Two pathways are concerned with the formation of purine nucleotides (Fig. 6.6).

I. *De novo* synthesis of purines.

The purine ring is assembled on a molecule of ribose-5-phosphate, therefore, the purines are synthesized as mononucleotides as opposed to free bases. The location of this pathway is in liver cells (hepatocytes) in the cell cytosol and there are two stages:

- The formation of inosine monophosphate. Eleven reactions are necessary to form inosine monophosphate (IMP), the nucleotide of hypoxanthine. The first reaction forms 5-phosphoribosyl-1-pyrophosphate (PRPP). The rest of the reactions are concerned with the construction of the purine ring by the addition of five carbon and four nitrogen atoms from amino acids (aspartate, glycine, and glutamine), CO_2, and THF derivatives to PRPP.
- The conversion of IMP to AMP and guanosine monophosphate (GMP).

II. Salvage pathways

The turnover of nucleic acids leads to the release of free purines. These free bases are recycled by the salvage pathway which re-attaches a sugar and a phosphate group to reform the nucleotide.

Breakdown of purines

AMP and GMP are broken down to the free bases hypoxanthine and xanthine, respectively (see Fig. 6.6). These are converted into uric acid, which is excreted by the kidneys. Uric acid is insoluble. When present at high levels in the blood it may precipitate out forming crystals which may cause gout. These pathways will now be considered in more detail.

Purine formation

De novo synthesis of purines

The sources of the carbon and nitrogen atoms for the synthesis of the purine ring are shown in Fig. 6.7.

Formation of IMP

This first stage of purine synthesis has 11 reactions (numbers refer to Fig. 6.8):

1. 5-phosphoribosyl-1-pyrophosphate (PRPP) synthesis: PRPP synthetase catalyses the phosphorylation of ribose-5-phosphate at the C1 position forming 5-phosphoribosyl-1-pyrophosphate. This irreversible reaction requires two molecules of ATP (as ATP is hydrolysed to AMP) and serves to 'activate' ribose-5-phosphate.

2. The synthesis of 5-phosphoribosylamine. PRPP amidotransferase catalyses the addition of an amide group from glutamine to the C1 position, displacing the pyrophosphate. This starts the formation of the purine ring at N9, and is the irreversible rate-limiting step of the pathway.

3. The addition of glycine requires ATP.

4. The addition of the formyl group from N^{10}-formyl THF produces C8 of the five-carbon ring.

5. The addition of the second amide group from glutamine requires ATP.

6. Closure of the five-carbon ring requires ATP.

7. Carboxylation at the C6 position.

8. The addition of aspartate. The whole molecule attaches at position C6, requiring ATP.

9. The removal of the carbon skeleton of aspartate as fumarate, leaving behind the amino group to form N1 of the six-carbon ring.

10. The addition of a second formyl group from N^{10}-formyl THF.

11. Closure of the six-carbon ring.

The formation of IMP requires six molecules of ATP in total.

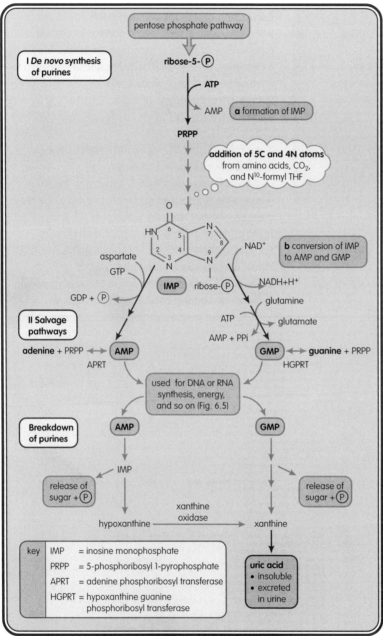

Fig. 6.6 Overview of purine metabolism. Two pathways are concerned with the formation of purine nucleotides:
I. *De novo* synthesis of purines where the purine ring is assembled on a molecule of ribose-5-phosphate. The pathway consists of two stages:
a. Formation of IMP, which occurs in 11 reactions. The purine ring is constructed by addition of C and N atoms from a number of sources: amino acids, CO_2, and THF derivatives.
b. IMP is then converted to either GMP or AMP.
II. Salvage pathways 'recycle' free purines released during nucleic acid turnover by reattaching a sugar phosphate unit to them.
There is only one pathway for purine breakdown, which converts the purines to the free bases hypoxanthine and xanthine; these are then oxidized to uric acid for excretion by the kidney.

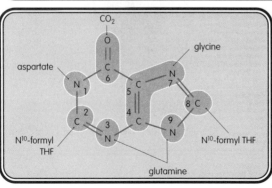

Fig. 6.7 Sources of the carbon and nitrogen atoms of the purine ring. (THF, tetrahydrofolate.)

In purine formation the five-carbon ring is synthesized first. The order of assembly is very useful to know:

1. N9 from glutamine
2. C4, C5, N7 from glycine
3. C8 from N^{10}-formyl THF
4. N3 from glutamine
5. C6 from CO_2
6. N1 from aspartate
7. C2 from N^{10}-formyl THF

Conversion of IMP to AMP and GMP

IMP is converted to GMP by the addition of an amino group at the C2 position; two steps are involved (Fig. 6.9):
1. Oxidation at C2 by IMP dehydrogenase forming xanthosine monophosphate (XMP).
2. Insertion of the amino group from glutamine by GMP synthase to form GMP.

The synthesis of GMP requires ATP, that is, the reciprocal nucleotide is required.

AMP is formed from IMP by converting the keto group at the C6 position to an amino group; again two steps are involved (see Fig. 6.9):
1. The addition of aspartate at the C6 position by adenylsuccinate synthase. This reaction requires GTP (again the reciprocal nucleotide).
2. The elimination of the carbon skeleton of aspartate as fumarate, leaving behind the amino group.

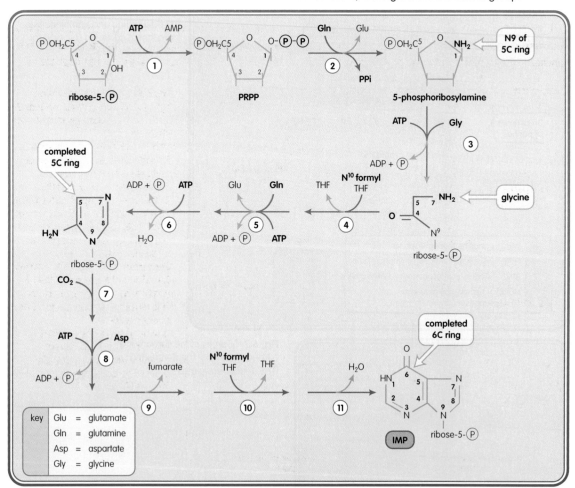

Fig. 6.8 Formation of inosine monophosphate (IMP). This first stage of purine synthesis has 11 reactions (numbers refer to text).

Regulation of purine biosynthesis

Purine synthesis is controlled allosterically by feedback inhibition at four major control sites:

- PRPP synthetase. This is inhibited by the end products GDP and ADP. As PRPP is also an intermediate in both the salvage pathway and pyrimidine synthesis (discussed later in this chapter), this is not the major control site.
- PRPP amidotransferase. This irreversible, rate-limiting reaction is unique to purine synthesis. It is allosterically inhibited by the end products IMP, AMP, and GMP.
- Adenylsuccinate synthase. This is inhibited by the end product AMP.
- IMP dehydrogenase. This is inhibited by the end product GMP.

If regulation is lost because of a defect in one of these four regulatory enzymes, this may lead to the overproduction of AMP and GMP, in excess of the requirements for nucleic acid synthesis and other functions. The excess purines are broken down to uric acid, which may become deposited in tissues, leading to symptoms of gout.

ATP yield of purine biosynthesis

The formation of IMP requires six molecules of ATP (see Fig. 6.8); the conversion of IMP to AMP uses one GTP; the conversion of IMP to GMP uses two molecules of ATP (see Fig. 6.9). Therefore, seven molecules of ATP are required to form one molecule of AMP and eight ATP are required to form a molecule of GMP.

Thus in terms of energy, the *de novo* pathway is an expensive process. The salvage pathway, however, provides an alternative way of forming purine nucleotides without using much ATP.

Salvage pathways

When nucleic acids and nucleotides are broken down, the free bases are released. The salvage pathway recycles these free bases by re-attaching ribose-5-phosphate to them (Fig. 6.10). It is a one-step pathway and the ribose-5-phosphate is transferred to the free bases from PRPP. The release of pyrophosphate

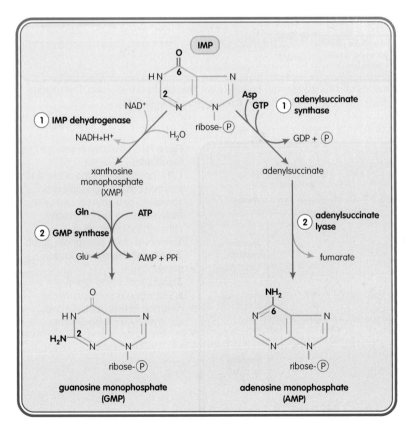

Fig. 6.9 Conversion of inosine monophosphate (IMP) to AMP and GMP. Both conversions involve two steps.
Conversion of IMP to GMP involves:
1. Oxidation at the C2 position by IMP dehydrogenase, forming xanthosine monophosphate.
2. The amino group of glutamine is then inserted at the C2 position by GMP synthase to form GMP. This reaction requires the reciprocal nucleotide, ATP.
Conversion of IMP to AMP involves:
1. addition of aspartate at the C6 position to form adenylsuccinate. This reaction requires the reciprocal nucleotide, GTP.
2. Adenyl succinate lyase then eliminates the C-skeleton of aspartate as fumarate, leaving behind the amino group at C6 to form AMP.

makes the reactions irreversible. Only two enzymes are necessary: adenine phosphoribosyl transferase (APRT) and hypoxanthine guanine phosphoribosyl transferase (HGPRT). The pathway is simple and requires much less ATP than *de novo* synthesis because the bases do not have to be made first.

Lesch–Nyhan syndrome
Lesch–Nyhan syndrome is a disorder caused by an almost total absence of HGPRT. The salvage pathway is virtually inactive for guanine and hypoxanthine (this is discussed fully in Chapter 12).

Breakdown of purines
The breakdown of purines has two stages: the breakdown of the nucleotide to a free base

hypoxanthine or xanthine, and the formation of uric acid (Fig. 6.11).

I. Breakdown of the nucleotide to a free base: hypoxanthine or xanthine
Three reactions are necessary (numbers refer to Fig. 6.11):
1. The removal of the phosphate group by a nucleotidase.
2. The removal of ribose as ribose-1-phosphate by nucleoside phosphorylase.
3. The release of the amino group.

Both AMP and GMP are degraded by the same three reactions; only the order differs (shown in Fig. 6.11). AMP and IMP form hypoxanthine and GMP forms xanthine.

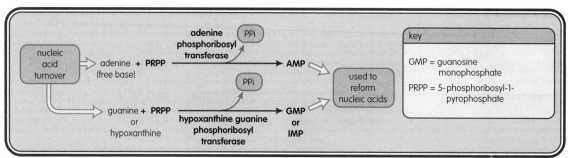

Fig. 6.10 Salvage pathways. When nucleic acids and nucleotides are broken down, free bases are released. The salvage pathway recycles these free bases by re-attaching ribose-5-phosphate to them by transfer from PRPP.

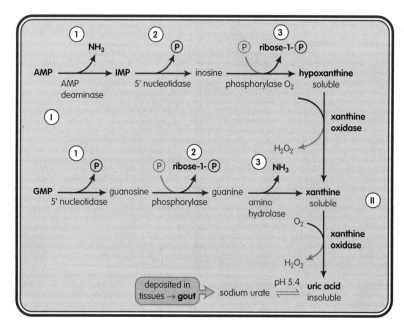

Fig. 6.11 Breakdown of purines has two stages:
I. The breakdown of the nucleotide to a free base, hypoxanthine or xanthine. For both AMP and GMP, three reactions are necessary, although the order differs:
1. removal of the phosphate group.
2. removal of ribose as ribose-1-phosphate.
3. release of amino group.
II. Formation of uric acid: by the oxidation of hypoxanthine and xanthine by xanthine oxidase.

II. Formation of uric acid

Only two steps are necessary, and are catalysed by the same enzyme (see Fig. 6.11):

1. The oxidation of hypoxanthine to xanthine by xanthine oxidase.
2. The oxidation of xanthine to uric acid by the same enzyme.

Xanthine oxidase is the key enzyme involved in purine degradation. It is unusual because it is a molybdenum and iron containing flavoprotein that uses molecular oxygen as an oxidizing agent.

In humans, the uric acid formed is excreted in the urine. Uric acid is insoluble. The acidic pH of urine allows it to precipitate out at high concentrations as sodium urate. Hyperuricaemia, that is, high serum levels of uric acid may lead to gout (discussed fully in Chapter 12).

Xanthine oxidase inhibitors

Xanthine oxidase is the key enzyme involved in controlling the amount of uric acid produced. Treatment with xanthine oxidase inhibitors decreases the amount of uric acid formed and increases the amounts of the soluble precursors hypoxanthine and xanthine, which are easily excreted in the urine. Therefore, xanthine oxidase inhibitors are used in the treatment of gout. Allopurinol, an analogue of hypoxanthine, is the most commonly used xanthine oxidase inhibitor. It has a number of actions:

- It is a competitive inhibitor of xanthine oxidase.
- The salvage enzyme can catalyse the addition of ribose-5-phosphate to allopurinol, forming allopurinol ribonucleotide. This can inhibit the rate-limiting enzyme of *de novo* purine synthesis, namely by PRPP amidotransferase leading to a decrease in the level of purines and also of the PRPP pool.
- Allopurinol can be metabolized by xanthine oxidase to oxypurinol, an even stronger inhibitor of xanthine oxidase.

Other breakdown products

In mammals other than primates, uric acid is further degraded by splitting of the purine ring to form allantoin, which is highly soluble. The reason why humans and monkeys have lost the ability to break down uric acid may be because it has some evolutionary advantage. It is possible that when we lost the ability to synthesize vitamin C, we also lost the enzyme uricase, which degrades uric acid to a soluble product. However, uric acid does have a beneficial effect: it is an effective scavenger of free oxygen radicals and can take over the role of vitamin C as an anti-oxidant. Remember, only humans and monkeys can get gout!

- What are the structures and the main functions of adenine and guanine?
- Name the stages involved in *de novo* purine synthesis and the four regulatory enzymes.
- Name the sources and the order of assembly of the carbon and nitrogen atoms of the purine ring.
- Describe the ATP yield of *de novo* synthesis.
- Describe the main functions of the salvage pathways.
- Give a basic outline of purine breakdown.
- What use do xanthine oxidase inhibitors have?

PYRIMIDINE METABOLISM

Structure and function of pyrimidines

Structure

There are three main pyrimidines: thymine, cytosine, and uracil. Like purines, the pyrimidines are mostly found associated with a five-carbon sugar attached at N1 to form the nucleosides thymidine, cytidine, and uridine (Fig. 6.12). The sugar may be mono-, di-, or tri-phosphorylated to form the corresponding nucleotides.

Functions

Pyrimidines are the building blocks of DNA and RNA: thymine and cytosine are present in DNA and cytosine and uracil are present in RNA.

Nucleotide derivatives are activated intermediates in a number of synthetic reactions, for example, UDP-glucose, the precursor of glycogen (see Chapter 2).

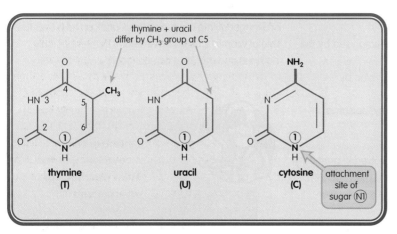

Fig. 6.12 Structure of pyrimidines. Like purines, the pyrimidines are mostly found associated with a five-carbon sugar attached at N1 to form nucleosides.

Biosynthesis of pyrimidines

There are three main stages in the biosynthesis of pyrimidines (Fig. 6.13 and 6.15):

a. The construction of the pyrimidine ring to form uridine monophosphate (UMP).

b. The conversion of UMP to uridine triphosphate (UTP) and cytidine triphosphate (CTP), the ribonucleotides found in RNA.

c. The formation of the deoxyribonucleotides dCTP and dTTP found in DNA (Fig. 6.15).

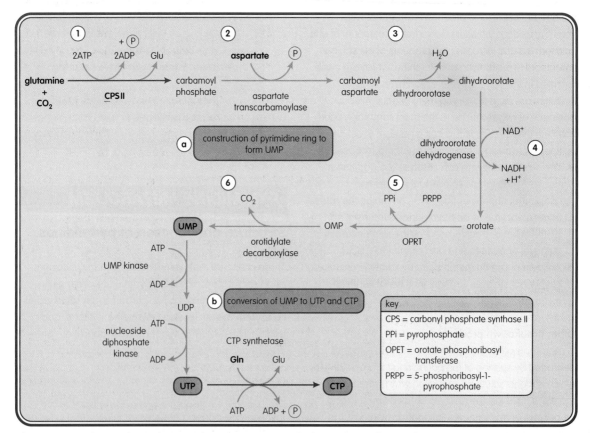

Fig. 6.13 Pyrimidine synthesis: there are three main stages in the biosynthesis of pyrimidines. Construction of the pyrimidine ring from glutamine, aspartate, and CO_2 to form uridine monophosphate. UMP can then be converted to UDP, UTP, and CTP, the ribonucleotides of RNA (numbers refer to text). The third stage of pyrimidine synthesis is shown in Fig. 6.15.

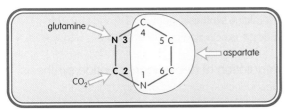

Fig. 6.14 The pyrimidine ring. The ring is derived from glutamine, aspartate, and CO_2.

All of the three stages take place in the cell cytosol and will now be considered in more detail.

Construction of the pyrimidine ring

Unlike purine synthesis, the pyrimidine ring is synthesized before attachment to ribose-5-phosphate, that is, it is formed as a free base. The ring is derived from glutamine, aspartate, and CO_2 (Fig. 6.14). There are six steps in the reaction sequence (numbers refer to Fig. 6.13).

1. The synthesis of carbamoyl phosphate by carbamoyl phosphate synthase II (CPSII). This is the rate-limiting step. Carbamoyl phosphate is also the precursor of urea, however, urea is formed by the mitochondrial enzyme, carbamoyl phosphate synthase I (see Chapter 5).

2. The addition of aspartate.

3. Closure of the ring by dihydroorotase.

The first three enzymes are actually present as a single, polypeptide chain forming a multi-functional enzyme,

CAD of carbamoyl phosphate synthase II, aspartate trans-carbamoylase, and dihydroorotase. In a similar way to fatty acid synthase, the enzymes are linked together to minimize side reactions and loss of substrate.

4. The oxidation of dihydroorotate to orotate using NAD^+.

5. Conversion of the free pyrimidine to a nucleotide by the addition of ribose-5-phosphate from PRPP. This is catalysed by orotate phosphoribosyl transferase (OPRT) and is driven by the hydrolysis of pyrophosphate to two free molecules of inorganic phosphate. PRPP is thus required for the synthesis of both purines and pyrimidines.

6. The decarboxylation of orotidine monophosphate (OMP) to UMP by orotidylate decarboxylase. Both OPRT and orotidylate decarboxylase are also found together as a single polypeptide.

Conversion of UMP to UDP, UTP, and CTP—ribonucleotides of RNA

UMP is phosphorylated to UDP and UTP as shown in Fig. 6.13. CTP is formed from UTP by amination, that is, the addition of an NH_2 group from glutamine to position 4 of the pyrimidine ring. Both UTP and CTP are used for RNA synthesis.

Formation of the deoxyribonucleotides dCTP and dTTP (see Fig. 6.15)

1. Formation of dCTP. Ribonucleotide reductase reduces CDP to dCDP by removing the C2-OH group on ribose,

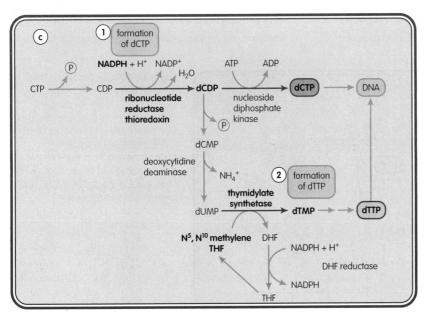

Fig. 6.15 Pyrimidine synthesis: the formation of deoxyribonucleotides.
1. Ribonucleotide reductase reduces CDP to deoxyCDP by removal of the C2-OH group on ribose, converting it to deoxyribose. The dCDP formed is phosphorylated to dCTP.
2. dTTP is formed by the methylation of dUMP. Thymidylate synthetase transfers a methyl group from N^5, N^{10}-methylene THF to position 5 of the pyrimidine ring, forming dTMP which can be phosphorylated to dTTP (numbers refer to text on pp.109–110).

converting it to deoxyribose. The enzyme requires thioredoxin as a co-factor. The actual mechanism is quite complicated but can be divided into three steps (not shown in Fig. 6.15):

- Ribonucleotide reductase contains two thiol (SH) groups and it is these that actually reduce the ribose.
- Thioredoxin also contains two thiol groups that are oxidized to enable the thiol groups on the enzyme to be reformed.
- NADPH then reduces the co-factor to regenerate the reduced form.

The dCDP formed is phosphorylated by nucleoside diphosphate kinase to dCTP.

2. Formation of dTTP. dTTP is formed by the methylation of dUMP. Dephosphorylation and deamination converts dCDP to dUMP, the precursor of dTMP. Thymidylate synthetase catalyses the transfer of a methyl group from N^5,N^{10}-methylene THF to position 5 of the pyrimidine ring, forming dTMP. The reaction is unusual because N^5,N^{10}-methylene THF undergoes oxidation itself to dihydrofolate, that is, it transfers the methyl group and two hydrogen atoms. Dihydrofolate reductase regenerates the THF. dTMP can be phosphorylated by dTMP kinase and nucleoside diphosphate kinase to dTTP.

Regulation of pyrimidine synthesis

The rate-limiting step in humans is the formation of carbamoyl phosphate by carbamoyl phosphate synthase II. CPSII is inhibited by the end products of pyrimidine synthesis, namely UDP and UTP. The reaction is activated by ATP and PRPP.

Regulation of deoxyribonucleotide synthesis

Ribonucleotide reductase actually catalyses the irreversible reduction of all four nucleoside diphosphates (ADP, GDP, CDP, and UDP) to their corresponding deoxy forms and is therefore subject to regulation. The enzyme has four subunits (two B1 and two B2). Each B1 subunit has two allosteric sites distinct from the active site: an activity site and a substrate specificity site. The binding of the product dATP to the activity site inhibits the enzyme. The binding of the substrate, a ribonucleotide, e.g. ATP, to the substrate specificity site, activates the enzyme.

Salvage pathways

The salvage pathways for pyrimidines are similar to those for purines (Fig. 6.16). The breakdown of nucleotides releases free pyrimidines that are salvaged by the enzyme uracil/thymine phosphoribosyl transferase (UTPRT), which re-attaches a ribose-5-phosphate to them, reforming the mononucleotides. PRPP donates the ribose-5-phosphate. The enzyme UTPRT cannot salvage cytosine. Therefore cytidine (nucleoside) is deaminated to uridine; this can then be converted to uracil, which can be salvaged.

Breakdown of pyrimidines

Purines are excreted with their ring still intact as uric acid. The pyrimidine ring, however, can be split and broken down to soluble structures (Fig. 6.17). Uracil and cytosine are broken down to β-alanine, which forms

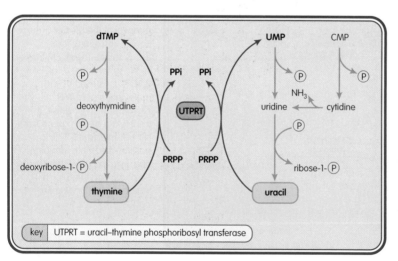

Fig. 6.16 Salvage pathway. The salvage pathways for pyrimidines are similar to those for purines. Breakdown of nucleotides releases free pyrimidines thymine and uracil. UTPRT transfers a ribose-5-phosphate unit from PRPP, to the free pyrimidine to reform the mononucleotide, for example, UMP or dTMP. Cytidine must be deaminated to uridine since it is not a substrate for UTPRT.

acetyl CoA. Thymine is degraded to β-aminoisobutyrate, which forms succinyl CoA. The carbon skeletons of the pyrimidines, namely, acetyl CoA and succinyl CoA, can be oxidized by the TCA cycle.

Anti-cancer drugs

These drugs inhibit the formation of nucleotides, leading to a decrease in DNA synthesis and cell growth. Cancer cells divide rapidly and have an increased demand for DNA synthesis. These drugs help to slow down the growth of cancer cells. However, they also affect normal cell replication, leading to serious side effects (Fig. 6.18).

Azidothymidine and other anti-viral drugs

Azidothymidine (AZT) is a nucleoside analogue of thymidine in which the 3'-OH group on the ribose is replaced by an azido group (N3). AZT can be phosphorylated to the nucleotide AZTTP, which is a potent inhibitor of reverse transcriptase, the enzyme found in retroviruses that is responsible for replication of the viral genome. Therefore, AZT inhibits viral replication. AZT has been used with some success in treatment of the retrovirus HIV. Host-cell DNA polymerase is relatively insensitive to AZT.

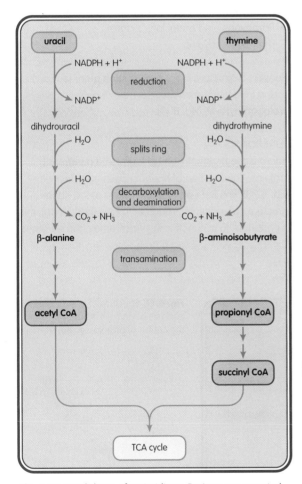

Fig. 6.17 Breakdown of pyrimidines. Purines are excreted with their ring still intact as uric acid. The pyrimidine ring, however, can be split and broken down to soluble structures such as acetyl CoA and succinyl CoA for oxidation by the TCA cycle. N.B. only the main reactions and substrates are shown here.

Action of anti-cancer drugs		
Drugs	**Action**	**Effect on pyrimidine and purine synthesis**
glutamine antagonists: azaserine, diazo-oxo-norleucine	analogues of glutamine: competitively inhibit enzymes that incorporate glutamine	↓pyrimidine synthesis: inhibits CPS II ↓purine synthesis: inhibits reaction 2 (PRPP amidotransferase) and reaction 5 (Fig. 6.8)
folate antagonists: methotrexate	inhibits DHF reductase leading to decreased available THF for transfer of one-carbon units	inhibits methylation of dUMP to dTMP causing ↓ dTMP synthesis ↓ purine synthesis (Fig. 6.8)
5-fluorouracil	analogue of dUMP: irreversibly inhibits thymidylate synthetase	inhibits synthesis of dTMP; no effect on purine synthesis

Fig. 6.18 Action of anti-cancer drugs.

Most anti-cancer drugs affect normal cell replication and proliferation, especially cells of the bone marrow, gastrointestinal tract, gonads, skin, and hair follicles. This results in severe side effects such as anaemia, neutropenia (making patients susceptibile to infection), hair loss, vomiting, infertility, impaired wound healing, and stunting of growth.

Acyclovir or acycloguanosine is an analogue of guanosine which is used in the treatment of herpes virus infections. Humans cannot use acyclovir as a substrate but the herpes virus can. It can be phosphorylated by a viral enzyme and incorporated into the DNA chain where it causes chain termination, preventing viral DNA replication.

- Describe the structure of the main pyrimidines and their function.
- Outline the three stages of pyrimidine synthesis, noting any differences from purine synthesis.
- What are the breakdown products of pyrimidines?
- Analyse the action of anti-cancer drugs and their effect on purine and pyrimidine synthesis.

HAEM METABOLISM

Structure and function of haem
Structure
It is very easy to get lost with the terminology used in haem metabolism; this is a basic 'all you need to know' approach.

- The basic structure is a four-ringed cyclic structure called a porphyrin.
- Each ring is called a pyrrole ring and the rings are linked together via methenyl bridges.
- Three types of side chains can be attached to the pyrrole ring, methyl, vinyl, or propionates, and the arrangement of these is important to the activity.
- Porphyrins bind metal ions to form metalloporphyrins.

Haem is a structure containing an iron atom (as Fe^{2+}) bound in the centre of a tetrapyrrole ring of protoporphyrin IX (Fig. 6.19).

Functions
Haem is the prosthetic group found in a number of proteins. The function of haem in each group can vary (Fig. 6.20). The Fe^{2+} atom at the centre of the haem structure can undergo oxidation to Fe^{3+} (ferric form); this is important to its function in cytochromes and enzymes,

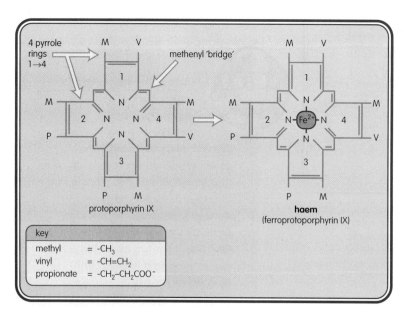

Fig. 6.19 Structure of haem. Haem consists of an Fe^{2+} atom bound in the centre of protoporphyrin IX.

Functions of haem	
Protein	**Function of haem**
haemoglobin and myoglobin	reversibly binds O_2 for transport
peroxidases and catalase	forms part of the active site of enzyme
cytochromes (a, b, c, and P_{450})	electron carrier: continually oxidized and reduced potentiating electron flow

Fig. 6.20 Main functions of haem.

enabling it to act as a recyclable electron carrier. However, in haemoglobin and myoglobin, Fe^{3+} cannot bind oxygen, and its function as an oxygen transporter is impaired (it forms methaemoglobin, see Chapter 3).

Haem biosynthesis

The main locations of haem biosynthesis are:
- Bone marrow erythroid cells, where haem is used to form haemoglobin.

- Liver hepatocytes, where haem is used for cytochrome synthesis, particularly cytochrome P_{450} which is involved in drug metabolism.

Humans make 40–50 mg/day of haem, about 80–85% of which is used for haemoglobin synthesis. Mature RBCs lack mitochondria and therefore they cannot make haem.

Site
Haem biosynthesis is 'partitioned' between mitochondria and the cytosol (Fig. 6.21).

An overview of the pathway
- There are eight reactions; the first and last three occur in mitochondria, the rest are in the cytosol.
- Protoporphyrin IX is derived totally from glycine and succinyl CoA.
- Eight moles of each are required to form eight moles of δ-aminolevulinic acid (ALA), which condenses to

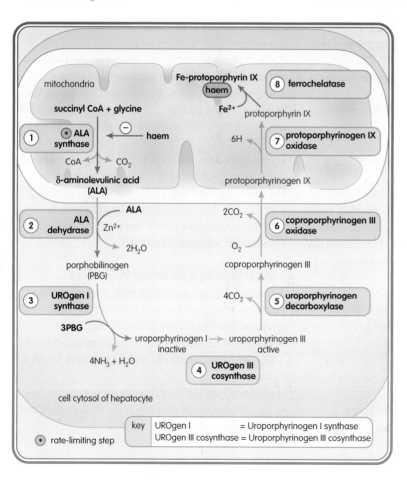

Fig. 6.21 Haem synthesis. The site of haem biosynthesis is 'partitioned' between mitochondria and the cytosol. The first and last three reactions occur in the mitochondria, the rest are in the cytosol. ALA synthase catalyses the condensation of glycine and succinyl CoA to form ALA. Two molecules of ALA condense to form PBG. Four molecules of PBG then condense to form uroporphyrinogen I, which is activated by UROgen III cosynthase, converting it to the asymmetrical active form, uroporphyrinogen III. The rest of the reactions modify the side chains and degree of unsaturation of the porphyrin ring. Ferrochelatase inserts the Fe^{2+} ion to form haem in the mitochondria.
(Numbers are explained in the text on p. 114.)

form four moles of porphobilinogen (PBG). These, in turn, condense to form 1 mole of uroporphyrinogen I (UROgen I).

- The rest of the reactions modify the side chains.
- If the side chains on porphyrins are arranged symmetrically then the molecules are physiologically inactive. When the side chains are arranged asymmetrically, the molecules are active.

The steps are now considered in detail (see Fig. 6.21).
1. The synthesis of ALA. ALA synthase catalyses the condensation of glycine and succinyl CoA in mitochondria. The reaction requires pyridoxal phosphate (PLP) as a co-factor. This is the irreversible, rate-limiting step of haem synthesis.
2. The formation of porphobilinogen (PBG). ALA dehydrase catalyses the dehydration of two molecules of ALA to form PBG. The enzyme is inhibited by heavy metals such as lead.
3. Formation of uroporphyrinogen I (UROgen I). UROgen I synthase catalyses the condensation of four molecules of PBG to form UROgen I (inactive).
4. UROgen III cosynthase produces the asymmetrical and therefore active uroporphyrinogen III (UROgen III). The rest of the reactions alter the side chains and the degree of unsaturation of the porphyrin ring.
5. The first decarboxylation results in the formation of coproporphyrinogen III.
6. The second decarboxylation forms protoporphyrinogen IX in the mitochondria.
7. Oxidation to protoporphyrin IX.
8. Ferrochelatase inserts the Fe^{2+} ion to form haem. Protoporphyrinogen IX is the colourless, unstable, easily oxidized precursor of porphyrin. Porphyrins are highly coloured (red), stable compounds that characteristically absorb ultra-violet light at a wavelength of 400 nm.

Lead poisoning

Lead inhibits three key enzymes of haem synthesis, resulting in the accumulation of intermediates:

- ALA dehydrase.
- Coproporphyrinogen III oxidase.
- Ferrochelatase.

Lead poisoning results in the inhibition of haem synthesis and anaemia (covered in detail in Chapter 12).

Porphyrias

Porphyrias are a rare group of inherited disorders caused by a defect in one of the enzymes of haem synthesis. They result in the accumulation and increased excretion of porphyrins and their precursors in urine and/or faeces and consequently the inhibition of haem synthesis. The diseases affect either the bone marrow (erythropoeitic porphyrias) or liver (hepatic porphyrias). Again, a full discussion can be found in Chapter 12.

Regulation of haem synthesis

The key rate-controlling enzyme of haem synthesis is ALA synthase. It is an ideal control point because the enzyme undergoes rapid turnover (has a half-life of 60–70 min). ALA synthase is inhibited by high levels of the end product haem (Fe^{2+}) and also haemin (Fe^{3+}), formed by the oxidation of haem.

In the liver, control of ALA synthase by haem is considered at three levels (numbers refer to Fig. 6.22):
1. Allosteric inhibition of the enzyme by haem. However, high concentrations of haem are necessary (10^{-5} M) and, therefore, this is not usually an important control mechanism.
2. Haem also inhibits the transport of newly synthesized enzyme from cytosol into mitochondria.
3. Repression of transcription of the ALA synthase gene by haem. This is probably the most effective regulation because it works at low concentrations (10^{-7} M).

In erythroid tissue, the same regulatory mechanisms apply as for the liver but additionally, under certain conditions, for example, chronic hypoxia or anaemia, erythropoeitin production is stimulated leading to an increase in red cell synthesis and thus number and, therefore, an increase in haem.

Induction of ALA synthase in the liver

A number of drugs such as steroids and barbiturates cause an increase in the amount of hepatic ALA synthase. The mechanism proceeds as follows:

- Drugs are metabolized by microsomal cytochrome P_{450} enzymes, which are haem-containing proteins themselves.
- Certain drugs induce the synthesis of cytochrome P_{450}, leading to an increase in the consumption and breakdown of haem.

- This leads to an overall decrease in the concentration of haem in the liver cells, which in turn stimulates or induces the transcription of ALA synthase and haem synthesis (see Fig. 6.22).
- Glucose blocks this induction.

Haem breakdown

About 80–85% of haem for breakdown comes from old RBCs; the rest comes from cytochrome turnover (Fig. 6.23).

Location/site

Kupffer cells and macrophages of the reticuloendothelial system (mainly liver, spleen, and bone marrow).

Pathway

The two steps in the pathway are (steps refer to Fig. 6.23):
1. Cleavage of the porphyrin ring to form biliverdin. Haem oxygenase found in microsomes splits the porphyrin ring by breaking one of the methenyl bridges between two pyrrole rings. This produces biliverdin, Fe^{3+}, and carbon monoxide (this is the only reaction *in vivo* that produces carbon monoxide).
2. The reduction of biliverdin to bilirubin in the cytosol. Bilirubin is an insoluble orange pigment, which is taken to the liver bound to albumin. In the liver it is conjugated with glucuronic acid by the enzyme bilirubin glucuronyl transferase, forming bilirubin diglucuronide. This increases its solubility, enabling its excretion in the bile.

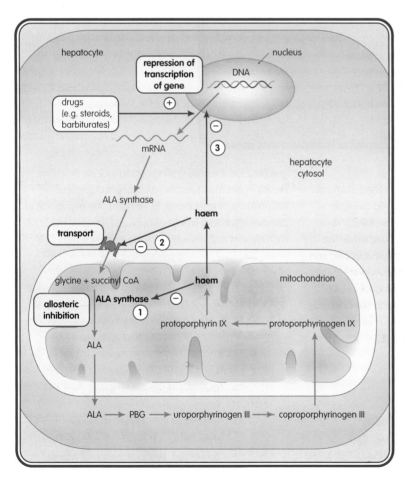

Fig. 6.22 Control of haem synthesis in the hepatocyte. In the liver, control of ALA synthase is considered at three levels:
1. Allosteric inhibition by end product, haem.
2. Inhibition of transport of newly made ALA synthase into the mitochondria by haem.
3. Haem also inhibits transcription of the ALA synthase gene.
Drugs, for example phenytoin or phenobarbitone, induce the activity of the cytochrome P_{450} enzymes which breakdown haem. This results in a decrease in the concentration of haem and thus stimulation of transcription of ALA synthase.

Purines, Pyrimidines, and Haem

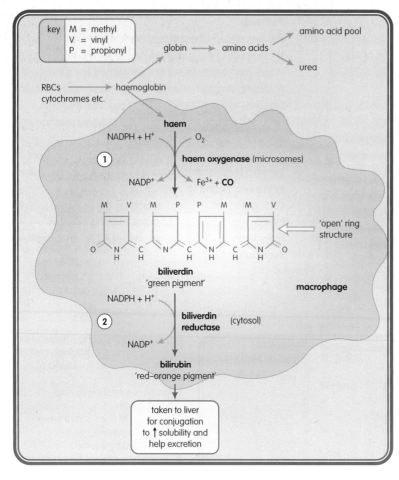

Fig. 6.23 Haem breakdown. About 80–85% of haem for breakdown comes from old RBCs; the rest comes from cytochrome turnover. The pathway consists of two steps: **1.** Cleavage of the porphyrin ring to form biliverdin by haem oxygenase. **2.** Reduction of biliverdin to bilirubin. Bilirubin is taken to the liver where it is conjugated to facilitate its excretion.(Numbers refer to text on p. 115.)

Haemolytic anaemia

Haemolytic anaemia is an anaemia resulting from an increase in RBC breakdown. Normally, red cell lysis releases haem for breakdown to bilirubin, which is taken to the liver to be conjugated and excreted. The liver has a large capacity to conjugate bilirubin and can cope with moderately elevated levels. However, massive red cell lysis that may occur in patients with severe haemolytic anaemia such as sickle cell anaemia (during a crisis) or thalassemia, leads to a very large increase in haem breakdown and high bilirubin levels,

greater than the conjugating capacity of the liver. This results in elevated plasma levels of unconjugated bilirubin, causing jaundice. In jaundice, the deposition of bilirubin leads to a yellow colouring of the skin, mucosal membranes and the whites of the eyes (sclerae).

Haem breakdown occurs at sites of minor trauma underneath the skin. The changing colours of a bruise represent the different pigments produced.

- Draw the structure of haem and give three of its functions.
- What are the main locations and sites of haem biosynthesis?
- Outline haem synthesis and the key regulatory step.
- What is the effect of lead poisoning on haem synthesis?
- Describe the pathway of haem breakdown and the effect of haemolytic anaemia.

116

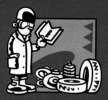

7. Metabolic Integration

Three stages of glucose homeostasis

Glucose homeostasis can be conveniently divided into three basic stages: the fed, fasted (post-absorptive), and starved states (Fig. 7.1). The starved state, however, can be subdivided into early and late since different fuels are available depending on the degree of starvation (Fig. 7.2).

It is important to realize that glucose homeostasis is a dynamic process. There are no well-defined boundaries between the states, instead, there is some degree of overlap between them, as the availability of substrates and hormonal influences is continually changing.

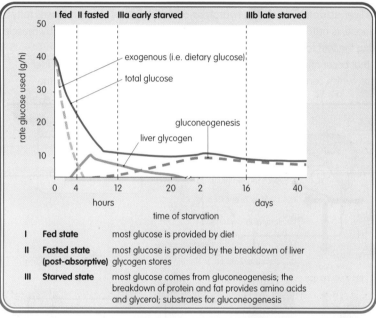

I	Fed state	most glucose is provided by diet
II	Fasted state (post-absorptive)	most glucose is provided by the breakdown of liver glycogen stores
III	Starved state	most glucose comes from gluconeogenesis; the breakdown of protein and fat provides amino acids and glycerol; substrates for gluconeogenesis

Fig. 7.1 Stages of glucose homeostasis. Glucose homeostasis can be conveniently divided into three stages: the fed, fasted (post-absorptive), and starved states. The starved state can be subdivided into early and late starvation.

Three stages of glucose homeostasis

State	Time course	Major fuels used	Hormonal control
I fed	following a meal 0–4 h	most tissues use glucose	↑ insulin results in: ↑ glucose uptake by peripheral tissues ↑ glycogen, TG, and protein synthesis
II fasted (post-absorptive)	4–12 h after feeding	brain: glucose muscle and liver: fatty acids	↑ glucagon and NA stimulates breakdown of liver glycogen and TG ↓ insulin
IIIa starved: early	12 h →16 days	brain: glucose and some ketone bodies liver: fatty acids muscle: mainly fatty acids and some ketone bodies	↑ glucagon and NA → ↑ TG hydrolysis and ketogenesis ↑ cortisol → breakdown of muscle protein, releasing amino acids for gluconeogenesis
IIIb starved: late	>16 days	brain: uses more ketone bodies and less glucose to preserve protein muscle: only fatty acids	↑ glucagon and NA

Fig. 7.2 Three stages of glucose homeostasis. (NA, noradrenaline; TG, triacylglycerol.)

The fed state

This is the period 0–4h after a meal and is summarized in Fig. 7.3. During the fed state (numbers refer to Fig. 7.3):

1. An increase in plasma glucose results in the release of insulin from the β cells in the pancreas. The availability of substrate and the increase in insulin stimulates glycogen, triacylglycerol, and protein synthesis by tissues; therefore this is an anabolic state.
2. Glucose is the sole fuel for the brain; uptake is insulin independent.
3. Muscle and adipose tissue also use glucose; uptake by these tissues is insulin dependent.

An increase in glucose and insulin in the liver activates glucokinase. Glucokinase, unlike hexokinase, is not inhibited by glucose-6-phosphate, enabling the liver to respond to the high blood glucose levels that occur after a meal. Glucokinase phosphorylates glucose, which can be used for synthesis of liver glycogen, therefore preventing hyperglycaemia (see Chapter 2).

Hexokinase, present in most cells, is maximally operational when the concentration of glucose in the blood is low.

The fasted state

This is the period 4–12h after a meal, that is, the post-absorptive state (Fig. 7.4). During the fasted state (numbers refer to Fig. 7.4):

1. The breakdown of liver glycogen stores provides glucose for oxidation by the brain. These stores are sufficient to last only between 12 and 24h.
2. The hydrolysis of triacylglycerol stores releases fatty acids, which are used preferentially as a fuel by muscle and liver.
3. Muscle can also use its own glycogen as a fuel. All these processes involved are activated by the

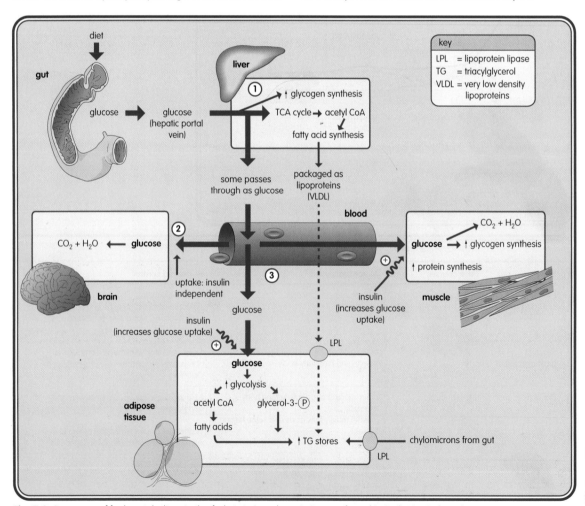

Fig. 7.3 Summary of fuel metabolism in the fed state (numbers 1–3 are referred to in the text above).

increase in the ratio of glucagon to insulin. This activates glycogen phosphorylase and hormone sensitive lipase by phosphorylation and thus glycogen breakdown and lipolysis.

The starved state

Early starved state

Once the liver glycogen has been used up, an alternative substrate is required to provide glucose (Fig. 7.5). In early starvation (numbers refer to Fig. 7.5):

1. Noradrenaline and cortisol activate protein breakdown in muscle which releases amino acids, particularly alanine and glutamine.

2. Hydrolysis of triacylglycerol stores (adipose tissue) releases glycerol.

Both amino acids and glycerol are used by the liver for gluconeogenesis.

3. The glucose produced is used by the brain.

'A comparison of the fed and the fasted state' is probably the most commonly examined question in metabolism because it requires overall knowledge of protein, fat, and carbohydrate metabolism and their regulation. The way to answer this for each state is to think: time-course; hormonal influences; main pathways active and substrates available; any special tissue requirements.

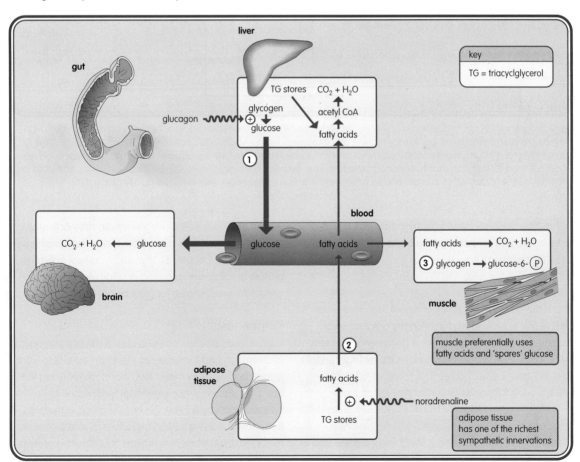

Fig. 7.4 Summary of fuel metabolism in the fasted state. This is the period 4–12 h after a meal. A high glucagon to insulin ratio activates the breakdown of liver glycogen, which provides glucose for the brain. Noradrenaline activates hydrolysis of triacylglycerol stores, releasing fatty acids which can be used as a fuel by muscle and liver. Muscle can use its own glycogen as fuel (numbers refer to text on pp. 118–19).

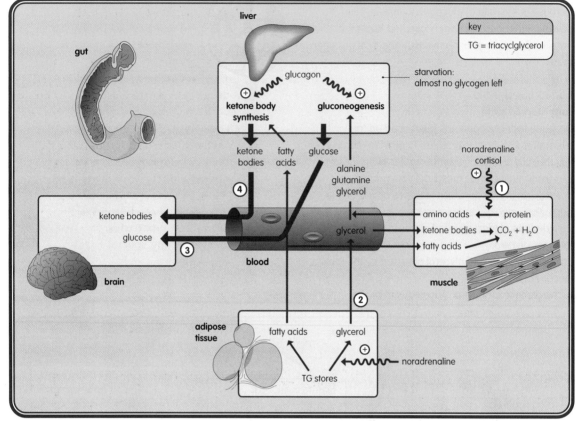

Fig. 7.5 Summary of fuel metabolism in the early starved state. Noradrenaline and cortisol activate the breakdown of muscle protein to release amino acids, particularly alanine and glutamine. Noradrenaline also activates hydrolysis of triacylglycerol to release glycerol. Glycerol, alanine, and glutamine are taken to the liver where they are oxidized to glucose by gluconeogenesis. Glucose is used by the brain mainly. Fatty acids released from hydrolysis of triacylglycerol can be taken to the liver and used to generate ketone bodies which can be used by brain and other tissues (numbers refer to text on pp. 119–20).

4. The fatty acids released from triacylglycerol are also used by the liver to make ketone bodies which can be used by peripheral tissues as well as the brain.

Late starved state

This is the period of starvation of longer than 16 days up until death. In prolonged starvation the breakdown of muscle protein slows down. This is because there is less need for glucose via gluconeogenesis as the brain adapts to using more ketone bodies. This is further helped by muscle using fatty acids almost exclusively as fuel.

Gluconeogenesis

Gluconeogenesis starts about 6–12 h after a meal and is the major source of glucose once the glycogen stores are depleted. The main role of gluconeogenesis is the maintenance of blood glucose and the provision of glucose for the brain and red blood cells (RBCs) during

fasting. An increased glucagon:insulin ratio activates gluconeogenesis and causes the reciprocal inhibition of glycolysis (see Chapter 5). In muscle, cortisol activates protein breakdown, releasing in particular alanine and glutamine—substrates for gluconeogenesis.

Ketogenesis

Ketone body synthesis begins during the first few days of starvation and increases as the brain adapts to using ketone bodies as its major fuel, therefore reducing the need for glucose. Once significant ketone body synthesis occurs, a fall in the level of gluconeogenesis from amino acids is seen. This results in a reduction in the breakdown of muscle protein, thus sparing protein.

After 2–3 weeks of starvation, muscle reduces its use of ketone bodies and uses fatty acids almost exclusively, leading to an increase in available ketone bodies for the brain.

Both ketogenesis and gluconeogenesis are balanced to ensure the efficient use of metabolic fuels during starvation. Gluconeogenesis activates ketogenesis: by depleting oxaloacetate which therefore ensures that the concentration of acetyl CoA exceeds the oxidative capacity of the TCA cycle. Acetyl CoA can therefore be used for ketone body synthesis.

Hormonal control of glucose homeostasis

Insulin is an anabolic hormone and it therefore increases the uptake and synthesis of glycogen, triacylglycerol, and protein. Glucagon, noradrenaline, adrenaline, and cortisol are all catabolic hormones. The main effects of glucagon are summarized in Fig. 7.6. Noradrenaline and adrenaline have some similar effects to glucagon:

- They increase glycogen breakdown (in muscle only).
- They increase lipolysis in adipose tissue.
- They stimulate protein breakdown.

Glucose homeostasis in exercise

Sprinters

Sprinting is an anaerobic excercise.

- In muscle during intense activity, there is only time for anaerobic glycolysis, resulting in the build-up of lactate.
- Lactate diffuses out of muscle and is taken to the liver where it is oxidized to pyruvate, which can then be converted back to glucose via gluconeogenesis.
- The glucose formed diffuses out of the liver and can return to the muscle to be further used as a fuel.

This series of reactions, which 'shift the metabolic burden from the muscle to the liver', is known as the Cori cycle (Fig. 7.7) (Compare it with the glucose–alanine cycle; see Fig. 5.27).

Long-distance running

Long-distance running is aerobic.

The body does not store enough glycogen to provide the energy necessary to run long distances. If the

Summary of the main effects of insulin and glucagon		
Pathway	**Insulin: anabolic**	**Glucagon: catabolic**
carbohydrate metabolism		
glycogen	increases glycogen synthesis in muscle and liver	increases glycogen breakdown in liver only (NA and adrenaline increase breakdown in muscle)
glycolysis/gluconeogenesis	increases glycolysis	Increases gluconeogenesis
glucose uptake	increases uptake by peripheral tissues, not liver	no effect
pentose phosphate pathway	increases PPP, producing NADPH for lipogenesis	
Lipid metabolism		
lipolysis and β oxidation	inhibits	activates
ketone body synthesis	inhibits	activates
lipogenesis	activates	inhibits
Protein metabolism		
uptake of amino acids by tissues	increases uptake by most tissues	increases uptake by the liver for gluconeogenesis
protein synthesis	increases rate by most tissues	decreases
protein breakdown	decreases rate	stimulates breakdown

Fig. 7.6 Summary of the main effects of insulin and glucagon. (NA, noradrenaline; PPP, Pentose phosphate pathway).

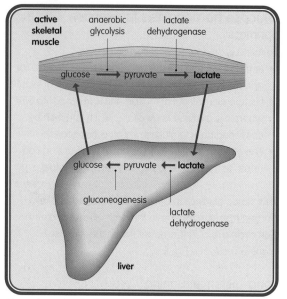

Fig. 7.7 Cori cycle shifts the metabolic burden from the muscle to the liver. Lactate which builds up in muscle during intense activity, is taken to the liver to be converted back to glucose via gluconeogenesis. This replenishes fuel supplies of muscle and prevents lactic acidosis.

respiratory quotient (RQ), the ratio of the amount of O_2 consumed to the amount of CO_2 released, is measured during a run, initially it is about 1.0, indicating that mainly carbohydrate is being used. However, the RQ falls during running to give a value of about 0.77 after about 1 h, indicating that mainly fats are being oxidized.

The type and amount of substrate used varies with the intensity and duration of exercise in a similar way to starvation. As glycogen stores are depleted, an increase in glucagon, noradrenaline, and adrenaline stimulates lipolysis, releasing fatty acids for muscle to use in order to try to conserve glucose. An increase in these hormones, along with an increase in cortisol, leads to stimulation of gluconeogenesis and protein degradation in muscle. These changes are similar to those of the fasting state, but the difference is that the level of ketone bodies in the blood is low. It is not understood if this is because they are not being synthesized or if they are being oxidized as soon as they are formed.

Glucose homeostasis in diabetes mellitus

Diabetes mellitus is a syndrome caused by the lack or diminished effectiveness of insulin. It results in a raised blood glucose, hyperglycaemia. There are two main types:

In every examination you will ever have in medicine, there will be a question on diabetes. Know the effects of an increased glucagon/insulin ratio—the rest is easy and can be worked out!

- Insulin-dependent diabetes mellitus (IDDM) in which there is an absolute failure of the pancreas to produce insulin (type 1).
- Non-insulin dependent diabetes mellitus (NIDDM) in which there is a failure of the tissues to respond normally to insulin (type 2).

IDDM

This is an absolute deficiency of insulin caused by the auto-immune destruction of the b cells of the islets of Langerhans in the pancreas (see Chapter 12). Insulin normally facilitates the uptake of glucose by peripheral tissues. In its absence, glucose remains in the blood resulting in a low tissue availability of glucose but a high plasma concentration of glucose. The phrase 'starvation in the midst of plenty' is frequently used to

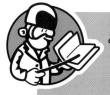

- Describe the three main stages of glucose homeostasis, their time course, and the major fuels used in each.
- Compare the fed, fasted, and starved states.
- Describe the main effects of insulin and glucagon on carbohydrate, protein, and lipid metabolism.
- Describe the use of fuels during sprinting and long-distance running.
- Describe the main metabolic effects of diabetes.

describe this state. The disease leads to the characteristic features of hyperglycaemia, ketoacidosis, and dehydration. As there is a low concentration of insulin, the metabolic effects of glucagon are unopposed (see Fig. 7.6).

Effect of an increased glucagon:insulin ratio in diabetes (Fig. 7.8)

Hyperglycaemia is caused by:
- A decreased uptake of glucose by the tissues, leading to a large increase in blood glucose.
- Glucagon increases the breakdown of liver glycogen and stimulates gluconeogenesis, leading to an increased hepatic output of glucose.

Ketoacidosis is caused by:
- An increase in triacylglycerol hydrolysis in adipose tissue, releasing fatty acids.
- An increase in ketone body synthesis in liver.

The release of fatty acids is much greater than in starvation, therefore, the rate of formation of ketone bodies is much greater than the rate of use, leading to ketoacidosis (see Chapter 4).

Hypertriglyceridaemia

Hypertriglyceridaemia is caused by:
- Some of the fatty acids released from triacylglycerol being packaged in the liver as very low density lipoproteins (VLDL). Dietary triacylglycerol is assembled into chylomicrons.
- In the absence of insulin, the activity of lipoprotein lipase being decreased, therefore, the very low density lipoproteins and chylomicroms remaining in plasma, leading to hypertriglyceridaemia (see Fig. 7.8).

NIDDM

The signs and symptoms of NIDDM are not usually as severe as those of IDDM and NIDDM is typically associated with older age of onset and obesity. Usually there is hyperglycaemia but ketoacidosis is normally absent (it may develop under stress). The clinical features and treatment of diabetes are discussed in Chapter 12.

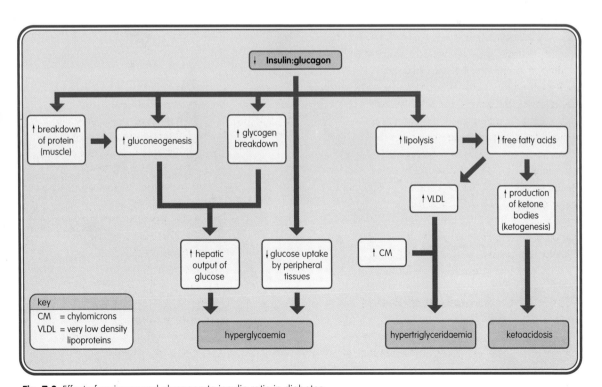

Fig. 7.8 Effect of an increased glucagon to insulin ratio in diabetes.

8. Nutrition

BASIC PRINCIPLES OF HUMAN NUTRITION

Some useful definitions

Nutrients
Nutrients are essential dietary factors, such as vitamins, minerals, essential amino acids, and essential fatty acids, that cannot be synthesized by the body at a sufficient rate. Sources of energy are not classed as nutrients and neither is water nor dietary fibre.

Staple foods
Staple foods are the principal sources of energy in the diet. They are specific to a particular country, for example, in parts of Africa and Asia cereals provide more than 70% of the energy in the diet. As countries become more prosperous, the percentage of energy derived from a single staple food declines. For example, in the UK, flour and flour products provide only about 25% of food energy.

Methods of estimating an individual's dietary intake
There are three main methods for estimating an individual's dietary intake:

- **Dietary recall.** Simply, ask the patient what he or she has eaten. This is the least accurate because it relies on the patient's recall and honesty.
- **Food diary.** This is slightly more accurate. To improve the accuracy, a 24-hour urine nitrogen measurement can be performed. This measures the amount of nitrogen excreted in the urine in 24 hours. From this the protein excretion can be calculated to see if it balances with the protein intake as recorded in the diary.
- **Complete chemical analysis.** This is the most expensive but the most accurate method.

Dietary reference values (Fig. 8.1)
The following definitions are in keeping with the dietary reference values (DRVs) for food energy and nutrients for the UK, 1991:

- **Estimated average requirement** (EAR). This is the average requirement of a group of people for energy or a nutrient (protein, vitamin, or mineral). About 50% of the population will need less than the EAR and 50% will need more.
- **Reference nutrient intake** (RNI). This is the amount of nutrient that is enough or more than enough for about 97% of people in the group (EAR + 2SD).
- **Lower reference nutrient intake** (LRNI). This is the amount of nutrient that is sufficient for only the few people in a group with low needs (EAR – 2SD).
- **Safe intake** is the amount of nutrient enough for almost everyone but not so much as to cause undesirable effects. This term is applied for nutrients for which there is not enough information known to estimate EAR, RNI, or LRNI, for example, vitamin E.

The DRVs for vitamin C are:

LRNI = 10 mg/day
EAR = 25 mg/day
RNI = 40 mg/day

Therefore below the LRNI, symptoms of vitamin C deficiency (scurvy) are seen and above the RNI, symptoms of excess may be seen.

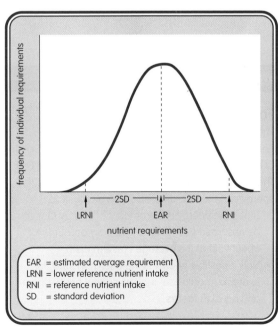

EAR = estimated average requirement
LRNI = lower reference nutrient intake
RNI = reference nutrient intake
SD = standard deviation

Fig. 8.1 Graph to show dietary reference values for food energy and nutrients for the UK in 1991.

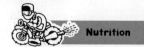

You may come across some other definitions that are now out of date:
○ Recommended daily amounts (RDA):
The levels of intake of essential nutrients considered to be adequate to meet the known needs of all healthy people in the population (RNI is now used).
○ Minimum daily requirement (MDR): The estimated minimum requirement of an individual for a particular nutrient to avoid the development of the symptoms of deficiency of that nutrient.
○ Do not learn these definitions.

○ Define the terms nutrient and staple food and give examples of each.
○ Give three methods for assessing dietary intake.
○ Give definitions for the DRVs: EAR, RNI, and LRNI.

ENERGY BALANCE

Food energy
The total energy content of food is the amount of energy released when food is completely burnt in air to CO_2 and H_2O, that is, the heat of combustion (Fig. 8.2). The total energy is equal to the sum of the digestible energy and the non-digestible energy (Fig. 8.3).
- Digestible energy is the amount of energy that can be absorbed from food and usually accounts for about 95% of the average Western diet.
- Non-digestible energy is the energy in food, for example in cellulose, that we cannot break down and is lost in faeces.

Metabolizable energy is the energy available to the body for use; it has three fates:

- 50% is lost as heat.
- 5–10% of energy is used up in digestion, absorption, and transport of food. This is known as either the thermic effect of food, diet-induced thermogenesis, or post-prandial thermogenesis (they all mean the same thing).
- Only about 25–40% of the energy is trapped as ATP, that is, the body is only 25–40% efficient.

From Fig. 8.2, it can be seen that protein has a higher total energy content than carbohydrate. However, protein is not as efficiently oxidized (it forms urea and requires ATP to do this [see Chapter 5]) and only about 4 kcal/g are available for the body to use as metabolizable energy. Carbohydrate is oxidized completely to CO_2 and H_2O and therefore all the available energy is obtained for use, that is, the metabolizable energy is 4 kcal/g.

Body composition
An average 72 kg man is composed of:
- 15% fat.
- 85% fat-free mass.

Fat-free mass or lean body mass (LBM) is made up of:
- 72% water.
- 20% protein.
- 8% bone mineral.

Women generally have a higher fat content than men; typically they consist of about 25% fat. Fat content tends to increase with age. An average 72 kg man can survive on his energy stores for about 50–60 days provided he is given water. This is mostly due to fat reserves because glycogen stores last only 12–24 h. Fig. 8.4 summarizes the methods available to measure body composition. However, most of the methods with the exception of anthropometry are rarely used in clinical practice.

Energy requirements
Energy is used by the body for three main processes.

Basal metabolic rate
The basal metabolic rate (BMR) is the energy used to carry out normal body functions such as blood flow, breathing, and so on, that is, it is the energy expended doing nothing! The units of BMR are kJ/h/kg of body weight. To calculate the BMR the patient must be:

- At rest, lying down but not asleep.
- At a constant, warm temperature.
- Assessed about 12 h after the last meal or any exercise.

The BMR is usually measured first thing in the morning. The BMR is proportional to LBM and, therefore, men have a higher BMR than women. Women have a greater percentage of fat which is less metabolically active. The BMR usually accounts for 50–70% of the total energy expended.

Thermic effect of food

This is the energy required for the digestion and absorption of food and accounts for 5–10% of the energy expenditure.

Physical activity

The amount of energy consumed depends on the duration and intensity of exercise. The physical activity ratio (PAR) can be measured for where activity is expressed as a multiple of the BMR (i.e. BMR = 1).

Major sources of energy in the diet		
Energy source	**Total energy/g**	
	kcal	kJ
fat: essential for absorption of fat-soluble vitamins (A, D, E, and K)	9.2	38.6
carbohydrate as either starch, sugar or non-starch polysaccharide (NSP) i.e. fibre	4.0	16.8
protein: 'empty calories'	5.4	22.7
alcohol	7.0	29.4

Fig. 8.2 Major sources of energy in the diet.

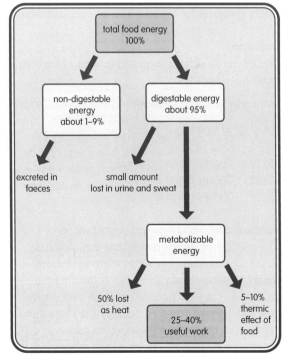

Fig. 8.3 The food energy chain.

Measurement of body composition	
Measurement	**Method**
body density	weigh in air to give fat content (density = 0.9 mg/mL) weigh in water to give lean body mass (density = 1.1 mg/mL)
body water	inject patient with a known volume of tritiated water and measure its concentration at equilibrium this is representative of lean body mass
total body potassium	inject $^{40}K^+$ and measure its distribution this is a measure of lean body mass as there is no potassium in fat
body fat	measure the uptake of a fat-soluble gas, e.g. xenon or cyclopropane biopsy to measure concentration
anthropometry	measure: • weight and height • mid-arm circumference (biceps and triceps) • skin-fold thickness (subscapular and suprailiac) compare with normograms for weight and height

Fig. 8.4 Measurement of body composition. Some of these methods are a little drastic and therefore, seldom used. Anthropometry is the most widely used method.

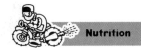

The PAR = metabolic rate during exercise ÷ BMR. For example:

Activity	PAR
Lying	1.0 (equal to BMR)
Sitting	1.2
Standing	1.7
Football	7.0

The physical activity level (PAL), can also be calculated. This is equal to the total energy expenditure in 1 day divided by the BMR.

Other factors can also affect energy requirements. For example:

- Environmental temperature changes. This is a very small effect unless the temperature is either extremely hot or cold.
- Pregnancy and lactation. For the first 6 months of pregnancy no extra energy is necessary, but for the last 3 months, an extra 0.8 MJ (200 kcal) are needed each day. During lactation, an extra 2.0 MJ (500 kcal) are required each day.
- Growth. The energy requirement in the first year of life is double that of adulthood.
- Age. The BMR decreases after the age of about 20 years.

How do we measure energy requirements?
Indirect calorimetry
The measurement of O_2 consumption allows measurement of the metabolic rate because 1 L (1 litre) of O_2 consumed at rest is equal to 20 kJ of energy expended from the oxidation of either fat, carbohydrate, or protein.

Indirect mass spectrophotometry
The incorporation of doubly labelled water ($^2H_2$$^{18}O$) into body fluids and its loss in the urine can be measured. ^2H is incorporated only into H_2O but ^{18}O is incorporated into both H_2O and CO_2. The difference between them is equal to the CO_2 produced.

Regulation of food intake
A number of systems are thought to participate in the regulation of food intake.

Overall control is thought to be at the level of the hypothalamus
There are two important areas for the control of food intake:

- The hunger or 'feeding' centre in the lateral hypothalamic area.
- The satiety centre in the ventromedial nucleus.

Lesions in the hunger centre have been shown to inhibit appetite and thus feeding and lead to anorexia. Lesions in the satiety centre cause overeating and obesity.

Gastric distension and gut hormones
Cholecystokinin (CCK) and calcitonin are known to decrease appetite. Cholecystokinin slows gastric emptying, thus maintaining gastric distension, which is thought to be an important satiety signal.

Blood concentration of glucose, insulin, and glucagon
Originally it was thought that low blood glucose levels had a direct stimulatory effect on the hunger centre. Now it is believed that it is the increased availability of glucose to tissues that produces satiety (the glucostatic hypothesis). Insulin therefore promotes satiety by stimulating the uptake of glucose by peripheral tissues.

Obesity
If energy intake is equal to energy expenditure, there is no change in body mass. Obesity results from an imbalance between the input, storage, and expenditure of energy; that is, energy intake is greater than energy expenditure.

Definition
Obesity can be defined or graded in terms of the body mass index (BMI).

$$BMI\ (kg/m^2) = weight \div (height)^2$$

The grading for BMI is:

20–25	Ideal weight.
25–30	Obesity grade I (overweight).
30–35	Obesity grade II (obese).
35+	Obesity grade III.

Obesity grades II and III are associated with an increased risk of various clinical disorders. A BMI of 20–25 is considered to be within the range for ideal weight. However, these ideal weights are obtained from tables compiled by a life insurance company in New York and are based on data obtained from upper middle class Caucasians; therefore, they are not accurate for everybody! The tables give ranges of ideal weights for height.

Causes of obesity		
Cause	**Evidence**	**Conclusion**
excessive intake of calories	due to psychological factors, stress, or social reasons	most common cause
genetic	identical twins are not always the same weight adopted children copy their new family weightwise	likely genetic predisposition but also intraction with environmental factors (diet, social-economic status) recent evidence suggests there is a 'gene' for obesity
socio-economic	in the West, low socio-economic class → obesity in the East, high socio-economic class → obesity	survey in Finland and Scotland showed obesity is associated with: • low education • high alcohol intake • giving up smoking • getting married!
endocrine	adrenal hyper function (Cushing's syndrome), hypothyroidism, and non-insulin dependent diabetes mellitus are all associated with obesity	but most obese people do not have endocrine problems
energy expenditure	DIT is greater in lean people (N.B. basal metabolic rate is not lower in obese people!)	maybe obese people are better at conserving energy
	80% of obese teenagers become obese adults hypothesis is that standard weight is set in infancy when fat people develop a greater number of fat cells than thin people	not true!

Fig. 8.5 Causes of obesity. There are a number of proposed causes of obesity; excessive calorie intake, genetic, endocrine, etc. However, evidence suggests that the major cause of obesity is excessive calorie intake usually due to an underlying social or socio-economic cause.

The main cause of obesity is probably an excessive intake of calories usually accompanied by a decrease in energy expenditure. It is not 'hormonal' as so many people often quote. Sad but true!

In the UK, 45% of men and 36% of women are overweight. Of these, about 8% of men and 12% of women are obese. The causes of obesity are discussed in Fig. 8.5.

Recent research has suggested that there is a 'gene' for obesity strengthening the evidence for a genetic cause. However, still the most obvious cause is an imbalance between energy input and expenditure.

Clinical consequences of obesity

The main clinical consequences of obesity are an increased risk of coronary heart disease, NIDDM, and hypertension. This is discussed further in Chapter 13.

Diets

Lots of different weight-reducing diets have been formulated; most do not work! For example, a low carbohydrate diet, where bread, potatoes, cakes and any starch-containing foods are cut out of the diet. Initially, weight loss is fast (0.5 kg/day) but most of the loss is water. Protein is also broken down to maintain the blood glucose, but is replaced as soon as the diet is stopped. However, the loss of fat is the same as for a normal mixed diet.

⊙ **What are the major energy sources in the diet?**
⊙ **Discuss the terms total energy, digestible energy, and metabolizable energy.**
⊙ **Name three methods for measuring body composition.**
⊙ **Define the BMR, and know how to measure it, and the main factors affecting it.**
⊙ **Define obesity in terms of BMI.**
⊙ **What are the causes of obesity and the problems of dieting?**

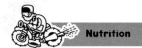

Why is it that 80–100% of obese people regain lost weight? During starvation, the metabolic rate falls by 15–30%. Therefore, after dieting, to remain at a lower weight, a lower energy intake must be maintained otherwise the weight will be put straight back on.

PROTEIN NUTRITION

More definitions

Reference proteins

Reference proteins contain all the amino acids in the exact proportions needed for protein synthesis. Albumin (found in egg white) and casein (milk) are the closest examples. Other proteins are compared with these reference or 'perfect' proteins.

Limiting amino acids

A limiting amino acid is the essential amino acid present in a protein in the lowest amount relative to its requirement for protein synthesis. Examples of proteins and their limiting amino acids are:
- Wheat limited by lysine.
- Meat and fish limited by methionine and cysteine.
- Maize limited by tryptophan.

Combining different protein-containing foods such as meat and the pulses ensures an adequate intake of all the amino acids, that is, protein complementation. This is particularly important in vegetarian diets. A diet of beans on toast provides adequate amounts of protein (you may not have many friends though!).

Protein quality

The quality of any protein can be assessed using a rating system based on a number of variables.

Chemical score

The chemical score is the ratio of the amount of limiting amino acid to its requirement. For example, if the amount of limiting amino acid in a 'test' protein is 2% and the amount of limiting amino acid in the reference protein is 5%; the chemical score is therefore 40%.

Biological value

The biological value is the proportion of the absorbed protein which is retained by the body for protein synthesis.

Net protein utilization

The net protein utilization (NPU) is the proportion of dietary protein which is retained by the body for protein synthesis. For example:
- For a typical mixed Western diet, NPU is 70% meaning 70% of the dietary protein is retained for protein synthesis.
- For a diet of mainly meat NPU would be 75%.
- For a diet of cereals NPU would be 50–60%.
- For a diet of eggs, NPU would be 100%.

Net dietary protein as a percentage of energy

Net dietary protein as a percentage of energy (NDPE%) is the proportion of total dietary energy provided by fully 'usable' protein. This method provides a way of comparing different diets. For example:
- Cereal-based diets provide 5–6%.
- Western diets provide 10–12%.
- In India, the diet provides 10%.

Children require an NDPE% of greater than 8%, that is, at least 8% of their diet must come from usable protein. Adults require an NDPE% of greater than 5%. In areas where the staple food is starch (e.g. yam, cassava), the diet provides only low levels of protein. It would be physically impossible to consume the amount of food necessary to satisfy the protein requirement, especially for children, and this leads to protein deficiency states. Cereal-based diets are adequate for adults but not children.

Protein requirement

Diet should provide the essential amino acids and enough amino acid nitrogen to synthesize the non-essential amino acids. These are required for:
- The maintenance of tissue proteins in adults.
- The formation of body proteins during periods of growth, pregnancy, lactation, infection, and after major trauma or illness such as cancer.

The recommended protein requirement for an adult in the UK is 0.8 g/kg/day of protein and should not be greater than 1.5 g/kg/day.

The RNI for protein is 55 g/day for men and 44 g/day for women.

Protein–energy deficiency states

Protein–energy malnutrition (PEM) arises when the body's need for protein or energy, or both, is not met by the diet. The physiological effects of severe prolonged

The bulk of excess protein is oxidized via gluconeogenesis to glycogen or fat and stored by the body.
Therefore protein is not a slimming food.
A famous diet is made of protein-supplemented modified fast (PSMF) which is hydrolysed gelatine and collagen, that is, it is cheap! However, in the hydrolysis process a lot of electrolytes are lost including potassium, which may lead to certain serious clinical consequences.

○ Explain the following terms: reference protein, limiting amino acid, protein quality, net protein utilization, and net dietary protein energy ratio.
○ Discuss protein requirements.
○ Define protein–energy malnutrition giving two examples.
○ Discuss the physiological effects of malnutrition.

malnutrition are discussed in Fig. 8.6. It is most commonly seen in developing countries. Two examples of PEM are:

- Marasmus, a lack of protein and energy (i.e. starvation).
- Kwashiorkor, a lack of protein but energy usually adequate.

These are discussed fully in Chapter 13.

In Western countries, a degree of PEM may be seen in hospitalized patients with the following conditions :

- Anorexia.
- Trauma, severe infection, major surgery, or burns.
- Cancer.

i.e. anything that causes a negative nitrogen balance (see Chapter 5).

Physiological effects of severe prolonged malnutrition	
Effect	**Consequence**
decreased brain development	permanent damage to both physical and mental development
defective immune system	decreased cell-mediated response immuno globulin production is maintained: this can have harmful effects as it depletes production of other proteins
loss of protein	firstly from muscle, then viscera → death
electrolyte losses	may effect Na^+/K^+ pump and the maintenance of ion gradients across cells
low haemoglobin	anaemia
low serum albumin (only kwashiorkor)	→ oedema
gastrointestinal function impaired	bacterial overgrowth and malabsorption
fatty liver (only kwashiorkor)	fat accumulates since its transport requires apolipoproteins that are deficient not seen in marasmus as no fat (energy) or protein

Fig. 8.6 The physiological effects of severe prolonged malnutrition.

VITAMINS

Definition

A complex organic substance required in the diet in small amounts compared with other components such as protein, carbohydrate, or fat and the absence of which leads to a deficiency disease. The vitamin deficiency diseases are covered in detail in Chapter 13.

Vitamins can be divided into two main groups, fat-soluble vitamins and water-soluble vitamins.

Fat-soluble vitamins

Vitamins A, D, E, and K. These are:

- Stored in the liver.
- Not absorbed or excreted easily.
- Sometimes toxic in excess (particularly A and D).

Water-soluble vitamins

The B group vitamins and vitamin C. These are:

- Not stored extensively.
- Required regularly in the diet.
- Generally non-toxic in excess (within reason).

All B vitamins are co-enzymes in metabolic pathways.

Fat-soluble vitamins
Vitamin A: retinol
RNI

700 μg/day for men; 600 μg/day for women.

Sources

Animal sources are butter, whole milk, egg yolk, liver, and fish liver oils; they contain retinol.

Plant sources are most green, yellow, or orange vegetables,and contain β-carotene, the precursor of retinol.

Absorption and transport of vitamin A

Retinol is absorbed in the intestinal mucosa and esterified to long chain fatty acids, forming retinyl esters. These are packaged in chylomicrons and transported to the liver for storage. When required, retinol is released and transported bound to retinol-binding protein. Retinol can be oxidized to other active forms, namely retinoic acid and retinal. β-Carotene is absorbed in the intestine and converted into retinal.

Functions

There are three active forms of vitamin A:

- Retinoic acid, which acts as a typical steroid hormone. It binds to chromatin to increase the synthesis of proteins controlling cell growth and differentiation of epithelial cells. Therefore, it increases epithelial cell turnover.
- Retinal. 11-*cis* retinal binds to opsin to form rhodopsin, the visual pigment of the rod cells in the retina involved in vision and dark adaptation to light. Low light intensity (scotopic vision) activates a series of photochemical reactions that bleach rhodopsin, converting it to all *trans* retinal, which triggers a nerve impulse in the optic nerve to the brain (Fig. 8.7).
- β-carotene is an anti-oxidant. Along with the other anti-oxidants, vitamins C and E, β-carotene is thought to help decrease the risk of heart disease and lung cancer.

Clinical manifestations of a deficiency or excess

Fig. 8.8 lists the symptoms of a deficiency and an excess of vitamin A. (These are discussed fully in Chapter 13.)

Vitamin D: cholecalciferol
RNI

There is no RNI for vitamin D because it is synthesized by the body.

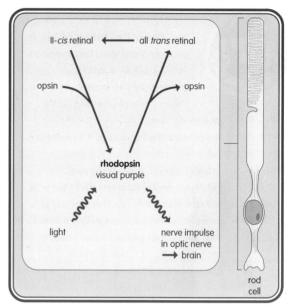

Fig. 8.7 Role of vitamin A in vision. 11-*cis* retinal binds to opsin converting it to rhodopsin, the visual pigment of the rod cells in the retina involved in vision and dark adaptation to light. Low light intensity (scotopic vision) activates a series of photochemical reactions that bleach rhodopsin, converting it to all *trans* retinal which triggers a nerve impulse in the optic nerve to the brain.

Deficiency and excess of vitamin A	
Deficiency	**Excess**
initially causes impaired dark adaptation and night blindness	excessive intake leads to a toxic syndrome called hypervitaminosis A
increased epithelial keratinization of the cornea leads to xerophthalmia	teratogenic
progresses to keratomalacia and cataracts	

Fig. 8.8 Deficiency and excess of vitamin A (see Chapter 13).

Sources

The sources of vitamin D include:

- Diet. In fish liver oils as cholecalciferol.
- Endogenous synthesis: most vitamin D is made by the body.

Vitamin D is a derivative of cholesterol and is therefore not present in plants; vegetarians must make their own.

Synthesis (Fig. 8.9)

Vitamin D is manufactured in the skin by the action of

sunlight of wavelength 290–310 nm. No radiation of this length is available between October and March in the UK, and therefore, the body relies on stores made during summer. Cholecalciferol undergoes two hydroxylation reactions, the first in the liver and the second in the kidney to form the active form, 1,25-dihydroxycholecalciferol (see Fig. 8.9). Vitamin D is mostly stored as 25-hydroxycholecalciferol in the liver.

Functions

The main role of vitamin D is in calcium homeostasis, which it controls in three ways:

- Increases uptake of calcium (and inorganic phosphate) from the intestine (main role).
- Increases the reabsorption of calcium from the kidney (minor role).
- Increases resorption of bone (when necessary) so that calcium is released.

Therefore, vitamin D increases the plasma concentration of calcium ions.

Mechanism of action

The active form, 1,25-dihydroxycholecalciferol, is a steroid hormone. In intestinal cells it binds to a cytosolic receptor. The resulting complex enters the nucleus and

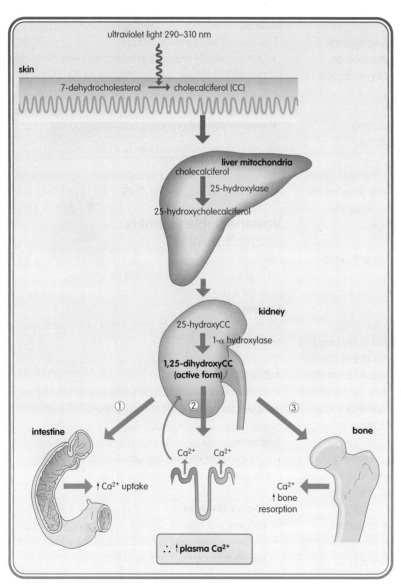

Fig. 8.9 Synthesis, metabolism, and functions of vitamin D.
Active form, 1,25-dihydroxycholecalciferol has 3 main effects which increase the plasma calcium concentration.
1. Increases uptake of Ca^{2+} from the intestine.
2. Increases reabsorbtion of calcium from the kidney.
3. Increases resorption of bone.

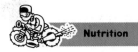

Deficiency and excess of vitamin D	
Deficiency	**Toxicity**
low plasma Ca^{2+} and impaired bone mineralization	most toxic of all vitamins
if severe, children develop rickets, adults develop osteomalacia	high levels lead to a large increase in calcium absorption and bone resorption resulting in **hypercalcaemia** and Ca^{2+} deposition in organs

Fig. 8.10 Deficiency and excess of vitamin D.

Functions of vitamin E	
Functions	**Deficiency**
• naturally occurring antioxidant which prevents oxidation of cell components by free radicals, e.g. PUFA present in cell membranes • may protect against the development of heart disease by preventing LDL oxidation	very rare except in premature infants in whom it can cause haemolytic anaemia of newborn

Fig. 8.11 Functions and effects of deficiency of vitamin E.

binds to chromatin at a specific site (enhancer region or response element) to increase the synthesis of a calcium-binding protein, calbindin, resulting in increased calcium reabsorption in the intestine.

Clinical manifestations of a deficiency or excess
Fig. 8.10 lists the symptoms of a deficiency and an excess of vitamin D. This is discussed fully in Chapter 13.

Vitamin E
Vitamin E consists of eight naturally occurring tocopherols; α-tocopherol is the most active.

RNI
None. A diet high in polyunsaturated fatty acids (PUFA) requires a high vitamin E intake.

Sources
Vegetable oils, especially wheatgerm oil, nuts, and green vegetables.

Absorption and transport
Tocopherol is found 'dissolved' in dietary fat and is therefore absorbed with it. It is transported in the blood by lipoproteins, initially in chylomicrons which deliver dietary vitamin E to the tissues. Vitamin E is transported from the liver with very low density lipoproteins (VLDL) and is stored in adipose tissue. Any malfunction in lipoprotein and fat metabolism may lead to a deficiency of vitamin E.

Functions
The functions of vitamin E are listed in Fig. 8.11. Its mechanism of action is described in Fig. 8.12.

Clinical manifestations of a deficiency or excess
Deficiency is very rare (see Fig. 8.11). No adverse effects are seen with doses as high as 3.2 g/day!

Vitamin K
RNI
None.

Sources
The sources of vitamin K include:
• Diet: especially green vegetables, egg yolk, liver, and cereals.
• It is mostly made by the normal bacterial flora of jejunum and ileum.
• Human milk only contains a small amount.

Functions and deficiency
The functions and clinical manifestations of a deficiency of vitamin K are listed in Fig. 8.13.

Water-soluble vitamins
Vitamin B_1: thiamin
RNI
1.0 mg/day for men. 0.8 mg/day for women.

Sources
Whole grain cereals, liver, pork, yeast, dairy produce, and legumes.

Active form
Thiamine pyrophosphate (TPP), which is formed by the transfer of a pyrophosphate group from ATP to thiamin.

Functions
The functions of thiamin are listed in Fig. 8.14, with its mechanism of action described in Fig. 8.15.

Deficiency diseases
A deficiency of thiamin causes:
• Beriberi. This occurs in two forms: wet beriberi, which results in oedema, cardiovascular symptoms, and

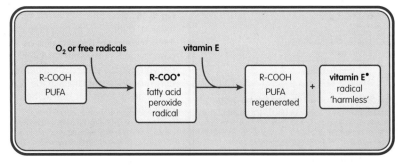

Fig. 8.12 The action of vitamin E as an anti-oxidant. Free radicals attack double bonds in polyunsaturated fatty acids to form a highly reactive fatty acid peroxide radical. This can attack other fatty acids, disrupting membrane structure and cell integrity. Vitamin E 'scavenges' fatty acid peroxide radicals to form a free radical itself. It is regenerated by other anti-oxidant nutrients (vitamins A and C).

Functions and deficiency of vitamin K	
Functions	**Deficiency**
vitamin K is a co-enzyme for the carboxylation of glutamate residues of blood clotting factors II, VII, IX, and X	true deficiency is rare because bacteria in gut usually produce enough
carboxylation activates clotting factors and thus clotting cascade	long-term antibiotic therapy leads to ↓bacteria and ↓vitamin K resulting in poor blood clotting and bleeding disorders
anticoagulants warfarin and dicoumarol inhibit vitamin K	may result in haemorrhagic disease of the newborn (see Chapter 13)

Fig. 8.13 Functions and deficiency of vitamin K.

Functions and effect of thiamin deficiency	
Functions	**Deficiency**
Thiamine pyrophosphate is co-factor for **four key enzymes:**	
• pyruvate dehydrogenase • α-ketoglutarate dehydrogenase (TCA cycle) • branched chain amino acid α-ketoacid dehydrogenase	decreased activity of pyruvate dehydrogenase and α-ketoglutarate dehydrogenase causes: • accumulation of pyruvate and lactate • decreased acetyl CoA and ATP formation and thus decreased acetylcholine and central nervous system activity
• transketolase (pentose phosphate pathway)	decreased activity of pentose phosphate pathway results in low levels of NADPH necessary for fatty acid synthesis; therefore this leads to a decrease in synthesis of myelin, which may cause a peripheral neuropathy

Fig. 8.14 The functions and effects of a deficiency of thiamin.

heart failure, and dry beriberi, which causes muscle wasting and peripheral neuropathy.
• Wernicke's encephalopathy, which is associated with alcoholism (alcohol is thought to impair the absorption of thiamin).
• Korsakoff's psychosis.

These diseases are discussed fully in Chapter 13.

Toxicity
Toxicity is rare but an excess causes headaches, insomnia, and dermatitis.

Vitamin B$_2$: riboflavin
RNI
1.3 mg/day for men. 1.1 mg/day for women.

Sources
Milk, eggs, liver. Riboflavin is readily destroyed by ultra-violet light.

Active forms
Riboflavin occurs in two active forms:
• Flavin mononucleotide (FMN).
• Flavin adenine dinucleotide (FAD).

Functions and deficiency
The functions and clinical manifestations of a deficiency of riboflavin are listed in Fig. 8.16. Riboflavin is not toxic in excess.

Niacin or nicotinic acid
RNI
17 mg/day for men. 13 mg/day for women.

Sources
Whole grain cereals, meat, fish, and the amino acid tryptophan.

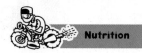
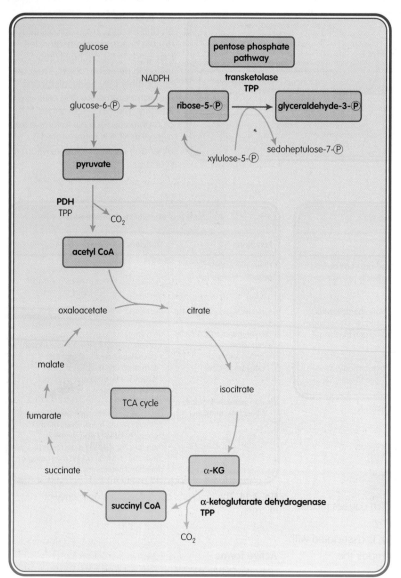

Fig. 8.15 Mechanism of action of thiamin. Thiamin pyrophosphate, the active form of thiamin, acts as co-enzyme for pyruvate dehydrogenase and α-ketoglutarate dehydrogenase reactions in the TCA cycle and for transketolase in the pentose phosphate pathway.

Functions and deficiency of riboflavin	
Functions	**Deficiency**
FAD and FMN are co-enzymes for a number of oxidases and dehydrogenases	rare except in elderly or alcoholic individuals no specific deficiency disease
they can accept two hydrogens to form $FADH_2$ and $FMNH_2$ respectively and take part in redox reactions, e.g. electron transport chain or act as antioxidants	symptoms of deficiency: • angular stomatitis (inflammation at sides of mouth) • cheilosis (fissures at corners of mouth) • cataracts • glossitis (inflamed tongue)

Fig. 8.16 Functions and effects of deficiency of riboflavin.

Synthesis of niacin from tryptophan

The synthesis of niacin from tryptophan is a very inefficient process: as much as 60 mg of tryptophan is needed to make 1 mg of niacin. Synthesis requires thiamin, riboflavin, and pyridoxine as co-factors, and only occurs after the needs of protein synthesis are met. This means in theory that niacin deficiency can be treated with a high protein diet, but lots would be needed!

Active forms

NAD^+ and $NADP^+$.

Functions and deficiency

The functions and clinical manifestations of a deficiency of niacin are listed in Fig. 8.17.

Toxicity

A high intake upsets liver function, carbohydrate tolerance, and urate metabolism. More than 200 mg/day will cause vasodilatation and flushing.

Vitamin B$_6$

Vitamin B$_6$ exists in three forms: pyridoxine, pyridoxal, and pyridoxamine.

RNI

1.4 mg/day for men. 1.2 mg/day for women.

Sources

Whole grains (wheat or corn), meat, fish, and poultry.

Active form

All three forms can be converted to the co-enzyme pyridoxal phosphate (PLP).

Functions and deficiency

The functions and clinical manifestations of a deficiency of vitamin B$_6$ are listed in Fig. 8.18. Toxicity is rare, in fact vitamin B$_6$ is actually used in the treatment of premenstual tension (PMT). An excess is however associated with the development of a sensory neuropathy.

Pantothenic acid

Sources

Most foods but eggs, liver, and yeast are very good sources.

Active form

Component of co-enzyme A (see Chapter 2).

Functions and deficiency

The functions and manifestations of a deficiency of pantothenic acid are listed in Fig. 8.19. Panthothenic acid is not toxic in excess.

Biotin

Sources

Most foods, especially egg yolk, offal, yeast, and nuts. A significant amount is synthesized by bacteria in the intestine.

Functions and deficiency of vitamin B$_6$	
Functions	**Deficiency**
• pyridoxal phosphate is a co-enzyme for many enzymes:	→ primary deficiency is very rare
• in amino acid metabolism: aminotransferases and serine dehydratase	→ abnormal amino acid metabolism
• in haem synthesis, ALA synthase (catalyses rate-limiting step)	→ hypochromic, microcytic anaemia
• glycogen phosphorylase	
• conversion of tryptophan to niacin	→ secondary pellagra
• indirect role in serotonin and noradrenaline synthesis as they are derived from amino acids	→ convulsions and depression

Fig. 8.18 The functions and effects of deficiency of vitamin B$_6$.

Functions and deficiency of niacin	
Functions	**Deficiency**
NAD$^+$ and NADP$^+$ are co-enzymes for many dehydrogenases in redox reactions	pellagra (see Chapter 13)
NAD is required for repair of UV light-damaged DNA in areas of exposed skin (nothing to do with redox state)	symptoms, the **3D's**: **d**ermatitis **d**iarrhoea **d**ementia leading to death
nicotinic acid is used for treatment of certain hyperlipidaemias because it inhibits lipolysis, leading to decreased VLDL and LDL (see Chapter 4)	

Fig. 8.17 Functions and effects of deficiency of niacin.

Functions and deficiency of pantothenic acid	
Functions	**Deficiency**
as co-enzyme A it is involved in the transfer of acyl groups, e.g. acetyl CoA, succinyl CoA, fatty acyl CoA	very rare; causes 'burning foot syndrome'
it is also a component of fatty acid synthase: acyl carrier protein (see Chapter 4)	N.B. can induce a deficiency in rats, which causes depigmentation of fur, i.e. they go grey; this is widely exploited by the shampoo industry; not toxic in excess

Fig. 8.19 Functions and effects of deficiency of pantothenic acid.

Active form

As a co-enzyme for carboxylation reactions, biotin binds to a lysine residue in carboxylase enzymes (Fig. 8.20).

Functions and deficiency

The functions and clinical manifestations of a deficiency of biotin are listed in Fig. 8.21.

Vitamin B_{12}: cobalamin

RNI

$1.5\,\mu g$/day.

Sources

Only animal sources: liver, meat, dairy foods; therefore vegans are at risk of deficiency.

Active form ——two active forms

Deoxyadenosylcobalamin and methylcobalamin.

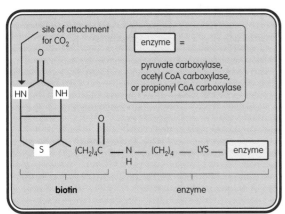

Fig. 8.20 Biotin. A co-enzyme for carboxylation reactions, biotin binds to a lysine residue in carboxylase enzymes.

Functions and deficiency of biotin	
Functions	**Deficiency**
it is an activated carrier of CO_2 it is a co-enzyme for: • pyruvate carboxylase in gluconeogenesis (see Chapter 5) • acetyl CoA carboxylase in fatty acid synthesis (see Chapter 11) • propionyl CoA carboxylase in β oxidation of odd-numbered fatty acids (see Fig. 8.23) • branched chain amino acid metabolism	very rare on a normal diet, may lead to dermatitis can be induced by: • eating lots of raw egg whites, which contain a glycoprotein avidin that binds to biotin in the intestine preventing its absorption • long-term antibiotic therapy which kills intestinal bacteria

Fig. 8.21 The functions and deficiency of biotin.

Absorption and transport (Fig. 8.22)

The absorption and transport of vitamin B_{12} occurs in several steps (numbers refer to Fig. 8.22):

1. Vitamin B_{12}, released from food in the stomach, becomes bound to a glycoprotein carrier, intrinsic factor (IF), produced by gastric parietal cells (see Fig. 8.22).

2. The complex of B_{12} and intrinsic factor binds to receptors on the mucosal cells of the terminal ileum.

3. B_{12} is absorbed and transported to tissues, attached to transcobalamin II. About 2–3 mg of B_{12} are stored by the body, mainly in the liver; this is relatively large compared with its daily requirement.

Functions

Vitamin B_{12} is a carrier of methyl groups. It is the co-enzyme for two enzymes:

• Methylmalonyl CoA mutase, as deoxyadenosylcobalamin, to assist in the breakdown of odd-numbered fatty acids (Fig. 8.23).

• Homocysteine methyltransferase, as methylcobalamin, to assist in the synthesis of methionine. This reaction also reverses the

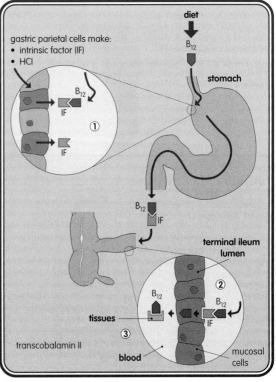

Fig. 8.22 The absorption and transport of vitamin B_{12}. Numbers refer to text below.

methylfolate trap, regenerating tetrahydrofolate (THF) from methyl-THF (discussed below with folate).

Deficiency and toxicity

A significant amount of vitamin B_{12} is stored; it therefore takes about 2 years for symptoms of deficiency to develop. Deficiency can cause two main problems:

- The accumulation of abnormal odd-numbered fatty acids, which may be incorporated into the cell membranes of nerves resulting in neurological symptoms, inadequate myelin synthesis, and nerve degeneration.
- Secondary 'artificial' folate deficiency since folate is 'trapped' as methyl-THF. This causes a decrease in nucleotide synthesis, resulting in megaloblastic anaemia.

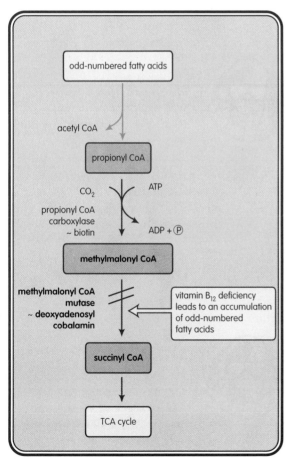

Fig. 8.23 β oxidation of odd-numbered fatty acids. B_{12} is a carrier of methyl groups. It is the co-enzyme for methylmalonyl CoA mutase, assisting in the breakdown of odd-numbered fatty acids.

The most common cause of vitamin B_{12} deficiency is pernicious anaemia, an autoimmune condition where antibodies are made by the body to intrinsic factor (this is discussed fully in Chapter 13). The toxicity of vitamin B_{12} is low.

Folate
RNI
200 μg/day.

Sources
Green vegetables, liver, and whole grain cereals.

Active form
5,6,7,8-THF, which is involved in the transfer of one-carbon units (see Chapter 6).

Absorption and storage
Folate is absorbed in the duodenum and jejunum. About 10 mg of folate is stored, mainly in the liver. The store is small relative to the daily requirement and therefore deficiency can occur quickly, usually within about 2–3 months.

The role of folate and vitamin B_{12}
All one-carbon THF units are interconvertible except N^5-methyl-THF; the THF cannot be released from it and is trapped, forming the 'methyl-folate' trap (see Chapter 6).

The only way to reform THF is via vitamin B_{12}-dependent synthesis of methionine: the methionine salvage pathway (Fig. 8.24).

Even if plenty of folate is present in the diet, if there is a deficiency in vitamin B_{12}, this will lead to secondary folate deficiency.

Functions and deficiency
The functions and clinical manifestations of a deficiency of folate are listed in Fig. 8.25. For a discussion of the use of folate in pregnancy see Chapter 13.

Vitamin C: ascorbate
RNI
40 mg/day.

Sources
Citrus fruits, tomatoes, berries, and green vegetables.

Active form
Ascorbate.

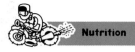

Functions and deficiency

The functions and clinical manifestations of a deficiency of ascorbate are listed in Fig. 8.26.

Toxicity

A high intake of vitamin C may lead to the formation of kidney stones, diarrhoea, and also cause systemic conditioning, that is, requirements increase as the body adapts to metabolizing more.

Functions and deficiency of ascorbate	
Functions	**Deficiency**
co-enzyme in hydroxylation reactions: • proline and lysine hydroxylases in collagen synthesis • dopamine β-hydroxylase in adrenaline and noradrenaline synthesis powerful reducing agent: • reduces dietary Fe^{3+} to Fe^{2+} in the gut, allowing its absorption (therefore deficiency can lead to anaemia) anti-oxidant and free radical 'scavenger': • inactivates free oxygen radicals which damage lipid membranes, proteins and DNA • also protects other anti-oxidant vitamins A and E	**scurvy** most symptoms are due to a decrease in collagen formation, leading to poor connective tissue formation and wound healing (see Chapter 13)

Fig. 8.26 Functions and effects of deficiency of ascorbate.

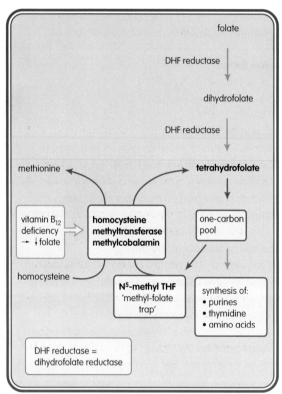

Fig. 8.24 Role of folate and B_{12}. The only way to reform tetrahydrofolate is via vitamin B_{12}-dependent synthesis of methionine: the methionine salvage pathway.

The role of ascorbate in hydroxylation reactions: Hydroxylase enzymes contain iron, which exists in two oxidation states: Fe^{3+} which is stable and inactive, and Fe^{2+} which is reduced and active. Ascorbate is necessary to maintain iron in its reduced and active state (Fe^{2+}).

Functions and deficiency of folate	
Functions	**Deficiency**
synthesis of: • amino acids, e.g. glycine and methionine • purines, AMP, and GMP (see Chapter 6) • thymidine (see Chapter 6)	**megaloblastic anaemia:** • decrease in purines and pyrimidines leads to a decrease in nucleic acid synthesis and cell division • shows up mostly in cells that are rapidly dividing, e.g. bone marrow and gut • large, immature red blood cells are present

Fig. 8.25 Functions and effects of deficiency of folate.

The best way to learn this sort of information is to take a large piece of paper and for each vitamin list only the main points mentioned above. Examiners love to ask about deficiency diseases. They are covered fully in Chapter 13.

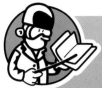

For each vitamin discuss:
- **Whether it is water- or fat-soluble and the implications for storage.**
- **The approximate RNI value and two or three examples of good sources.**
- **Its active form and main functions.**
- **The result of deficiency; try to relate this to function (the signs and symptoms of each deficiency disease are covered in Chapter 13).**
- **The effect of toxicity when relevant.**

MINERALS

Classification of minerals

There are 103 known elements. Living organisms are composed mainly of 11 of these. Namely carbon, hydrogen, oxygen, nitrogen, and the seven major minerals:
- Calcium, phosphorus, and magnesium, which are used mainly in bone.
- Sodium, potassium, chloride, which are electrolytes.
- Sulphur, which is used mainly in amino acids.

The RNI is greater than 100 mg/day for each of these (the exception is sulphur for which no RNI is published).

In addition, there are at least 12 other elements that are required in the diet in smaller quantities. These are known as the essential 'trace' elements, for which the RNI is less than 100 mg/day: iron, zinc, copper, cobalt, iodine, chromium, manganese, molybdenum, selenium, vanadium, nickel, and silicon.

The major minerals
Calcium

Calcium is the most abundant mineral in the human body. There is about 1.2 kg of calcium in the average 70 kg adult, of which 99% is in bone.

RNI

The RNI of calcium is 700 mg/day; it is higher during periods of growth, pregnancy, lactation, and after the menopause.

Sources

Milk and milk products; a lot of foods are fortified with calcium, for example, bread.

Absorption

Absorption of calcium from the diet is variable, usually 32% ± 14%.

Factors affecting absorption:
- Lactose and basic amino acids increase absorption because they form complexes with calcium.
- Fibre decreases absorption, therefore vegans need a lot more calcium.

Active forms

Calcium phosphate and the ionic form, Ca^{2+}.

Main functions

The main functions of calcium are listed in Fig. 8.27.

Regulation of calcium

Calcium levels are controlled by three hormones which also regulate plasma phosphate levels:
- Parathyroid hormone, which increases plasma calcium but decreases levels of inorganic phosphate.
- Vitamin D, which increases both plasma calcium and inorganic phosphate levels.
- Calcitonin, which decreases both plasma calcium and inorganic phosphate levels.

For further information refer to an endocrinology text.

Main functions of calcium	
Function	**Examples**
structural role	bone and teeth calcium is present as calcium phosphate (hydroxyapatite) crystals
muscle contraction	calcium binds to troponin C
nerve impulse transmission	calcium is released in response to hormones and neurotransmitters
blood clotting	co-enzyme for coagulation factors
ion transport and cell signalling	intracellular second messenger

Fig. 8.27 Main functions of calcium.

141

Deficiency and toxicity

The clinical manifestations of a deficiency and excess of calcium are listed in Fig. 8.28.

Phosphorus
RNI
550 mg/day.

Sources

Most foods; a dietary deficiency has not been described.

Functions

Phosphorus works in conjunction with vitamin D and calcium:

- It has a structural role in bones and teeth.
- Required for the production of ATP and other phosphorylated metabolic intermediates. It is therefore fundamental to the maintenance of the function of all the cells of the body.

Deficiency and toxicity

The clinical manifestations of a deficiency and excess of phosphorus are listed in Fig. 8.29.

Deficiency and excess of calcium	
Deficiency	**Excess**
in children leads to rickets	hypercalcaemia Ca^{2+} is deposited in many organs, particularly arteries, heart, liver, and kidneys, leading to tissue calcification
in adults leads to osteomalacia, that is defective mineralization of bone	
in post-menopausal women it may contribute to osteoporosis, i.e. loss of bone mass (see Chapter 13)	this may interfere with organ function and in the kidney, results in the formation of renal stones

Fig. 8.28 Effects of calcium deficiency and excess.

Deficiency and excess of phosphorus	
Deficiency	**Excess**
if severe (< 0.3 mmo/L), will affect the function of all cells causing: • muscle weakness • in RBC leads to a decrease in formation of 2,3–bisphosphoglycerate and therefore reduces unloading of oxygen to tissues • rickets and osteomalacia	may combine with calcium to produce calcium phosphate and be deposited in tissues (see Fig. 8.28)

Fig. 8.29 Deficiency and excess of phosphorus.

Magnesium
RNI
270 mg/day.

Sources

Most foods, especially green vegetables.

Functions

The functions of magnesium are:

- Structural role in bones and teeth.
- Co-factor for more than 300 enzymes in the body, that is, those enzymes that catalyse ATP-dependent reactions. Magnesium binds to ATP, forming a magnesium–ATP complex which is the substrate for enzymes such as kinases.
- Interacts with calcium to affect the permeability of excitable membranes and neuromuscular transmission.

Deficiency

Seen in alcoholics; patients with liver cirrhosis; following diuretic therapy; and in renal disease. The symptoms are:

- Muscle weakness.
- Secondary calcium deficiency.
- Confusion, hallucinations, convulsions and other neurological symptoms.

Excess

Extremely rare.

Sodium, potassium, and chloride

Sodium, potassium, and chloride function together to regulate the osmolality of intracellular and extracellular fluids. For further information refer to a physiology text. The characteristics of sodium and potassium are listed in Fig. 8.30.

Sulphur

The dietary intake of the sulphur-containing amino acid methionine is essential for synthesis of cysteine (see Fig. 5.5); both can then be incorporated into proteins and enzymes.

Trace elements
Iron
RNI

The daily loss of iron from the body is 0.5–1.0 mg/day and is due to:

- Gastro-intestinal tract turnover, about 0.5 mg/day.

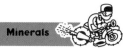

Characteristics of sodium and potassium		
	Sodium	**Potassium**
RNI	1.6 g/day	3.5 g/day
sources	salt, most foods	most foods
functions	principal cation of ECF: concentration maintained between 135 and 145 mmol/L; necessary for: • control of ECF volume • Na^+/K^+ ATPase and uptake of solutes by cell • Na^+ gradient provides driving force for secondary active transport • neuromuscular transmission	principal cation of ICF: fundamental to: • Na^+/K^+ ATPase and uptake of molecules by cell • neuromuscular transmission • acid–base balance
deficiency	• common in hospitalized patients; causes include: vomiting, diarrhoea, use of diuretics, Addison's disease, hypothyroidism, hyperglycaemia (causing an osmotic diuresis) or renal failure • usually accompanied by water loss leading to decrease in plasma volume and signs of circulatory failure and collapse	• may be secondary to vomiting, use of diuretics, diarrhoea, excess steroids, hyperaldosteronism (e.g. Conn's syndrome), Cushing's syndrome or alkalosis • high chance of cardiac arrhythmias and neuromuscular weakness • severe hypokalaemia is dangerous and requires immediate treatment
excess	role in hypertension	kills → ventricular fibrillation and cardiac arrest

Fig. 8.30 The characteristics of sodium and potassium.

• Desquamation of intestinal mucosal cells and biliary excretion, about 0.3 mg/day.
• Sweat and desquamation of skin cells, about 0.1 mg/day.
• Urinary losses, about 0.1 mg/day.

Small daily losses are accounted for by the absorption of dietary iron in the duodenum. The demand for iron increases during growth, pregnancy, and menstruation (1 ml of blood loss is equal to 0.5 mg of iron). The daily iron requirements are:

• Adult male   1.0 mg.
• Child   1.5 mg.
• Menstruating woman   2.0 mg.
• Pregnant woman   3.0 mg.

However, only about 10% of dietary iron is absorbed, and therefore, the amount ingested daily is equal to the daily requirement × 10. Therefore, the RNI = 10–20 mg/day.

Sources
Liver, meat, green vegetables, and cereals. Dietary iron exists in two forms:
• Haem iron, which is derived from haemoglobin or myoglobin in meat and is rapidly absorbed.
• Non-haem iron, which is present in vegetables and cereals and is absorbed slowly (see Chapter 13).

Absorption, transport, and storage
A summary of the absorption, transport, and functions of iron is given in Fig. 8.31. Total body iron is about 3–5 g About 60% is in haemoglobin and most of the rest is stored, mainly as ferritin with a small amount as haemosiderin. Ferritin is a protein–iron complex. The protein part, apoferritin, has 22 subunits which form a hollow protein shell and it is capable of binding about 4300 Fe^{3+} ions.

Dietary iron is more readily absorbed in the Fe^{2+} state and ascorbic acid, alcohol and other reducing substances favour its absorption (see Chapter 13). Iron is transported in the blood bound to transferrin; each molecule of transferrin binds two Fe^{2+} ions. This transports iron from sites of absorption and haemoglobin breakdown to storage sites: mainly the reticuloendothelial cells (bone marrow, spleen), hepatocytes (liver), and muscle cells. These cells have transferrin receptors enabling iron to be taken up by receptor-mediated endocytosis. Iron is also transported to these sites for production of haemoglobin (bone marrow), myoglobin (muscle) or production of enzymes (liver). Fig. 8.32 summarizes the functions of body iron.

Deficiency
A deficiency of iron results in a reduction in haemoglobin production and anaemia (see Chapter 13).

143

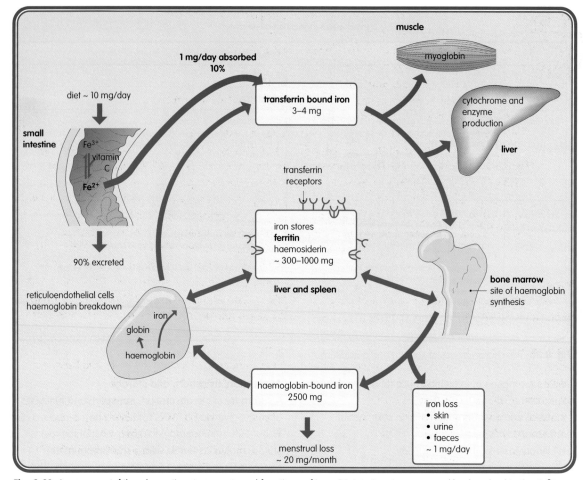

Fig. 8.31 A summary of the absorption, transport, and functions of iron. Dietary iron is more readily absorbed in the Fe^{2+} state. Only about 10% is absorbed. Iron is transported in the blood bound to transferrin, which takes iron either 'newly absorbed' from the diet or released from haemoglobin breakdown to muscle, liver, bone marrow or spleen either for production of haemoglobin, myoglobin, or other enzymes, or for storage. About 60% of total body iron is in haemoglobin.

Distribution and function of total body iron (3500–5000 mg)			
Site	**Function**	**Amount of iron (mg)**	**Percentage total body iron**
haemoglobin	oxygen transport	2500	60–70
ferritin (2/3) and haemosiderin (1/3)	iron storage: mainly liver, spleen and bone marrow	1000	27
myoglobin	oxygen transporter in muscle	130	3.5
uncharacterized iron-binding molecules	storage	80	2.2
cytochromes and other iron-containing enzymes	electron transport chain cytochrome P_{450} (drug metabolism) catalase (H_2O_2 breakdown) peroxidase	8	0.2
transferrin	transports iron from intestines to tissues	3	0.08

Fig. 8.32 The distribution and function of total body iron.

Bioavailability is the efficiency (%) with which any dietary nutrient is used in the body. A number of factors can influence the absorption and use of nutrients. For example:
1. The chemical form of the nutrient.
2. Antagonistic or facilitatory ligands.
3. The breakdown of the nutrient.
4. The pH and redox state.
5. Anabolic requirements, endocrine influences, infection, and so on.

Excess

Iron overload leads to iron deposition in the tissues, which may interfere with their function (see Fig. 13.19).

Iron damaging effects

People with iron overload are at risk of iron-catalysed free radical formation which can cause cell damage. At normal iron levels, a very reactive superoxide radical $O_2^{\bullet-}$ is removed effectively by the enzyme superoxide dismutase as shown in the reaction below:

$$2O_2^{\bullet-} + 2H^+ \rightarrow H_2O_2 + O_2^{-}$$

However, in iron overload, Fe^{3+} reacts with the superoxide radical to form an extremely reactive hydroxyl radical, $OH^{\bullet}$ (this is known as the Fenton reaction). This hydroxyl radical is capable of damaging biological molecules, particularly lipids, leading to lipid peroxidation and membrane damage (especially of lysosomal membranes).

$$O_2^{\bullet-} + Fe^{3+} \rightarrow Fe^{2+} + O_2$$
$$Fe^{2+} + H_2O_2 \rightarrow Fe^{3+} + OH^- + OH^{\bullet}$$

Zinc

The daily zinc requirement is 2–3 mg/day but absorption is only approximately 30% effective. Therefore, the RNI is 10 mg/day. Zinc can be found in most foods. The total body zinc is 2–3 g. It is found in all tissues but high concentrations are present in the liver, kidney, bone, retina, muscle, and prostate. The role of zinc in the body is described in Fig. 8.33.

Copper

RNI

1.2 mg/day.

Sources

Liver is a very good source.

Copper metabolism

The total body copper is about 75–150 mg. High copper concentrations are found in the liver, brain, heart, and kidneys. Dietary copper is absorbed in the stomach and duodenum and transported to the liver loosely bound to albumin; the absorption is about 30% effective. It is incorporated into caeruloplasmin, a glycoprotein synthesized by the liver, which transports copper to the tissues where it can be used for the synthesis of other copper-containing enzymes. Normally, it is excreted in the bile (daily loss is approximately 2–3 mg/day). In the blood, 80–90% of the copper present is bound to caeruloplasmin.

Function

Copper is required for the synthesis of a number of copper-containing enzymes (Fig. 8.34).

Inherited disorders of copper metabolism

These are discussed fully in Chapter 13.
- Menke's disease is due to a defective absorption of copper from the intestine.
- Wilson's disease is due to excessive copper deposition in tissues.

Other trace elements

The characteristics of some of the other trace elements not covered here are listed in Fig. 8.35.

Role of zinc in the body	
Functions	**Deficiency**
co-factor of over 100 enzymes , e.g.: • dehydrogenases, e.g. LDH • peptidases • carbonic anhydrase • enzymes of DNA and protein synthesis • superoxide dismutase transcription factors are thought to contain 'zinc fingers' that enable them to bind DNA	causes: growth retardation, hypogonadism, and delayed wound healing these effects are mainly a result of decreased activity of the enzymes of DNA synthesis

Fig. 8.33 The role of zinc in the body.

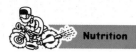
Role of copper and effects of deficiency		
Enzyme	**Functional role**	**Effect of deficiency**
caeruloplasmin	promotes absorption of iron	iron deficiency anaemia
lysyl oxidase	cross-links collagen and elastin	weak walled blood vessels
tyrosinase	melanin production	failure of pigmentation
dopamine β-hydroxylase	catecholamine production	neurological effects
cytochrome c oxidase	electron transport chain	decreased ATP formation
superoxide dismutase	scavenges the superoxide radical and prevents lipid peroxidation and membrane damage	tissue damage

Fig. 8.34 The role of copper and the effects of copper deficiency.

Characteristics of some of the other trace elements								
Element	**Iodine**	**Chromium**	**Cobalt**	**Manganese**	**Molybdenum**	**Selenium**	**Silicon**	**Fluoride**
Source	salt RNI = 140 μg	meat, liver, yeast, whole grains	foods of animal origin			meat, green vegetables RNI = 60 μg	green vegetables	drinking water
Main function	synthesis of thyroid hormones	constituent of factor which binds to insulin to potentiate its action	constituent of vitamin B_{12} as cobalamin	co-factor for enzymes: decarboxylases, transferases, superoxide dismutase	constituent of xanthine oxidase: involved in purine breakdown	co-factor of glutathione peroxidase	bone calcification, glycosamino-glycan metabolism in connective tissue	increases hardness of teeth
Deficiency	• goitre in adults • cretinism in babies	impaired glucose tolerance (seen in patients on parenteral nutrition)	as for vitamin B_{12} deficiency	unknown	decreased uric acid synthesis	endemic in parts of China → cardio-myopathy (Keshan disease)	decrease in normal growth	low intake leads to increased dental caries
Excess	toxic goitre hyperthyroidism	non-specific: nausea, diarrhoea and irritability		inhalation poisoning leading to psychotic symptoms and parkinsonism (rare)		leads to hair loss, dermatitis, and irritability	silicosis: long-term inhalation of silicon dust leads to pulmonary fibrosis	fluorosis: where fluorine infiltrates enamel causing pitting and discoloration of teeth

Fig. 8.35 The characteristics of some of the other trace elements.

○ **For each of the main minerals and trace elements covered here describe:**
○ **The major sources, functions, transport, and storage forms.**
○ **The effects of deficiency and excess (refer to Chapter 12 for deficiency diseases).**
○ **Have a rough idea of the RNI. Examiners usually ask about iron,**

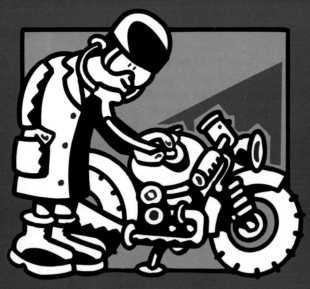

CLINICAL
ASSESSMENT

9. Taking a History

THINGS TO REMEMBER WHEN TAKING A HISTORY

The purpose of this section is to remind you of the main points involved in taking a history from a patient.

The history is usually the most important part of the consultation.

Before you start:

- Always introduce yourself and shake hands. Make sure the patient is comfortable and there are no large obstacles, for example, a desk in-between you.
- Stand back and look around the bedside for clues. Is the patient being monitored, for example, for blood pressure, oxygen saturation, blood glucose? Look for inhalers, sputum pots, walking sticks, or frames; all of these provide indicators to the patient's condition.
- Observe the patient. Is he or she agitated or distressed either physically or emotionally? Are there any obvious signs, for example, tremor, squint, hyperactivity?

Structure of a history

This is a basic plan designed for you to photocopy and take with you when you first start clerking patients.

Personal info:

- Name/sex
- Age/date of birth
- Occupation

Presenting complaint (PC)

This should be a short statement of the symptoms the patient is complaining of in his or her own words, for example, pain, thirst, poor appetite, tiredness, weight loss, vomiting, and so on. Remember, symptoms not diagnoses: patients do not complain of coronary heart disease, diabetes, or acute intermittent porphyria!

History of presenting complaint (HPC)

Try to get the patient to tell the story in his or her own words from when he or she thought it began. For most symptoms you will need to know:

- What is the time course? When did the problem start or when did you first feel unwell?
- Was the onset rapid or slow?
- What is the nature of the complaint? If it is pain: site, radiation, and so on; if it is vomiting: how much? Colour? Is there any blood in it?
- Is there a pattern? Is it continuous, intermittent or continuous with acute exacerbations?
- Are there any precipitating or relieving factors? For example, is it related to meals or the type of food eaten or stress? Is it helped by painkillers?
- Are there any other relevant or associated symptoms? For example, for chest pain, ask about palpitations, sweating, nausea, to exclude a possible heart attack.
- Has it happened before? Ask about any previous treatment or investigations for the complaint.

For any pain, you need to know the site, radiation, onset, timing, character (e.g. sharp, dull, colicky), precipitating or relieving factors, and associated symptoms.

Previous medical history (PMH)

Ask the patient about previous illnesses, operations, and investigations with dates. Ask specifically about diabetes, asthma, anaemia, jaundice, high blood pressure, previous heart attacks, strokes, angina, epilepsy, tuberculosis infection, rheumatic fever.

Ask about the patient's nutritional history, if you think it is relevant. A lot of metabolic and nutritional diseases present in infancy. When dealing with children, ask the parents specifically about problems during the pregnancy or birth, or when their child was a neonate; for example, problems with feeding, bowels, or a failure to thrive. Enquire about developmental milestones: smiling, sitting, walking, talking, playing.

Drug history (DH)

Is the patient on any medication at present, either over the counter or prescription?

Allergies

Is the patient allergic to any medicines or foods that they know of? Ask specifically about penicillin.

Smoking

How many per day and how long ago did the patient start?

Alcohol

How many drinks or units each week?

Family history (FH)

Ask about any known illnesses in first degree relatives, in particular, diabetes and heart disease. It may help you to make a quick sketch of the family tree.

A number of inborn errors of metabolism are inherited as autosomal recessive disorders and have a high incidence amongst races where marriages between first cousins are quite common, for example Ashkenazi Jews.

Social history (SH)

Ask about marital status, number of children if any, and the type of accommodation. Ask about the patient's occupational history: current and previous jobs, exposure to chemicals or asbestos and any time off work due to illness. Ask about financial and personal worries and any risk-related behaviours, for example, taking illegal drugs or any history of risky homosexual or heterosexual contacts.

Review of symptoms

Some of these symptoms may have already been covered in the history of the presenting complaint. You need to use your discretion about the extent of this enquiry.

Cardiovascular system, ask specifically about:
- Chest pain.
- Palpitations.
- Exercise tolerance.
- Shortness of breath (SOB) at rest, when lying down flat (orthopnoea) or waking up at night breathless (paroxysmal nocturnal dyspnoea, PND).

- Claudication (calf pain on walking).
- Leg pain at rest.

Respiratory system, ask specifically about:
- Persistent cough or wheeze.
- Sputum: amount, colour.
- Haemoptysis (coughing up blood).
- Shortness of breath.

Gastrointestinal system, ask specifically about:
- Appetite or weight loss.
- Nausea or vomiting.
- Difficulty swallowing (dysphagia).
- Heartburn or indigestion.
- Change in bowel habit: diarrhoea, constipation, frequency, consistency, colour.

Urinary system, ask specifically about:
- Frequency.
- Nocturia.
- Urine stream: hesitancy, dribbling.
- Dysuria (pain on passing water).
- Haematuria.
- Incontinence.

Skin, ask specifically about:
- Rashes or sensitive skin.
- Dermatitis.
- Eczema/Psoriasis.

Musculoskeletal system, ask specifically about:
- Painful joints.
- Stiffness.
- Swelling.
- Arthritis.

Nervous system, ask specifically about:
- Headaches or migraines.
- Fits or faints.
- Changes in vision, hearing, speech, or memory.
- Anxiety, depression, or suicidal thoughts.
- Sleep.

Menstruation and obstetric history
This should only be taken when relevant.

Summary

This should be a brief recall of the main points. For

example: Jonathan Brown, a 4-year-old boy referred by his general practitioner, presenting with a 6-week history of increasing thirst, polyuria, and weight loss. His mother has insulin-dependent diabetes mellitus. On examination . . . .

- When talking to patients, try to maintain appropriate eye contact throughout and look interested.
- Take brief notes and write them up afterwards—you will be surprised at how much you can remember!

- Describe the main points and headings of history taking.

Main metabolic causes of fatigue	
Causes	Examples and notes
anaemia	this may be secondary to: • iron/B_{12}/folate deficiency • haemolytic anaemia, e.g. G6PDH or pyruvate kinase deficiency (see Fig. 9.3 for other examples)
hypothyroidism	this may be due to an iodine defeciency or an autoimmune disease, Hashimoto's thyroiditis
malnutrition	• PEM: marasmus or kwashiorkor (see Chapter 13) • general vitamin deficiencies
obesity	these people tire easily because of 'carrying' so much extra body weight
diabetes mellitus	see types of diabetes (Fig. 9.4)
Ca^{2+} or vitamin D deficiency	osteomalacia (weak, easily deformed bones)
glycogen storage disorders	e.g. McArdles' syndrome (see Chapter 12)

Fig. 9.1 Main metabolic causes of fatigue.

COMMON PRESENTING COMPLAINTS

This section deals with some examples of common presenting complaints, i.e. symptoms of metabolic diseases. For each complaint, the major metabolic causes are considered.

Remember, for each symptom there are also lots of non-metabolic causes which are probably more common but are beyond the scope of this book. For further discussions of these, refer to a clinical medicine textbook.

Fatigue

Fatigue covers a wide range of symptoms reported by patients, for example, tiredness, weakness, exhaustion, lack of energy, sleepiness, or weariness.

Causes of fatigue

Fatigue is a very common complaint and there are many causes. It is important to obtain a clear history of the complaint in terms of when it started, its progression, precipitating and relieving factors, and any associated symptoms that clearly help to eliminate other causes. The main metabolic causes of fatigue are described in Fig. 9.1.

Weight loss

Weight loss is a symptom of a great many diseases; here, only the main metabolic causes are considered.

Working definition

A loss of 5% or more of the usual body weight over a period of 6 months.

It is essential to take a clear, well-documented history from the patient because it is difficult to verify the true amount of weight lost, unless the patient is continually weighed and monitored over a period of time. Ask about:

- Changes in clothing or belt size.
- Verification from friend or relative.

Involuntary weight loss is often a clue that the patient has a serious underlying disease such as cancer. Fig. 9.2 lists the common metabolic causes of weight loss.

Symptoms of anaemia

Anaemia is defined as a reduction in the level of haemoglobin in the blood, resulting in a reduction in oxygen supply to the tissues.

The symptoms of anaemia depend on the severity of the anaemia; a small reduction in haemoglobin is usually asymptomatic. Most symptoms are non-specific and result from a decreased oxygen supply to the tissues:

- Fatigue.
- Headaches.
- Fainting
- Breathlessness.
- Angina of effort (i.e. brought on by exercise, relieved by rest).
- Palpitations.
- Intermittent claudication.

As these symptoms are relatively non-specific, to find out the cause of the anaemia a number of laboratory tests may be performed including:

- Full blood count. This measures the concentration of haemoglobin, the red cell count, and other indices, for example, mean cell volume, mean cell haemoglobin (see Fig. 11.1).
- Blood film. This looks at the morphology of cells.
- Reticulocyte count.
- Serum iron and total iron-binding capacity.
- Serum ferritin.
- B_{12} and folate levels.
- Schilling test. This is specific for pernicious anaemia.

These tests and their results are discussed fully in Chapter 11.

Causes of anaemia

There are many causes of anaemia ranging from acute blood loss to hereditary haemolytic anaemias such as sickle cell anaemia. The main metabolic causes of anaemia are listed in Fig. 9.3.

Common metabolic causes of weight loss	
Main cause	**Differential diagnosis**
decreased calorie intake	• malnutrition: common in developing countries, and in the UK may be seen in the elderly • cancer • alcoholism: alcohol replaces normal food intake with 'empty calories' • anorexia nervosa • depression
increased loss or energy expenditure	• hyperthyroidism • poorly controlled IDDM • cancer

Fig. 9.2 Common metabolic causes of weight loss.

Metabolic causes of anaemia	
Cause	**Notes**
iron deficiency	decrease in haem and red blood cell production leading to microcytic, hypochromic cells (see Chapter 13)
folate/B_{12} deficiency	macrocytic, megaloblastic anaemia (see Chapter 13)
pernicious anaemia	autoimmune condition in which antibodies are made to intrinsic factor, preventing vitamin B_{12} absorption; results in deficiency of B_{12} and folate (see Chapter 13)
vitamin C deficiency	vitamin C is required for absorption of Fe^{2+} (see Fig. 8.26)
haemolytic anaemia	deficiency of RBC enzymes of, e.g. pyruvate kinase or G6PDH deficiency (see Chapter 12)
lead poisoning	lead inhibits three enzymes of haem synthesis, leading to anaemia (see Chapter 12)

Fig. 9.3 Metabolic causes of anaemia.

Symptoms of diabetes mellitus

The presentation of the symptoms of diabetes mellitus may be acute or insidious in onset (types are listed in Fig. 9.4).

Acute

Young people often present with a brief 2–4 week history of the classical symptoms, namely polyuria, polydipsia, and weight loss, accompanied by tiredness. These patients usually have insulin-dependent diabetes mellitus.

Subacute

The onset of symptoms is usually over months to years. Patients may still present with the classical symptoms although quite often, tiredness is the prominent symptom. These patients usually have NIDDM.

Asymptomatic

Glycosuria or raised blood glucose is detected during a routine medical examination.

Diabetic ketoacidosis

If these early symptoms are not recognized, patients can present with ketoacidosis (Fig. 12.4) where:

- Severe hyperglycaemia causes an osmotic diuresis. The loss of fluid and electrolytes results in

Types of diabetes mellitus	
Type	**Notes**
Diabetes mellitus:	overall incidence, approximately 2% in Western World
type I, insulin-dependent diabetes mellitus	patients are usually younger than 25 years
type II, non-insulin-dependent diabetes mellitus	patients are usually older and often obese
impaired glucose tolerance	affects about 5% of population; these patients are more likely to develop diabetes when they are older
secondary diabetes	either due to pancreatic damage e.g. chronic pancreatitis, haemochromatosis or Wilson's disease, or due to endocrine disease, e.g. acromegaly, Cushing's

Fig. 9.4 Types of diabetes mellitus.

dehydration. If this is severe, the patient may be confused and be in shock.

- The increased production of ketone bodies results in metabolic acidosis. This typically causes nausea and vomiting and further loss of fluid and electrolytes. Respiratory compensation results in hyperventilation (Küssmaul breathing). Failure to treat a patient in ketoacidosis may result in coma and death.

Complications

Patients may also present with diabetic complications such as retinopathy, neuropathy, or nephropathy (Fig. 12.5). For example,they may present after visits to the opticians (diabetic retinopathy), or with tingling and numbness in the leg, or with leg or foot ulcers (neuropathy).

The diagnosis of diabetes is discussed fully in Chapter 12 but is based on measurement of the fasting plasma glucose. A confirmed fasting plasma glucose of greater than 7.8 mmol/L is diagnostic of diabetes.

Symptoms of amino acid disorders

Amino acid disorders are all rare (see Chapter 12). Most present in infancy with developmental delay, vomiting, failure to thrive, mental retardation, and seizures. The symptoms are all non-specific making the differential diagnosis vast. All neonates are now screened for phenylketonuria at a few days of age using the Guthrie test. The other amino acid disorders must be considered

and eliminated when infants present with these symptoms without other adequate explanation, for example, in the absence of infection (Fig. 9.5). Their diagnosis depends on the measurement of metabolites in the blood and urine.

Symptoms of porphyrias

There are two main types of symptoms (Fig. 9.6).

- Neuropsychiatric symptoms with abdominal pain. These present acutely and there is usually some obvious precipitating factor, for example, drugs, infection, stress. Acute attacks are separated by long periods of remission.
- Photosensitivity. This is a non-acute presentation in which the skin burns or itches on exposure to light. Usually no neurological symptoms are observed.

The diagnosis is based on:

- Clinical features.
- The presence of increased levels of porphyrins and their precursors in the blood, urine, and faeces.
- All 6 porphyrias are very rare (roughly 1 in 100 000).

Symptoms of gout

Gout initially presents as recurrent, acute attacks of arthritis usually affecting only one joint (monoarthropathy). The patient complains of a warm, swollen, and exquisitely tender joint, usually a big toe. Eventually, the attacks fail to resolve completely and persistent symptoms occur because of the permanent deposition of urate crystals, leading to chronic tophaceous gout. Persistent symptoms may also be due to the presence of kidney stones, which can cause abdominal pain or renal colic. The most common

Differential diagnosis of amino acid disorders in infants
phenylketonuria
inborn errors of carbohydrate metabolism, e.g. galactosaemia, glycogen storage disorders
neurological disorders, e.g. febrile convulsions, infantile spasms
infections (common), e.g. gastroenteritis, urinary tract infection
coeliac disease (1 in 2000 in the UK)
acute abdomen.

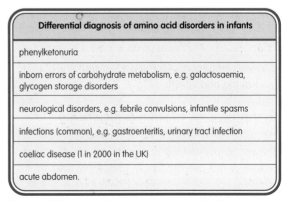

Fig. 9.5 Differential diagnoses of amino acid disorders in infants.

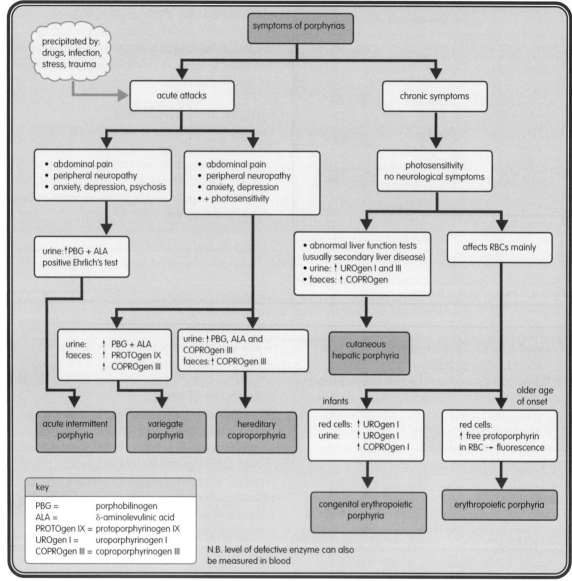

Fig. 9.6 Diagnostic approach to the symptoms of porphyrias.

differential diagnoses for the acute symptoms of gout are trauma and infection (Fig. 9.7).

Symptoms of vitamin deficiencies
Fat-soluble vitamins: A, D, E, and K
The symptoms and signs of each individual vitamin deficiency are covered fully in Chapter 13 and therefore will only be covered briefly here (Fig. 9.8). General causes of deficiency are:

- Decreased intake which may either be due to

generalized malnutrition, mainly seen in developing countries; poor diet, commonly seen in the elderly and the housebound in developed countries; or a vegan diet with specifically no vitamin D.
- Fat malabsorption, for example, due to liver and biliary tract disease or obstruction meaning that no bile salts are available to facilitate absorption.

Vitamin E deficiency is very rare.

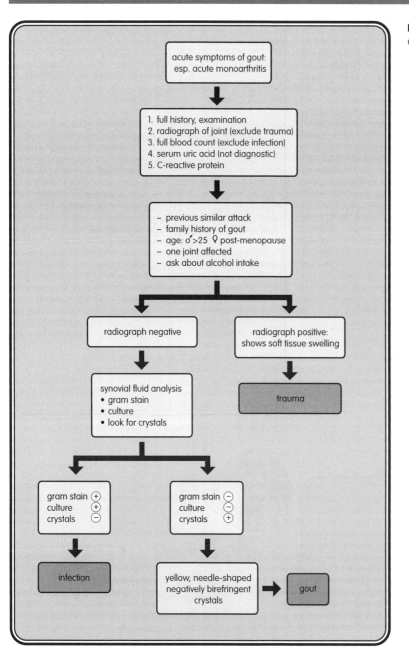

Fig. 9.7 Simplified diagnostic approach to gout.

Water-soluble vitamins (B and C)

The symptoms of a deficiency of vitamins B and C are listed in Fig. 9.9.

Symptoms of mineral deficiencies

The symptoms and signs of each individual mineral deficiency are covered in detail in Chapter 13. The symptoms of the more important mineral deficiency disorders are listed in Fig. 9.10. The differential diagnosis is biased towards metabolic causes.

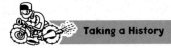
Differential diagnosis of fat-soluble vitamin deficiency diseases	
Vitamin deficiency	**Differential diagnosis**
vitamin A: night blindness and keratomalacia	other causes of degenerative eye changes, e.g. infections such as syphilis, gonorrhoea, chlamydia in neonates (rare)
vitamin D: rickets or osteomalacia	• Ca^{2+} deficiency • renal disease – causing ↓ activity of 1-α hydroxylase • liver disease: causing ↓ activity of 25-α hydroxylase
vitamin K: increased bleeding produces clotting problems (in newborn babies, causes haemorrhagic disease of the newborn)	• inherited coagulation disorders, e.g. haemophilia, von Willebrand's disease • anticoagulant therapy: warfarin/ dicoumarol • antibiotic therapy which knocks out vitamin K producing bacteria in gut

Fig. 9.8 Differential diagnosis of fat-soluble vitamin deficiency diseases.

Symptoms of water-soluble vitamin deficiencies	
Vitamin deficiency	**Main symptoms**
vitamin B₁—thiamin wet beriberi	oedema, tachycardia, shortness of breath and other signs of heart failure (see Fig. 13.10)
dry beriberi	ascending peripheral neuropathy: initially weakness and numbness of legs that ascends to involve trunk, arms, and eventually brain
Wernicke–Korsakoff syndrome	confusion, ataxia, ophthalmoplegia, and peripheral neuropathy
niacin deficiency: pellagra	3 D's: dermatitis, dementia, and diarrhoea
vitamin B₆: secondary pellagra	very rare
vitamin B₁₂: megaloblastic, macrocytic anaemia	see 'symptoms of anaemia' earlier
folate: megaloblastic, macrocytic anaemia	see 'symptoms of anaemia' earlier
vitamin C: scurvy	failure of wound healing hypochromic, microcytic anaemia swollen, sore, spongy gums with bleeding

Fig. 9.9 Symptoms of water-soluble vitamin deficiencies.

Symptoms of mineral deficiencies	
Symptoms	**Cause**
iron deficiency: anaemia (symptoms of anaemia covered earlier)	may be due to: ↓ dietary intake ↓ absorption caused by: ↑ phosphates and phytates in diet or vitamin C deficiency ↑ blood loss: either acute or chronic ↑ requirement: periods of growth
calcium deficiency (and phosphate): • in children: rickets; present with soft easily deformed bones, short stature, and failure to thrive • in adults: osteomalacia, ('brittle bones')	• ↓ dietary intake • secondary to vitamin D deficiency: vitamin D is necessary for intestinal absorption of calcium and phosphate (see Chapter 8) • intestinal malabsorption • renal failure • hypothyroidism
iodine deficiency: goitre can lead to symptoms of hypothyroidism: tiredness, weight gain, anorexia, cold intolerance, constipation	• autoimmune: Hashimoto's thyroiditis • after surgery for hyperthyroidism

Fig. 9.10 Symptoms of mineral deficiencies.

- Describe the main symptoms of anaemia, gout, acute and chronic porphyrias, and diabetes mellitus.
- What are the main diagnostic criteria for each of the above?
- Describe the main symptoms of vitamin and mineral deficiencies (these are covered in detail in Chapter 13).

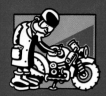

10. Examination of the Patient—Metabolic Signs

This chapter deals with the main signs that may be observed on examination of a patient that are caused by an underlying metabolic disease. Some of the signs mentioned are relatively non-specific and may be related to several types of disease which may indeed be a lot mare common than the metabolic cause. Others may be specific to and in fact be diagnostic of a metabolic disease. Just remember, a lot of metabolic diseases are very rare and you may 'go all your working life without seeing them', as many a clinician will indeed tell you.

The chapter also provides some 'guidelines' on how to examine certain parts or areas of the body and the best or simplest way to elicit signs. A lot of the diseases mentioned here are covered in detail in Chapters 12 and 13.

GENERAL INSPECTION

This section considers the main signs that may be observed on general inspection that are indicative of an underlying metabolic cause. These signs are reasonably non-specific and therefore there may be other possible, non-metabolic causes that must be considered and eliminated in the differential diagnosis. In any clinical examination it is important that you are seen to 'generally inspect' the patient and often the best way to do this is stand at the foot of the bed and ask them to take a breath in and out and observe.

> Before you examine any patient stand back and observe. Look at their general appearance, their level of consciousness, any obvious colour (anaemic or jaundiced), and whether the patient looks tired or distressed; these comments earn you extra marks.

The four main signs you need to look for are:

Wasting, cachexia, and obesity
The term wasting is usually used to describe a mild to moderate, generalized loss of muscle and thus weight. Cachexia however is reserved for severe, generalized muscle wasting, which usually implies a serious underlying cause, for example, cancer or AIDS. An assessment of wasting and obesity in patients and the underlying metabolic causes are set out in Fig. 10.1.

Pallor or jaundice
Pallor is usually associated with anaemia. Jaundice refers to the yellow pigmentation of skin or sclerae of the eyes due to a raised plasma bilirubin level. Jaundice has many causes, which are often classified into three main ones: pre-hepatic where there is excess bilirubin, for example due to increased haemolysis; hepatocellular where there is diminished liver cell function, for example due to a viral infection; and post-hepatic or obstructive jaundice. Both pallor and jaundice are common signs, which have a number of possible causes (Fig. 10.2). However, the best way to observe them is by observation of the eyes (see Fig. 10.9).

Respiratory distress
This is often best assessed by inspection (Fig. 10.3).

Tremors
The four common tremors are (Fig. 10.4):
- Essential or physiological tremor.
- Flapping tremor.
- Resting, 'pill-rolling' tremor of parkinsonism.
- Intention tremor of cerebellar disease.

Assessment of wasting and obesity in patients with its underlying metabolic causes		
Physical examination	**Symptoms and signs**	**Possible diagnosis**
wasting: look for generalized muscle wasting	• when severe, patient has a thin emaciated appearance, almost skeletal and it is referred to as cachexia • skin is wrinkled and there may be hair loss (see Fig. 13.1)	• implies serious disease, principally cancer • in developing countries: probably due to malnutrition caused by marasmus • in children also consider malabsorption e.g. coeliac disease
obesity: observe; can also: • measure weight and height and calculate body mass index (BMI) • compare with tables of ideal weight for height (mid-arm circumference and skin-fold thickness are rarely useful in practice)	• when severe it is obvious on inspection • BMI > 30 kg/m^2 is regarded as obese (see Chapter 8)	usually energy input is greater than energy output obesity is also seen in: • Cushing's syndrome • hypothyroidism • drug-induced, e.g. corticosteroids • consider the possibility of NIDDM

Fig. 10.1 An assessment of wasting and obesity in patients with the underlying metabolic causes.

Assessment of pallor and jaundice in patients and its underlying metabolic causes		
Physical examination	**Symptoms and signs**	**Possible diagnosis**
pallor: observe skin colour N.B. best way to assess pallor is to observe conjunctivae of eyes (see Fig.10.9)	• normal skin colour varies according to skin thickness, circulation and pigmentation • paleness may be normal for patient or indicative of anaemia N.B. poor indicator of anaemia	• iron deficiency anaemia • B$_{12}$/folate deficiency often secondary to pernicious anaemia causes pale-lemon skin as result of anaemia and increased haemolysis
jaundice: observe skin colour N.B. best way to assess jaundice is to observe sclerae of eyes (see Fig. 10.9)	• yellow colour of skin is fairly insensitive indicator of mild to moderate jaundice • with severe jaundice, skin is yellow-green	three basic causes of jaundice: • pre-hepatic: haemolytic anaemia e.g.G6PDH deficiency • hepatocellular: problem with liver itself e.g. viral hepatitis, paracetamol overdose • obstructive: obstruction of bile duct because of gallstones or carcinoma gallstones or carcinoma of head of pancreas

Fig. 10.2 Assessment of pallor and jaundice in patients with its underlying metabolic causes.

Assessment of respiratory distress and its metabolic significance to diabetes		
Physical examination	**Symptoms and signs**	**Possible diagnosis**
respiratory rate, rhythm, and depth of breathing are observed	• hyperventilation • 'Kussmaul respiration': deep, sighing breathing with rapid respiratory rate • smell of ketones on breath heightens suspicion	• accumulation of ketone bodies → metabolic acidosis • respiratory compensation → hyperventilation • untreated → severe diabetic ketoacidosis (see Chapter 12) • also seen in uraemia

Fig. 10.3 Assessment of respiratory distress and its metabolic significance to diabetes.

Assessment of tremors in patients and their significance to metabolic disease		
Physical examination	**Symptoms and signs**	**Possible diagnosis**
patient holds arms outstretched in front of them with hands flat place a piece of paper on them	look for fluttering of paper → tremor present	**essential tremor:** normal tremor associated with anxiety, ↑caffeine, and ↑ exercise also seen in: hypoglycaemia, alcoholics, thyrotoxic patients (hyperthyroid), and Wilson's disease
ask patient to hold arms outstretched with wrists hyperextended	observe flapping motion of hands	**flapping tremor:** CO_2 retention caused by hyperventilation may be seen in people with diabetes
finger–nose test	tremor arises on movement associated with cerebellar lesions	**intention tremor:** seen in chronic alcoholics with Wernicke–Korsakoff syndrome

Fig. 10.4 An assessment of tremors in patients and their significance to metabolic disease.

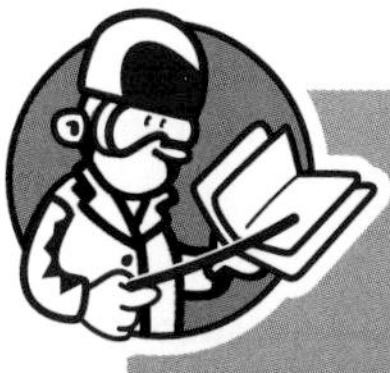

○ **Name the four main signs observed on general inspection. For each, know how to interpret them and their possible, underlying metabolic causes. Remember they are only rough guides to disease.**

LIMBS

Hands

There are a number of signs on the hands and nails indicative of underlying metabolic disease. They are often subtle (Fig. 10.5). Clubbing shown in Fig. 10.6 may be indicative of liver cirrhosis due to a number of causes, some of which are listed in Fig. 10.5. However it is most commonly caused by suppurative lung disease or infective endocarditis and therefore these must always be uppermost in your differential diagnosis. It may also be congenital.

Limbs

Examination of the limbs for underlying metabolic disease can be conveniently divided into assessment of vascular supply (Fig. 10.7) and skin and joint problems associated with metabolic disease (Fig. 10.8).

Main metabolic signs observed on examination of the hands		
Physical examination	**Symptoms and signs**	**Possible diagnosis**
nails:	**clubbing:** • loss of the angle between the nail and nail-bed • underlying nail feels soft, fluctuant and 'boggy' • increased curvature in all directions	liver cirrhosis caused by: • haemochromatosis (↑ iron) • Wilson's disease (↑ copper) • glycogen storage disorders (very rare) • alcohol
	koilonychia spoon-shaped brittle nails, may be ridges	iron-deficiency anaemia
palms:	**palmar erythema** reddening of palms indicative of a hyperdynamic circulation	liver cirrhosis caused by: • increase in either alcohol, iron, or copper • thyrotoxicosis

Fig. 10.5 Main metabolic signs observed on examination of the hands.

Examination of the limbs should include:

○ **Assessment of the vascular supply. The quickest way to do this is to feel the pulses (Fig. 10.7). If you are doing a full cardiovascular examination, you should also observe colour, assess capillary filling time, feel temperature, and look for oedema.**
○ **Skin: look for any obvious lesions (Fig. 10.8).**
○ **Neurological assessment. Both motor and sensory systems are important in patients with diabetes.**

Main metabolic problems to consider in examination of the limbs

Diabetic patients

Look specifically for ischaemic and neuropathic damage leading to ulceration and deformity of limbs (see Chapter 12).

Patients with peripheral vascular disease secondary to hyperlipidaemias

Look for arterial ulceration and, in extreme disease, gangrene.

Skin manifestations of hyperlipidaemias

Tendon xanthomata which are observed usually on the achilles tendon, or extensor tendons on the back of the hand, are often diagnostic of hyperlipidaemias.

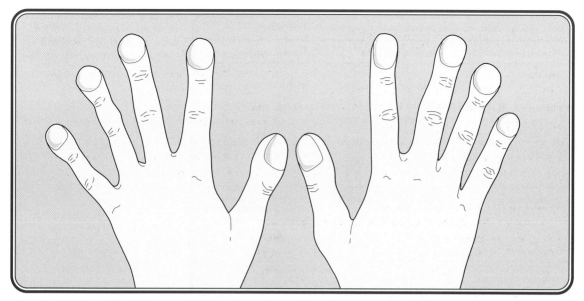

Fig. 10.6 Clubbing of the nails observed in liver cirrhosis, suppurative lung disease, or infective endocarditis.

Main metabolic signs observed on examination of the limbs		
Physical examination	**Symptoms and signs**	**Possible diagnosis**
arm pulses: • radial: assess rate, rhythm and volume • brachial	↑ rate: tachycardia	• anaemia, acute blood loss/shock • thyrotoxicosis • hypoglycaemia
	↓ rate: bradycardia	• hypothermia • hypothyroid
	irregular rhythm	atrial fibrillation: hyperthyroidism
legs pulses: • femoral • popliteal • posterior tibial • dorsalis pedis	↓ or absent peripheral pulses (may also hear bruit over the femoral artery, indicating turbulent blood flow caused by stenosis of arteries)	peripheral vascular disease seen in diabetes or patients with hyperlipidaemias
blood pressure (b.p.)	high	may occur secondary to endocrine or renal disease or to obesity in 95% of cases, cause of high b.p. is unknown; 'essential' hypertension
	low	• severe anaemia, acute blood loss/shock • diabetic ketoacidosis • hypothyroidism

Fig. 10.7 Main metabolic signs observed on examination of the limbs. Pulses provide a quick assessment of vascular supply.

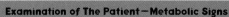

Main metabolic signs observed on examination of the limbs		
Physical examination	**Symptoms and signs**	**Possible diagnosis**
skin lesions: • ischaemic skin ulcers • note position, size, tenderness, edge of ulcer and note any discharge	• usually found over pressure areas: tips of toes/fingers • painful • discharge usually serum or pus, rarely blood-stained because of impaired blood supply • surrounding tissues pale and cold	ischaemic damage seen in: • diabetes • atherosclerosis
neuropathic ulcers	• usually found over pressure areas • painless (as lack of sensation) • surrounding tissues are healthy because of good blood supply	peripheral nerve lesions: chronic complication of diabetes
gangrene – dead tissue	• brown/black tissue usually found on extremities and pressure points • painless and senseless	ischaemic damage
tendon xanthomata: look especially on Achilles tendon and finger extensors on back of hand	• fatty deposits on tendons leading to thickening • may see fat deposition in palmar creases of hand called palmar xanthomata	characteristic of hyperlipidaemias (see Chapter 12)
gouty tophi	• deposits of urate crystals around joints, tendons, and cartilage of ear lobes • causes yellow discoloration of overlying skin	gout
joint problems: • arthropathy • observe joints for signs of inflammation, especially big toe	painful, red, hot, inflamed joint acute onset	acute gout pseudogout

Fig. 10.8 Main metabolic signs observed on examination of the limbs: skin and joint problems associated with metabolic disease.

Gout

This can affect any joint in the body. In an acute attack, look for a red, inflamed, painful joint. In chronic gout, look for gouty tophi: deposits of urate crystals around joints, tendons, and the cartilage of ear lobes, causing yellow discoloration of the overlying skin.

HEAD AND NECK

Face

A number of metabolic and nutritional diseases result in clinical signs evident on the face. For ease, the signs observed are divided into those affecting either the eyes (Fig. 10.9) or the lips and mouth (Fig. 10.10).

- **Name two or three clinical signs observed on the hands and nails and their possible metabolic causes.**
- **Name four main metabolic diseases that result in skin or joint lesions in the limbs. Describe the types of lesions produced.**

Observation of the eyes for signs associated with metabolic disease		
Physical examination	**Symptoms and signs**	**Possible diagnosis**
jaundice: observe colour of sclerae	yellow discoloration of sclerae is a more sensitive indicator of jaundice than skin colour (sclerae turn yellow first)	• liver disease • haemolytic anaemia (e.g. due to G6PDH or pyruvate kinase deficiency) (see Chapter 12)
anaemia: observe colour of conjunctiva (pull down the lower eyelid)	pale/pink colour N.B. the best way to look for anaemia is by the colour of mucous membranes particularly, conjunctiva (also buccal mucosa)	• acute blood loss/infection • iron/B_{12}/folate deficiency • pernicious anaemia • haemolytic anaemia • hypothyroidism
xanthelasma: look for yellow fatty lumps in skin of eyelids	yellow fatty masses confined to the skin non-tender	• one or two may be normal or indicate abnormality of cholesterol metabolism • hyperlipidaemia—especially familial hyperlipidaemia (FH) (see Chapter 12)
arcus senilis: corneal arcus	observe white rim around outer edge of iris due to cholesterol deposition sclerosis in cornea	• common in elderly people • significant in patients < 35 years old, as it may indicate hyperlipidaemia, such as FH or familial combined hyperlipidaemia (see Chapter 12)
Kayser–Fleischer rings: examine corneal–sclera junction for ring	green-brown ring due to copper deposition in periphery of cornea	Wilson's disease: copper overload (see Chapter 13)
observe cornea and conjunctiva for dryness and ulceration	• dryness and ulceration: xerophthalmia • white plaques on conjunctiva: Bitot's spots • opaque scar tissue: keratomalacia → cataracts	all due to vitamin A deficiency
progressive deterioration of vision	loss of visual acuity and cataracts	diabetes mellitus N.B. in neonates, cataracts may be the result of galactosaemia (Chapter 12)

Fig. 10.9 Observation of the eyes for signs associated with metabolic disease.

Observation of the mouth and tongue for signs associated with metabolic disease		
Physical examination	**Symptoms and signs**	**Possible diagnosis**
observe colour of lips and tongue	central cyanosis: purple-blue colour because of excess, haemoglobin in the tissues (at least 2.5 g/dL)	• inadequate perfusion of tissues, methaemoglobinaemia • since methaemoglobin cannot carry oxygen, this leads to poor perfusion of tissues and cyanosis (see Chapter 3)
observe colour of tongue and atrophic changes	glossitis: (red, smooth, sore tongue) loss of filiform papillae:	• iron/folate/B_{12} deficiency • other B vitamin deficiencies: niacin, B_6—pyridoxine
angular stomatitis observe corners of mouth for cuts and infection	angular stomatitis: inflamed, cracked corners of mouth cracks may become infected with *Candida albicans*	common in elderly due to iron deficiency or deficiency of B group vitamins

Fig. 10.10 Observation of the mouth and tongue for signs associated with metabolic disease.

163

Neck

With the exception of iodine deficiency and thyroid disease, there are very few metabolic or nutritional diseases that manifest as signs in the neck.

Thyroid disease

Look at the patient's neck and ask the patient to swallow. You will often observe a prominent goitre (a diffuse enlargement of the thyroid gland). Goitres, however, can also be seen in other thyroid diseases such as Grave's disease and Hashimoto's thyroiditis. All thyroid lumps ascend on swallowing because they are attached to the trachea.

> In your clinical career you will encounter 'lumps' on examination of every body system. It is crucial that you know the characteristics to elicit for any lump from benign hernias to malignant cancer. For every lump define the site, size, shape, surface, colour, temperature, tenderness, edge, composition, reducibility, and state of overlying and adjacent tissues.

> ○ Give four or five examples of clinical signs that can be observed in the eyes that may be related to metabolic diseases. (Remember most of these are rarely seen.)
> ○ Describe the metabolic causes of central cyanosis, glossitis, angular stomatitis, and goitre.

THORAX

The thorax is divided into the respiratory and cardiovascular systems.

Respiratory system

Very few metabolic diseases result in obvious respiratory signs. Therefore, only a brief discussion is included here for completion.

Check list for examination of the respiratory system

This is only a brief list to help you get started.
- Introduce yourself.
- The patient should be undressed to the waist so that the appropriate part of the body is exposed.
- Position the patient so that he or she is comfortable and at the correct angle for examination (45° for respiratory and cardiovascular examinations).
- Observe any respiratory distress, the level of consciousness, expansion (is it uniform between the two sides?), tachypnoea, and so on.

Begin any examination by observing the hands of the patient and work your way up the arms to the head, to the neck, and then down the chest. Remember for examination of any system follow the sequence: observation (Fig. 10.11), palpation, percussion, and auscultation (Fig. 10.12).

Cardiovascular system

As with the respiratory system, few metabolic diseases manifest as cardiovascular signs. However, anaemia of any cause can eventually cause shock and heart failure.

Percussion

Percussion is of no value in the cardiovascular examination.

Observation and palpation

Metabolic signs that can be observed during a cardiovascular examination are listed in Fig. 10.13.

Auscultation

Anaemia of any cause can lead to an innocent ejection systolic murmur. For heart failure, you may hear a third heart sound. Check-list for auscultation:

Examination of the respiratory system in metabolic disease		
Physical examination	**Symptoms and signs**	**Possible diagnosis**
signs of respiratory distress	e.g. tachypnoea, use of accessory muscles of respiration, nasal flare and sternal recession	in starvation, severe muscle wasting can eventually cause wasting of the diaphragm leading to respiratory distress and death
shape of chest wall	• pigeon chest, *pectus carinatum*: prominent sternum often accompanied by indrawing of softened ribs along attachment of diaphragm; Harrison's sulcus • rickety rosary: expansion or swelling of ribs at costochondral junctions	rickets in children
cyanosis	• central cyanosis: observe purple-blue colour of lips • peripheral cyanosis: observe purple-blue colour of extremities (fingers and toes) caused by increased level of deoxygenated blood	methaemoglobinaemia (see Fig. 10.10) inadequate perfusion of tissues caused by peripheral vascular disease seen in diabetics and hyperlipidaemias
respiratory rate: count rate for about a minute fast or laboured? normal 15–20/min	• hyperventilation • deep Küssmaul respiration • breath smells of ketone bodies • severe dehydration	• metabolic acidosis in diabetics leading to diabetic ketoacidosis • respiratory compensation for the acidosis results in hyperventilation

Fig. 10.11 Examination of the respiratory system in metabolic disease.

Auscultation of the respiratory system		
Physical examination	**Symptoms and signs**	**Possible diagnosis**
breath sounds	↓ breath sounds	in obese people these may be difficult to hear
crepitations/crackles	pulmonary oedema, often due to heart failure	heart failure may be secondary to: • anaemia from iron/folate/B$_{12}$/vitamin C deficiency • kwashiorkor

Fig. 10.12 Auscultation of the respiratory system: metabolic signs.

Clinical signs that can be observed during cardiovascular examination		
Physical examination	**Symptoms and signs**	**Possible diagnosis**
signs of shock and heart failure	pallor, tachycardia, heart murmur, and cardiac enlargement untreated progresses to heart failure	severe anaemia (haemoglobin<8 g/dL) causes: • blood loss • iron/folate/B$_{12}$ deficiency • acute haemolytic crisis • hypothyroidism
apex beat	visible on inspection	thin, wasted individuals
impalpable apex beat	normally felt fifth intercostal space, mid-clavicular line	obesity
displaced apex beat	heart failure → cardiomegaly	anaemia of any cause kwashiorkor hypercalcaemia

Fig. 10.13 Clinical signs that may be observed during a cardiovascular examination.

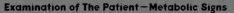

- Always begin at the apex.
- Are there two heart sounds present? The first heart sound is due to the closure of the mitral and tricuspid valves. The second heart sound is due to the closure of the aortic and pulmonary valves. Listen over all four areas (mitral, triscupid, aortic, and pulmonary.)
- Listen for extra third and fourth heart sounds.
- Listen for murmurs. Murmurs are caused by turbulent blood flow. They are classified into systolic, diastolic, or continuous depending on their timing with the cardiac cycle.
- Listen over the carotid, renal, and femoral arteries for bruits. These indicate turbulent blood flow caused by stenosis of arteries; they are heard in peripheral vascular disease caused by diabetes or hyperlipidaemias.

○ **Describe the metabolic causes of respiratory distress and cyanosis.**
○ **Name the clinical signs found in shock and heart failure.**

ABDOMEN

Most metabolic diseases that produce clinical signs in the abdomen do so as a result of excessive deposition of a metabolite or nutrient in organs such as the liver or in arteries or the skin. This interferes with the correct functioning of the organ. For example:

- In haemochromatosis, iron is deposited in the liver leading to liver cirrhosis.
- In glycogen storage disorders, the deposition of glycogen in the liver causes hepatomegaly and eventually liver failure.
- In hyperlipidaemias, the deposition of fat in the walls of arteries leads to atherosclerotic plaque formation and peripheral vascular disease.

Useful points for the examination of the abdomen

When examining the abdomen:

- The patient should be lying as flat as possible, with arms by his or her sides.
- The patient should be exposed from the nipples to knees, however, in the interest of privacy, it is best to expose in stages, beginning with xiphisternum to pubis.
- Kneel beside the bed so that you are at the same level as the patient.
- As with any system of the body, go through the sequence of observation, palpation, percussion, and auscultation.

Observation

Observe the general summetry and shape of the abdomen. The clinical signs and their underlying metabolic causes that can be observed during an abdominal examination are listed in Fig. 10.14.

Fig. 10.14 Clinical signs and the underlying metabolic causes that can be observed during an abdominal examination.

Clinical signs and the underlying metabolic causes that can be observed during an abdominal examination		
Physical examination	**Symptoms and signs**	**Possible diagnosis**
abdominal distension: note shape, symmetry, size of any bulge or mass	general/localized swelling	obesity ascites; kwashiorkor
	asymmetrical enlargement	e.g. liver enlargement due to glycogen storage disorders, hyperlipidaemias, kwashiorkor
striae (stretch marks)	purple abdominal striae	Cushing's syndrome obesity
spider naevi	single, central arteriole feeding a number of small branches in a radial manner, which blanche (turn white) on pressure	chronic liver failure and cirrhosis in: • alcoholics • haemochromatosis • Wilson's disease (copper overload) • vitamin A toxicity (see Chapter 13)
pigmentation	slate-grey colour	iron overload

Palpation

Points to remember when palpating the abdomen:

- Before you start, ask the patient 'Have you any pain anywhere in your abdomen?' If the answer is 'yes', begin your palpation furthest from the pain.
- The abdomen is divided either into nine areas or simply into quadrants (Fig. 10.15).

The clinical signs with their underlying metabolic causes that can be detected on palpation of the abdomen are listed in Fig. 10.16.

Percussion

Abdominal percussion has two main roles:

- To outline the liver. The liver is 'dull' to percussion and therefore it is useful in determining the degree of hepatomegaly.
- In the presence of abdominal distension, to determine whether it is due to solid, gas, or free fluid (ascites) in the abdomen.

Ascites is seen in congestive heart failure, liver cirrhosis and secondary to wet beri-beri and kwashiorkor (Chapter 13).

Auscultation

The clinical signs with their underlying metabolic causes that can be detected on auscultation of the abdomen are listed in Fig. 10.17.

Remember to check the patient's urine for glucose and protein.

- Name the main metabolic diseases that produce clinical signs in the abdomen.
- Give a general outline for the examination of the abdomen.
- Describe the metabolic causes of abdominal distension, spider naevi, striae, hepatomegaly, and splenomegaly.

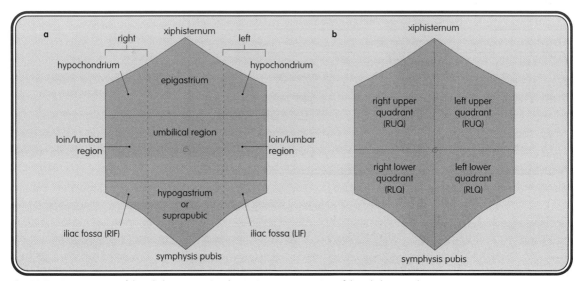

Fig. 10.15 Examination of the abdomen. **a.** A schematic representation of the abdomen showing nine areas. **b.** The four quadrants simplified.

Clinical signs with the underlying metabolic causes that can be detected on palpation of the abdomen		
Physical examination	Symptoms and signs	Possible diagnosis
abdominal pain: determine site, position, radiation, onset, timing etc.	acute, severe upper abdominal pain ± guarding and rebound tenderness	• acute pancreatitis seen in type I familial lipoprotein lipase deficiency or apo C-II hyperlipidaemia (see Chapter 12) • acute porphyria (see Chapter 12)
liver enlargement (hepatomegaly)	• liver edge is not normally palpable below costal margin • gross hepatomegaly can fill whole abdomen	causes: • heart failure • alcohol induced liver disease • haemolytic anaemia, e.g. G6PDH deficiency • porphyrias • iron overload: haemochromatosis • hyperlipidaemias • glycogen storage disorders (see Fig. 2.36) • galactosaemia (see Chapter 12)
spleen enlargement (splenomegaly)	spleen supposedly has a palpable notch on its medial side but very difficult to feel	causes: • pernicious anaemia • galactosaemia • hyperlipidaemias • haemolytic anaemia
kidneys	they are usually impalpable	• lower pole of right kidney can be felt in very thin or wasted people • renal disease and stones are found in gout

Fig. 10.16 Clinical signs with their underlying metabolic causes that can be detected on palpation of the abdomen.

Clinical signs with the underlying metabolic causes that can be detected on auscultation of the abdomen		
Physical examination	Symptoms and signs	Possible diagnosis
bowel sounds	absent if there is mechanical obstruction	• paralytic ileus • gallstones
bruits	listen along course of aorta, usually over femoral and renal arteries	• aortic aneurysm • renal artery stenosis • peripheral vascular disease, e.g. patients with diabetes or hyperlipidaemias

Fig. 10.17 Clinical signs with the underlying metabolic causes that can be detected on auscultation of the abdomen.

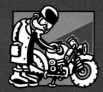

11. Further Investigations

ROUTINE INVESTIGATONS

This section serves as a summary of the main tests used every day to assess metabolic function. They can be conveniently divided into:

- 'First line' tests, that is, the tests most frequently requested.
- 'Second line' tests.

Haematology

The simplest, first line test is the full blood count (FBC). This measures red cell count and indices, white cell count (increased in infection), and platelets. Other 'second line' tests include clotting studies and assessment of bone marrow iron stores (Fig. 11.1).

Clinical chemistry

First line tests include blood glucose, liver function tests (LFTs), and urea and electrolytes (U and Es) (Fig. 11.2). Second line tests include serum iron, B_{12}, and lipid profile, and also more infrequently performed tests such as red cell transketolase (Fig. 11.3).

> **Figs 11.1–11.3 are here for you to refer to; you do not need to learn all the values for different enzymes. In any exam, or for any set of blood test results, either the abnormal results are highlighted or the normal ranges are quoted.**

Haematological investigations		
Test	**Normal range**	**Low/high**
Full blood count (FBC)		
haemoglobin g/dL	men 13–17 women 12–15	low: anaemia high: polycythaemia
red cell count ($\times 10^{12}$/L)	men 4.5–6.8 women 4.0–5.2	high: polycythaemia low: anaemia
mean cell volume (MCV)	80–100 fL	low: 'microcytic RBC'-in iron deficiency anaemia high: macrocytic RBC in B_{12}/ folate deficiency
mean cell haemoglobin (MCH)	27–32 pg	low: iron deficiency high: B_{12}/folate deficiency
reticulocyte count	1–2%	low: Fe/B_{12}/folate deficiency anaemia thalassemia high: haemolytic anaemia
bone marrow iron stores		low: iron deficiency high: thalassemia sideroblastic anaemia
clotting studies: • prothrombin time • activated partial thromboplastin time (APTT)	12–16 s 35-50 s	both high—vitamin K deficiency
blood film	normocytic, normochromic red blood cells (RBC)	microcytic, hypochromic: iron deficiency macrocytic: B_{12}/ folate deficiency sickle cells: sickle cell anaemia irregular 'blister' cells: G6PDH deficiency (very rare)

Fig. 11.1 Haematological investigations.

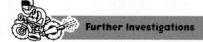

a	First line biochemical investigations on blood or serum		
Test	**Normal range**	**Low/high**	
fasting blood glucose	2.5–5.5 mmol/L	low: hypoglycaemia high: hyperglycaemia → diabetes	
liver function tests			
AST **ALT**	< 35 U/L < 55 U/L	high: hepatitis cirrhosis fatty liver	
alkaline phosphatase (ALP)	< 120 U/L (different isoenzymes present in liver, bone, placenta and intestine)	high: cirrhosis cholestasis	
γ-glutamyl transferase (GGT)	< 80 U/L	high: alcoholics obstructive liver disease carcinoma of head of the pancreas	
serum total bilirubin	< 22 μmol/L	high: liver disease haemolytic anaemia	

b	First line biochemical investigations on blood or serum		
Urea and electrolytes (U and Es)			
urea	2.5–7.5 mmol/L	high: renal disease catabolic state	
creatinine	0.06–0.12 mmol/L	high: renal failure increased muscle bulk e.g. athletes	
sodium	132–144 mmol/L	high: dehydration renal failure Cushing's syndrome low: water excess due to heart failure or liver cirrhosis	
potassium (U and Es also includes chloride and bicarbonate)	3.3–4.7 mmol/L	high: diabetic ketoacidosis renal failure K+ sparing diuretics	
total protein	75 g/L	high: malnutrition	
albumin	37–47 g/L	low: chronic liver disease myeloma	
calcium	2.2–2.67 mmol/L	low: vitamin D deficiency high: hypercalcaemia	
free T4 (thyroxine)	10–25 pmol/L	high: hyperthyroidism	
free T3 (triiodothyronine)	5–10.2 pmol/L	low: hypothyroidism	
thyroid stimulating hormone (TSH)	0.3–5.5 mU/L	low: hyperthyroidism high: hypothyroidism	

Fig. 11.2 (a and b) First line biochemical investigations on blood or serum. (AST, Aspartate aminotransferase; ALT, Alanine aminotransferase.)

Second line biochemical investigations on blood or serum		
Test	**Normal range**	**Low/high**
serum iron	13–32 μmol/L	low: iron deficiency high: haemochromatosis thalassemia
total iron binding capacity (TIBC)	42–80 μmol/L	low: iron deficiency
serum B12	160–925 ng/L	low: pernicious anaemia
folate	4–18 μg/L	low: pregnancy, cancer, drugs, e.g. methotrexate
serum urate	<0.48 mmol/L	high: hyperuricaemia and gout
lipid profile: total cholesterol triacylglycerol	<6.0 mmol/L 2.5 mmol/L	high: hyperlipidaemias chronic liver disease
red cell transketolase	no normal range	low: thiamin deficiency chronic alcoholics
vitamin D: 25-hydroxyCC 1, 25-dihydroxyCC	37–200 nmol/L 60–108 pmol/L	low: rickets or osteomalacia
copper caeruloplasmin	12–25 μmol/L 0.20–0.45 g/L	high: Wilson's disease

Fig. 11.3 Second line biochemical investigations on blood or serum.

Urine
Urine is commonly tested for glucose, protein, and ketones (dipstick tests). Although not as sensitive as blood tests, urine tests provide a quick and easy method of investigation (Fig. 11.4).

Histopathology
These tests are very specific and are therefore only performed to confirm a diagnosis, usually after simpler biochemical tests have been done (Fig. 11.5).

Immunopathology
Some examples of immunopathological investigations are listed in Fig. 11.6.

Examples of urine tests	
Test	**Low/high**
glycosuria	high: diabetes, pregnancy, renal tubular damage
ketones	high: diabetic ketoacidosis
proteinuria	high: urinary tract infections, renal failure, and diabetes
Porphobilinogen (PBG) and δ-aminolevulinic acid (ALA)	high: acute porphyrias (see Chapter 12)—very rare
bilirubin	high: hepatocellular or obstructive jaundice
urobilinogen	high: haemolytic or hepatocellular jaundice low: obstructive jaundice

Fig. 11.4 Examples of urine tests.

Examples of histopathology investigations	
Test	**Result**
liver biopsy	Wilson's disease: increased copper deposition leading to liver cirrhosis haemochromatosis: iron deposition may cause cirrhosis which may progress to hepatocellular carcinoma
synovial joint fluid analysis	gout: yellow, needle-shaped negatively birefringent monosodium urate crystals observed

Fig. 11.5 Examples of histopathology investigations.

Medical imaging

There are many medical imaging tests used, from simple radiographs and ultrasound to magnetic resonance imaging and positron emission tomography scanning. Fig. 11.7 illustrates some examples.

Remember, any patient presenting to casualty will probably require a combination of first line tests. For example:

- Full blood count.
- Urea and electrolytes.
- Liver function tests.
- If there are obvious signs of infection, blood and urine must be taken for culture.

Examples of immunopathology investigations		
Test	**Normal range/ result**	**Result**
Schilling test: patient given radioactive B_{12} and its excretion is monitored (see Chapter 13)	excrete > 10% radioactive B_{12}	< 10% excretion is indicative of B_{12} deficiency; if then repeat with intrinsic factor and excretion is within normal range, this confirms the diagnosis of pernicious anaemia
Direct Coombs' test (detection of antibodies to red blood cells)	usually no antibodies present and therefore no agglutination of RBCs	+VE = agglutination of RBCs e.g. in haemolytic disease of the newborn or autoimmune haemolytic anaemia

Fig. 11.6 Examples of immunopathology investigations.

Examples of medical imaging investigations	
Test	**Result**
chest X-ray (CXR)	anaemia of any cause, ischaemic heart disease, hypercalcaemia, or iron overload, can all result in heart failure; on X-ray this can show up as: • an enlarged heart (cardiomegaly) • pleural effusion • increased perihilar shadowing (bat wings) due to oedema • prominent upper lobe veins • Kerley B lines
other X-rays	in rickets and osteomalacia: defective mineralization seen in pelvis, long bones and ribs in the early stages → see soft tissue swelling late stages → well-defined 'punched out' lesions in juxta-articular bone
ECG	abnormalities of ECG pattern can be related to specific damage or disease e.g.: • ischaemic damage • myocardial infarction • heart block • bradycardia • arrhythmias
CT scans	used to observe abnormalities and to exclude focal lesions due to tumour or infection before considering a metabolic pathology

Fig. 11.7 Examples of medical imaging investigations.

- Bedside blood glucose. This can be life-saving if a patient comes in unconscious or in a stupor: they may be drunk or they may be severely hypoglycaemic.
- Electrocardiogram and chest radiograph if necessary.

Investigation of glucose homeostasis
Measurement of blood glucose
Use
The measurement of blood glucose is used to confirm or reject a diagnosis of diabetes mellitus and to monitor the control of blood glucose in diabetic patients. Reference ranges for blood glucose levels are shown in Fig. 11.8.

Test
The estimation of blood glucose uses the glucose oxidase and peroxidase reaction.

Method
The test is based on the reaction catalysed by the enzymes glucose oxidase, peroxidase, and a peroxidase substrate (a dye). Glucose oxidase oxidizes glucose present in a deproteinized blood sample to gluconolactone and hydrogen peroxide. The hydrogen peroxide reacts with a dye to form a coloured complex whose absorbance is read in a spectrophotometer. Under standard conditions, the amount of glucose in the unknown blood sample is equal to the amount of coloured product formed. Standardized solutions of glucose are processed at the same time in order to construct a calibration curve. Therefore, the amount of glucose in the unknown blood sample can be read off from the curve.

Advantages
The test is specific for glucose. A similar enzyme reaction is found in commercially available self-monitoring reagent strips: the dextrostix/glucometer system commonly used by patients with IDDM at home.

Oral glucose tolerance test
Use
The oral glucose tolerance test (OGTT) is sometimes used to diagnose diabetes. However, its use is often restricted to the detection of borderline cases and patients with impaired glucose tolerance (IGT), that is, those patients who are likely to develop diabetes when they are older.

Method
Patients should make sure that they eat a normal diet, containing adequate carbohydrate, for the preceding 3 days. This ensures the enzymes involved in glucose metabolism are present at normal levels. After an overnight fast, an initial basal blood sample is taken and the blood glucose concentration is determined. A drink containing 75 g of glucose in 250–300 mL of water is drunk and the blood glucose is measured every 30 min for the next 2 h. The blood glucose concentration is determined by the glucose oxidase method. Patients must rest during the test because stress can lead to cortisol release, which increases blood glucose. Figs 11.9 and 11.10 illustrate the results of an OGTT.

Assessment of glycaemic control: glycosylated haemoglobin
Use
The amount of glycosylated haemoglobin (HbA_1 or HbA_{1C}) provides a measure of the average blood glucose concentration over the preceding 6–8 weeks, that is, the lifetime of a haemoglobin molecule. This is useful for patients with diabetes to show how well their blood glucose concentration is being controlled. The value is high in poorly controlled diabetics.

Reference ranges: based on WHO diagnostic criteria			
	Normal (mmol/L)	IGT (mmol/L)	Diabetic (mmol/L)
fasting blood glucose	< 7.8	< 7.8	> 7.8
2 h post-load blood glucose	< 7.8	7.8–11.1	> 11.1
IGT= impaired glucose tolerance			

Fig. 11.8 Reference ranges for blood glucose levels based on World Health Organisation diagnostic criteria.

Results of oral glucose tolerance test	
Result	Reference range
normal	returns to fasting level within 2 h
IGT	fasting blood glucose < 7.8 mmol/L and 2 h value between 7.8 and 11.1 mmol/L
diabetic	fasting blood glucose > 7.8 mmol/L and/or 2 h value > 11.1 mmol/L

Fig. 11.9 Results of an oral glucose tolerance test.

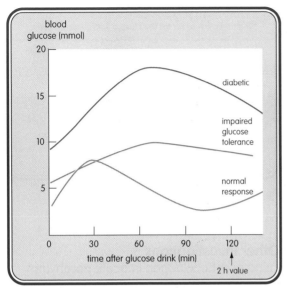

Fig. 11.10 Graph showing the results of an oral glucose tolerance test.

Method

Glucose attaches non-enzymatically to adult haemoglobin (HbA) over the lifetime of a RBC. The rate at which this occurs is proportional to the blood glucose concentration. The amount of glycosylated HbA_{1C} present in blood can be measured by a number of methods, including high-pressure liquid chromatography, electrophoresis, or immunoassay. It is then expressed as a percentage of total HbA (Fig. 11.11).

Assessment of glycaemic control: serum fructosamine concentration

Use

The serum fructosamine concentration is a measure of glycaemic control over the previous 2 weeks. It is cheaper and quicker than HbA_{1C} estimation but HbA_{1C} is often preferred. Serum fructosamine concentration is useful for patients with abnormal haemoglobin (e.g. thalassemia) and in pregnancy when haemoglobin turnover is very changeable from week to week.

Reference values	
Result	**Reference values for HbA_{1c}**
normal	4–8%
poorly controlled	> 10%

Fig. 11.11 Reference values for HbA_{1C} expressed as a percentage of HbA.

Enzyme assays
Glucose-6-phosphate dehydrogenase
Use

An enzyme assay is used for the diagnosis of glucose-6-phosphate dehydrogenase deficiency, the most common RBC enzyme defect (see Chapter 12). It allows patients with glucose-6-phosphate dehydrogenase deficiency to be detected between haemolytic attacks, such that diagnosis is not just dependent on the blood picture during an attack. An enzyme activity of <2% of the normal level may be seen in very severe cases.

Pyruvate kinase assay
Use

Pyruvate kinase assay is used for the diagnosis of RBC pyruvate kinase deficiency (see Chapter 12).

Test

The production of pyruvate is coupled to the reduction of a dye with the colour change monitored spectrophotometrically. A decreased production of ATP can also be observed when radioactively labelled ^{32}P is added to RBCs and its incorporation into ATP is monitored.

Reference values

Patients typically need to have an enzyme level of 5–25% of the normal level to show clinical features.

Galactose and fructose

Both galactose and fructose are reducing sugars and are detected in the urine of patients, using alkaline copper (II) reagents, such as Benedict's reagent.

Galactosaemia

Galactosaemia is usually caused by a deficiency of the enzyme galactose-1-phosphate uridyl transferase.

Tests

Screening test are performed in infants with suspicious symptoms:

- Test for galactosuria: Clinitest tablets or reagent strips contain copper citrate, which is reduced by galactose. The colour change observed is clear blue to green to brown to a brick red precipitate if the reduction is complete. The presence of galactose in the urine and positive symptoms leads to the withdrawal of galactose and lactose from the diet

until a diagnostic test can be performed.
- Diagnostic test: assay RBCs for decreased galactose-1-phosphate uridyl transferase activity.

Fructokinase deficiency: essential fructosuria

The absence of fructokinase leads to a combination of a high fructose concentration in the blood and fructose accumulation in the urine. Both must be present to form a diagnosis. Fructose, like galactose, is a reducing sugar and its presence in urine can be detected with Clinitest tablets.

Investigation of lipid metabolism
Cholesterol and triacylglycerol concentration
Uses

Coronary heart disease is a major cause of death in the UK and therefore cholesterol levels are monitored routinely in 'at risk' groups and when necessary in the rest of the population. 'At risk' groups include:
- Patients with coronary heart disease (angina, post-myocardial infarction, post-angioplasty or coronary artery bypass graft) and patients with peripheral or cerebrovascular disease.
- Patients with hyperlipidaemias and their families.
- Patients with multiple risk factors; for example, patients with diabetes, high blood pressure, or high cholesterol (a full list of risk factors can be found in Chapter 12).

Investigations

Screening measures cholesterol levels only. If a raised cholesterol is found, a full fasting lipid profile may be performed which measures the total cholesterol, high density lipoprotein (HDL)-cholesterol, and triacylglycerol. Blood taken for lipid studies is obtained after an overnight fast. Reference values for fasting plasma lipid concentrations are shown in Fig. 11.12.

Low density lipoprotein (LDL) cholesterol levels can also be obtained by calculation using the Friedwald equation. This is only valid if triacylglycerol levels are less than 4 mmol/L.

$$LDL = total\ cholesterol - HDL - (triacylglycerol \div 2.13)$$

Triacylglycerol levels of greater than 10 mmol/L cause an increased risk of pancreatitis.

Reference values for fasting plasma lipid concentrations	
Lipid	Plasma concentration (mmol/L)
total cholesterol	< 5.2
LDL cholesterol	< 3.5
HDL cholesterol	> 1.0
triacylglycerol (TG)	< 2.0

Fig. 11.12 Reference values for fasting plasma lipid concentrations.

Other investigations
Urine porphobilinogen in acute porphyrias
Use

Porphobilinogen can be detected in the urine during acute attacks of porphyrias for example in acute intermittent, variegate, and hereditary coproporphyrias are discussed in Chapter 13. In unexplained acute abdominal pain, peripheral neuropathy, and neuropsychiatric symptoms, especially if there is a family history of porphyrias, urine should be tested for porphobilinogen by a simple screening test.

Test

Porphobilinogen in urine is detected by adding one part Ehrlich's aldehyde reagent to one part urine, which causes a pink–red colour to appear. If very high levels of porphobilinogen are present, the pink colour persists on the addition of two parts chloroform. In the presence of excess porphobilinogen, urine will darken on standing, 'auto-oxidizing' to a red colour without the addition of Ehrlich's reagent. This is only a screening test because porphobilinogen is only present in urine during acute attacks. Accurate diagnosis depends on the measurement of defective enzyme levels.

Diagnosis of phenylketonuria

Every neonate is now screened for phenylketonuria as part of the Guthrie test. Diagnosis is based on a high concentration of phenylalanine in the blood (see Chapter 12 for a full discussion).

Screening test

A sample of capillary blood is taken from a heel-prick at 5–10 days after birth. The delay allows sufficient time for feeding, and therefore for protein intake to be established and for the effect of the mother's metabolism to subside. This test used to be based on a microbiological technique, using a strain of *Bacillus subtilis* which only grows if excess phenylalanine is present. However, it is now based on chromatography. Increased plasma phenylalanine levels are indicative of phenylketonuria. The Guthrie test also screens all babies for hypothyroidism.

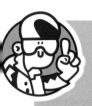

Lipoproteins in the blood can be separated by electrophoresis. Electrophoresis is useful in the detection of hyperlipidaemias because each one gives a characteristic separation pattern (Fig. 11.13), but this is rarely used now.

Know about the oral glucose tolerance test because this is frequently examined.

○ **Name the important first line haematological and clinical chemistry tests that are performed routinely and describe why they are used.**
○ **Describe the variation of results obtained with metabolic diseases.**
○ **Describe the Schilling test and its diagnostic use in pernicious anaemia.**
○ **Describe the tests available for the investigation of glucose homeostasis.**
○ **For each test describe the main use, reference values and, when applicable, the method.**

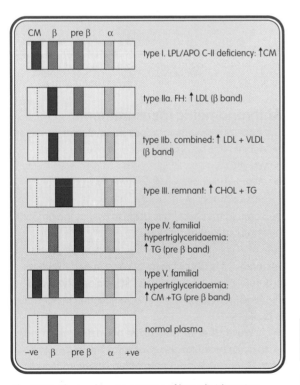

Fig. 11.13 Electrophoretic patterns of hyperlipidaemias. Lipoproteins in the blood can be separated by electrophoresis. This is useful in the detection of hyperlipidaemias because each gives a characteristic separation pattern. (APO C-II, apolipoprotein C-II; CHOL, cholesterol; CM, chylomicron; FH, familial hypercholesterolaemia; LDL, low density lipoprotein; TG, triacylglycerol; VLDL, very low density lipoprotein.)

ASSESSMENT OF NUTRITIONAL STATUS

For any individual, adequate nutrition is essential to maintain growth and development. It is especially important in newborn babies, infants, and during pregnancy when nutritional deficiency can lead to wasting, severe mental retardation, and even death. Malnutrition must be recognized and accurately assessed to enable decisions to be made about

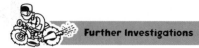
treatment and re-feeding methods. Assessment is divided into:

- Dietary history.
- Anthropometry.
- Physical examination.
- Laboratory and biochemical tests.

Medical, social, and dietary history

The main aspect of this is the dietary history but often weight loss and poor nutrition are related to a medical, psychological, or financial origin (see Fig. 9.2).

Medical history

Ask specifically about:

- Loss of appetite.
- How much weight loss or gain? The time course of the weight change.
- Dysphagia, nausea, vomiting.
- Periods of weight loss in the past; use of laxatives.
- Symptoms of hyperthyroidism: weight loss, increased appetite, irritability, eye signs, and so on.
- Psychiatric history, especially if there is the possibility of depression or an eating disorder (e.g. anorexia nervosa).

Social history

In developed countries:

- Malnutrition may be related to the poor socio-economic status of a family.
- Enquire about housing, social support, and income support.

In the UK, nutritional deficiency is particularly seen in:

- Elderly people ('tea and biscuit brigade') living alone who are unable to cook or shop.
- Young pregnant mothers who live off a staple diet of chips, pizzas, and so on.
- Chronic alcoholics.

In developing countries, nutritional deficiency may be related to war, poor crops, and the poor socio-economic status of the entire country.

Dietary history

Dietary recall

Ask specifically:

- What do you eat in a typical day?
- What do you like and dislike eating (important in children)?
- Access to food or presence of financial problems?

Patients are often asked to keep a food diary. This is usually more accurate than simply questioning the patient, although it relies on the patient's compliance to fill the diary in, and also honesty (patients with eating disorders are not usually honest).

The reason for weight loss or poor nutrition is often not as simple as 'not eating enough'. You must eliminate serious underlying illnesses such as cancer before you move on to diagnoses of psychiatric illness (depression or anorexia nervosa) or poor socio-economic status.

Anthropometric measurements

The basic anthropometric measurements are:

- Height.
- Weight.
- Mid-arm circumference: a measure of skeletal muscle mass.
- Skin-fold thickness. This helps to assess the amount of subcutaneous fat stores.

For infants, it is difficult to measure skin-fold thickness accurately and it is therefore of little value. The World Health Organization recommends that nutritional status is expressed as:

- % Weight/height: a measure of wasting as an index of acute malnutrition.
- % Height/age: a measure of growth retardation as an index of chronic malnutrition.

In infants, regular growth measurements are of extreme value in assessing their nutritional status. Therefore, all infants have their height and weight plotted on a growth chart (Fig. 11.14), which allows a decrease in the rate of growth to be easily recognized and monitored as an early sign of malnutrition.

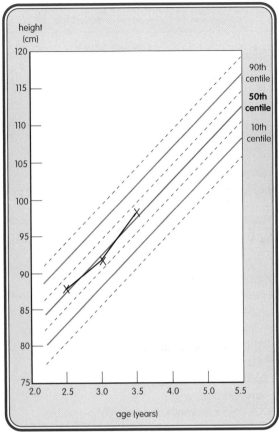

Fig. 11.14 Example of a growth chart often used to help in assessment of nutritional status in children. The line plotted shows the patient's height lies along the 50th centile, i.e. average height.

Physical clinical examination

Physical examination is a non-specific method useful in severe malnutrition, for example, marasmus or kwashiorkor, when obvious signs are present.
However, it only detects about 25% of moderate cases of malnutrition.

Clinical signs

These can be a combination of any of the following:
- Wasting or cachexia.
- Pallor indicates anaemia, possibly caused by an iron, vitamin B_{12}, or folate deficiency.
- Specific effects of vitamin deficiency, for example, of vitamin A causing Bitot's spots on the eyes, or of vitamin D and calcium causing rickets .
- Oedema.
- Bruising, for example, in vitamin D or K deficiency.

Biochemical tests

Biochemical tests are useful in the detection of early or mild to moderate malnutrition, that is, before clinical signs become evident. The tests for individual nutrients, vitamins, and minerals are dealt with in Chapter 13. Here, the different types of tests are considered.

Types of biochemical tests
Direct measurement

Direct measurement of the concentration of a nutrient or a metabolite in the body fluid, usually in the serum or urine.

Functional test

Thiamin is a co-factor for RBC transketolase. In thiamin deficiency, the RBC enzyme activity can be measured before and after the addition of thiamine pyrophosphate (the active form of thiamin). Addition of thiamine pyrophosphate to RBCs should lead to an increase in enzyme activity, proving thiamin deficiency.

Measurement of stores

The best way to measure the level of a nutrient is to measure its stores because:
- A decrease in the dietary intake of a nutrient leads to the mobilization of that nutrient from its stores to maintain a normal plasma concentration.
- Usually, only in severe deficiency does the plasma concentration drop significantly.
- Therefore, by measuring a decrease in the body stores we can detect a deficiency earlier.

For example, the best way to assess iron deficiency is to measure a decrease in bone marrow iron stores, and the best way to assess vitamin C deficiency is to measure a decrease in white cell vitamin C content (Fig. 11.15).

A plasma albumin of less than 30 g/L is often used as an index of malnutrition but it is not definite. The diagnosis of severe malnutrition is usually made on clinical assessment.

Parenteral nutrition

Nutritional support is provided for all patients who are severely malnourished or are unable to eat because of physical illness. Whenever possible enteral nutrition is used, that is, via a nasogastric tube, because it is more natural, cheaper, and far less hazardous in terms of the

Some biochemical tests for nutrients	
Nutrient	**Tests**
protein	serum protein, albumin
fat	total cholesterol and triglyceride
carbohydrate	blood glucose
vitamin A	plasma vitamin A, retinol binding protein
vitamin D	$\downarrow Ca^{2+}$, $\downarrow PO_4^{3-}$, $\uparrow$ alkaline phosphatase measure vitamin D levels and parathyroid hormone
vitamin K	$\uparrow$ prothrombin time
vitamin C	white cell vitamin C content (storage site)
B$_1$ (thiamin)	red blood cell (RBC) transketolase
B$_{12}$	FBC, serum B$_{12}$, MCV
folate	RBC folate
iron	FBC, ferritin, MCV etc. best estimate is a fall in bone marrow iron stores

Fig. 11.15 Some biochemical tests for nutrients, (FBC, full blood count; MCV, mean cell volume.)

effects on fluid and electrolyte balance than parenteral nutrition. Enteral nutrition is always given in preference if the gastrointestinal tract is functional.

Indications for parenteral nutrition
Indicators for parental nutrition include:
- Intestinal failure, either as the result of surgery (gut resection) or because of a fistula.
- Patients with a very high energy requirement i.e. hypercatabolic state, for example, severe trauma or burns patients and patients unable to eat.

Administration
Administration is usually via a central venous catheter into the superior vena cava or sometimes into a peripheral vein. It involves the intravenous infusion of glucose, fat emulsion, amino acids, vitamins, electrolytes, and trace elements.

Complications of total parenteral nutrition (TPN)
• infection and sepsis associated with the central catheter (the most important complication)
• hyperglycaemia
• hypokalaemia, hyponatraemia
• hypophosphataemia
• abnormal liver function
• acidosis
• long-term: metabolic bone disease and vitamin deficiency states

Fig. 11.16 Complications of total parenteral nutrition.

Monitoring the patient
Patients require careful daily clinical monitoring to avoid complications (Fig. 11.16).
- Fluid balance. The patient requires a fluid balance chart which is reviewed twice daily.
- Plasma electrolytes are monitored daily: sodium, potassium, chloride, biocarbonate, urea, creatinine, and glucose.
- Glucose intolerance and hyperglycaemia are common side effects.
- Regular haematological measurements (full blood count and so on) are necessary to monitor iron, vitamin B$_{12}$, or folate deficiencies.
- In a patient with stable renal function, 24 h urinary urea excretion can provide an index of the body's protein status.
- Liver function tests should be checked about three times a week.

- Give four methods for assessing nutritional status. For each, know the main principles involved, the uses, and any disadvantages.
- Describe the indications for parenteral nutrition and its main complications.

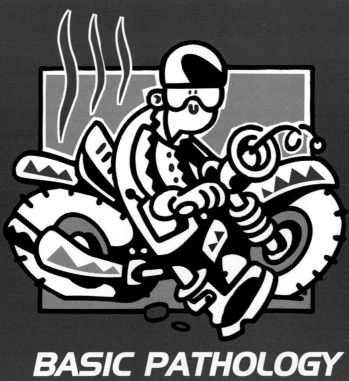

BASIC PATHOLOGY

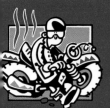

12. Important Metabolic Disorders

DISORDERS OF GLUCOSE AND ENERGY METABOLISM

Diabetes mellitus
Classification
There are two major types of diabetes mellitus.

Type I: Insulin-dependent diabetes mellitus (IDDM)
Insulin-dependent diabetes mellitus is often referred to as juvenile onset diabetes because it typically presents in childhood or puberty. It accounts for only 10–20% of the total number of people with diabetes and has an incidence rate of about about 1 in 3000.

The aetiology of the disease is a complete deficiency of insulin that can only be corrected by life-long insulin treatment. There are three theories as to its cause:
- Auto-immune destruction of the β cells in the islets of Langerhans in the pancreas by islet cell auto-antibodies, resulting in insulin deficiency.
- Genetic factors. The evidence for a genetic cause is that firstly there is a 50% concordance between identical twins, which implies a mixture of both genetic and environmental factors. Secondly, there is a positive family history in 10% of patients. Thirdly, more than 90% of IDDM patients carry HLA DR3 and DR4 antigens compared with 40% of the general population.
- A viral cause, for example, mumps or coxsackie B has also been considered. However, it is likely that viral infections provide the stimulus for autoimmune destruction rather than actually initiating diabetes.

Therefore, the cause is probably a mixture of all three: 'an auto-immune destruction of the β cells in genetically susceptible patients which may be precipitated by a viral infection'.

The presentation of the disease is usually of rapid onset: weeks or days with the characteristic symptoms of polyuria, polydipsia, and weight loss. These patients are prone to ketoacidosis, which can be life-threatening.

Type II: Non-insulin-dependent diabetes mellitus (NIDDM)
This is also known as maturity onset diabetes because it typically presents after the age of 35 years. The incidence is more common, and it accounts for 80–90% of the total number of people with diabetes.

NIDDM is caused by:
- Impaired insulin secretion from the β cells, that is, they fail to secrete enough insulin to correct the blood glucose level.
- Insulin resistance in the tissues, that is, cells fail to respond adequately to insulin.

Genetic factors are very important; there is almost 100% concordance between identical twins and about 30% of patients have a first degree relative with NIDDM. There is no auto-immune or viral involvement.

The presentation is of an insidious onset and more than 80% of patients are obese. Sufferers are not normally prone to ketoacidosis but it can develop under stress.

Other types of diabetes
There are a number of other types of diabetes, which usually occur secondary to a predisposing factor, e.g.:
- Gestational diabetes which has its onset during pregnancy.
- Secondary diabetes: this may be the result of damage to the pancreas itself, for example, in chronic pancreatitis or haemochromatosis, where iron may be deposited in the pancreas (see Chapter 13). It may also occur secondary to the excessive secretion of catabolic hormones, resulting in hyperglycaemia and insulin resistance. For example, in acromegaly where there is over-secretion of growth hormone or in Cushing's syndrome where there are high levels of glucocorticoids such as cortisol.

These other types of diabetes are covered in more detail in endocrinology or clinical medicine textbooks.

Metabolic effects of diabetes mellitus
IDDM
In IDDM, the absence of insulin leads to the unopposed action of glucagon and the other catabolic hormones, which results in high levels of catabolic processes, that is, the breakdown of carbohydrate, protein, and fat (see Fig. 7.8). This leads to hyperglycaemia, ketoacidosis,

hypertriglyceridaemia and also weight loss. The tissues are glucose deficient despite lots of glucose in the blood: 'starvation in the midst of plenty'. As cells cannot obtain glucose from the diet they have to obtain it by the breakdown of body stores or by synthesizing it from non-carbohydrate precursors (gluconeogenesis).

 A lot of people liken diabetes to starvation but there are some very important differences that can lead to fatal consequences for a diabetic patient (Fig. 12.1).

Important differences between diabetes and starvation		
Feature	IDDM	Starvation
insulin	absent or very low	low, i.e. not stimulated
blood glucose	hyperglycaemia	normal blood glucose is maintained
ketone body formation (see Chapter 4)	uncontrolled: ↑↑production of ketone bodies where rate of formation >> rate of use; this can lead to life-threatening, severeketoacidosis as the pH of blood can fall to dangerously low levels	controlled and regulated; usually rate of formation = rate of use

Fig. 12.1 Important differences between diabetes and starvation.

NIDDM

The metabolic effects are essentially the same as for IDDM but usually they are milder because insulin is present, but:

- The amount of insulin secreted from the pancreas may be inadequate to cope with the blood glucose level.
- Tissues or 'target organs' fail to respond correctly to insulin, that is, they become resistant to it.

In NIDDM, insulin resistance may be due to a number of defects, for example, an abnormal insulin receptor or a defect in a glucose transporter. Insulin resistance by the liver results in uncontrolled glucose production and a decreased uptake by the peripheral tissues. Both lead to hyperglycaemia. Hyperglycaemia leads to increased insulin secretion by the pancreas. A lot of these patients

are obese and it is thought that overeating leads to a constantly elevated blood glucose, which overstimulates insulin secretion. The elevated levels of insulin cause a down-regulation in the number of insulin receptors on adipose cells and thus a decreased response to insulin. In fact, the number of insulin receptors has been shown to increase if weight is lost but this is only a proposed mechanism.

Clinical features

IDDM

The clinical features and diagnosis of IDDM are covered in Fig. 12.2. The treatment consists of:

- Diet, ensuring the correct content and timing of meals. The diet should be high in fibre and unrefined carbohydrate, low in saturated fat and refined carbohydrate.
- Insulin. There are three main types of insulin: short acting, which is soluble and used in emergencies, intermediate acting, and long-acting. The duration of action of insulin is increased by complexing it with a protamine salt and/or varying the size of the crystals.
- Education: it is crucial that patients understand their disease.

Clinical features and diagnosis of IDDM	
Main clinical features	Diagnostic criteria
classically:	presence of symptoms
• acute onset of symptoms (2-4 weeks) polyuria, polydipsia, accompanied by weight loss and tiredness	raised random blood glucose, >11.1 mmol/L
	fasting blood glucose: venous plasma ≥7.8 mmol/L or whole blood ≥6.7 mmol/L
• ketoacidosis: may present in diabetic coma	(oral glucose tolerance test is not necessary—reserved for borderline cases; glycosuria is not diagnostic due to variation in renal threshold in population)

Fig. 12.2 Clinical features and diagnosis of insulin-dependent diabetes mellitus.

There are a number of possible methods for monitoring the control of diabetes and these are covered in detail in Chapter 11. They include:

- Measuring blood glucose levels, using reagent strips based on the glucose oxidase reaction.
- Monitoring the percentage of glycosylated haemoglobin (HbA$_{1c}$). This provides a measure of the average blood glucose control over the last 6–8 weeks.

- Measuring the serum fructosamine concentration, which measures glycaemic control over the preceding two weeks (rarely used).
- Presence of ketones in blood or urine.
- Long-term monitoring for chronic complications.

NIDDM
The diagnosis, management, and treatment of NIDDM are covered in Fig. 12.3.

Complications of diabetes
These arise when diabetes is poorly controlled.

Acute
- **Hypoglycaemia.** The aim of treatment of IDDM with insulin is to maintain a normal blood glucose level, which decreases the long-term effects of diabetes. However, too much insulin or infrequent 'top ups' of blood glucose because of insufficient intake of

Diagnosis, management, and treatment of NIDDM	
Clinical features	**Management**
• insidious onset: tiredness, polyuria, thirst, weight loss	**diet**: often the only treatment necessary
• usually older and may be obese	**oral hypoglycaemic drugs:** 2 main types:
• may be asymptomatic — detection of ↑ blood glucose on routine check-up	• sulphonylureas, e.g. glibenclamide: ↑ insulin secretion by islet cells (inhibits ATP-sensitive K$^+$ channels in b cell membranes)
diagnosis: as for IDDM — symptoms usually less severe	• biguanides, e.g. metformin: ↑ glucose uptake by peripheral tissues and ↓ glucose production by liver
	N.B. new drug —acarbose inhibits intestinal enzyme, glucosidase and therefore delays the digestion of starch
	insulin sometimes necessary when poorly controlled

Fig. 12.3 Diagnosis, management, and treatment of NIDDM.

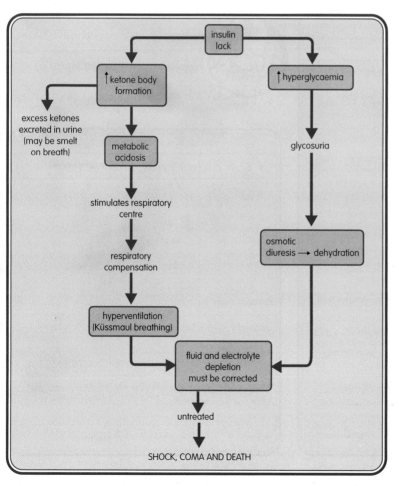

Fig. 12.4 Diabetic ketoacidosis. In the absence of insulin, hyperglycaemia causes an osmotic diuresis. The loss of fluid and electrolytes results in dehydration. Increased ketogenesis causes a metabolic acidosis. Respiratory compensation results in hyperventilation. The dehydration is more life-threatening than the acidosis and must be corrected first.

carbohydrate lead to a low blood glucose (hypoglycaemia). Hypoglycaemia causes unpleasant autonomic symptoms such as sweating, nausea, palpitations, and more severe neuroglycopenic symptoms as a result of a decrease in glucose supply to the brain: drowsiness, unsteadiness, confusion, and coma (these patients look almost drunk). This is a very serious condition and must be treated without delay with an intravenous 50% dextrose infusion. Mild hypoglycaemia can be treated with sugar or sweet drinks.

- **Diabetic ketoacidosis**. In the absence of insulin, effects of glucagon are unopposed. Decreased uptake of glucose by tissues, coupled with an increased hepatic glucose production leads to hyperglycaemia. This causes an osmotic diuresis, and the resulting loss of fluid and electrolytes results in dehydration. An increase in lipolyisis leads to increased ketogenesis and a metabolic acidosis.

Respiratory compensation results in hyperventilation. Failure to treat a patient in ketoacidosis may result in coma and death. The dehydration is more life-threatening than the hyperglycaemia and must be corrected first (Fig. 12.4).

Chronic
Well-controlled diabetes (i.e. when the blood glucose is strictly controlled) decreases the frequency and progression of microangiopathy (not macroangiopathy) (Fig. 12.5).

Enzyme deficiencies of the glycolytic and pentose phosphate pathways
Red cell enzyme deficiencies
Some enzyme defects are only expressed in red blood cells (RBCs) (Fig. 12.7). RBCs lack mitochondria and rely on glycolysis for ATP production. ATP is necessary for:

- The maintenance of RBC membrane flexibility and shape, enabling their passage through small vessels.

Some long-term complications of diabetes mellitus	
Complications	**Mechanism**
diabetic microangiopathy affects small blood vessels: in eyes: causes retinopathy and cataracts kidneys: causes nephropathy peripheral and autonomic nervous system: causes neuropathy	**1. sorbitol (polyol) pathway** (see Fig. 2.42): glucose is converted to sorbitol by aldose reductase found particularly in lens, retina, Schwann cells of peripheral nerves, and kidney in diabetes, hyperglycaemia leads to increased sorbitol formation in these tissues as they do not require insulin for glucose entry sorbitol cannot be metabolized further or leave these cells and therefore it accumulates; it exerts a strong osmotic effect causing cells to swell causing damage **2. glycation of proteins** haemoglobin is non-enzymatically glycosylated to form HbA_{1c} other proteins may also be glycated, which may mediate some of the damage as glycation may increase their oxidative potential
diabetic macroangiopathy affects large blood vessels causing accelerated atherosclerosis	precise mechanism is unknown increased formation of athero-sclerotic plaques leads to increased risk of myocardial infarction, stroke, and peripheral vascular disease

Fig. 12.5 Some long-term complications of diabetes mellitus.

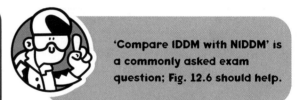

'Compare IDDM with NIDDM' is a commonly asked exam question; Fig. 12.6 should help.

Comparison of IDDM and NIDDM		
	IDDM type I	**NIDDM type II**
usual age of onset	young < 25 years	> 35 years
autoimmune factors	yes	no
genetic factors	risk associated with certain HLA types	yes—polygenic inheritance
concordance identical twins	50%	almost 100%
symptoms	polyuria, polydipsia, weight loss	similar but usually less severe presentation
signs	wasting, dehydration, loss of consciousness	obesity
ketosis	prone	rarely; precipitated by stress
obesity	infrequent	frequent

Fig. 12.6 Comparison of IDDM and NIDDM.

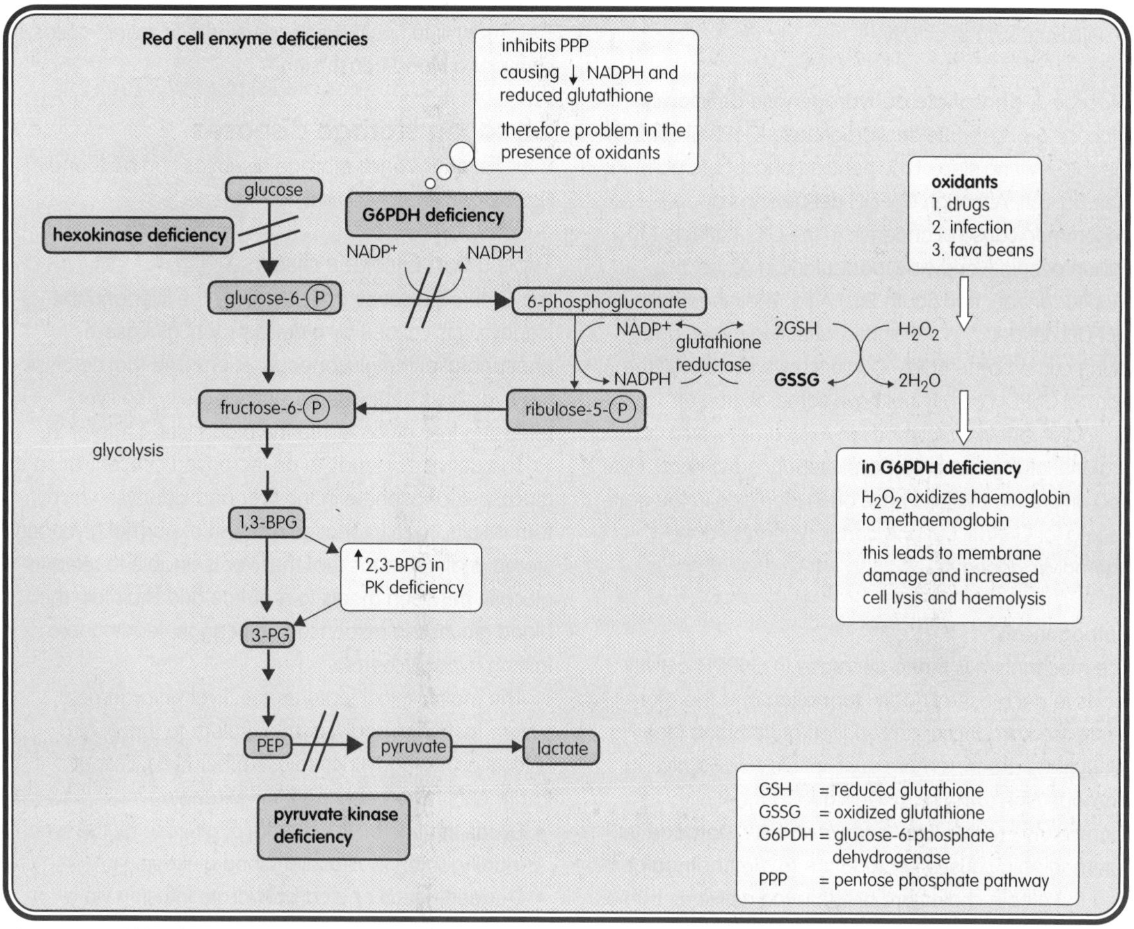

Fig. 12.7 Red blood cell enzyme deficiencies.

- The maintenance of ATP-dependent pumps in RBC membranes for osmotic equilibrium.

The pentose phosphate pathway in RBCs provides the NADPH necessary to keep glutathione in a reduced state; glutathione protects RBCs from oxidative damage (see Chapter 3). A failure of these pathways leads to:

- Decreased membrane flexibility and 'leakiness' of RBCs.
- The oxidation of haemoglobin and an increase in RBC breakdown, leading to haemolysis and a haemolytic anaemia.

Pyruvate kinase deficiency

This is a rare, autosomal recessive disorder. In homozygotes, pyruvate kinase activity in RBCs is about 5–20% of normal. It is the most common glycolytic enzyme defect and causes a chronic haemolytic anaemia.

Pathogenesis

In pyruvate kinase deficiency the rate of glycolysis and production of ATP is inadequate to maintain the energy requirements of the cell and the membrane structure. Alteration in cell shape creates distorted 'prickle' shaped cells, which are rigid and more sensitive to phagocytosis by cells of the reticuloendothelial system, mostly macrophages. Therefore, RBCs have a shorter life span leading to increased haemolysis. Inhibition of pyruvate kinase leads to an accumulation of earlier glycolytic intermediates, especially 2,3-bisphosphoglycerate (2,3-BPG). 2,3-BPG decreases the affinity of haemoglobin for oxygen, allowing greater unloading of oxygen to the tissues, which therefore decreases the severity of the anaemia (see Chapter 2). A diagnosis is based on:

- Presence of anaemia.
- Blood film showing prickle cells and an increased number of reticulocytes (red cell precursors).

- Pyruvate kinase activity.

Glucose-6-phosphate dehydrogenase deficiency

Glucose-6-phosphate dehydrogenase (G6PDH) controls the rate-limiting step of the pentose phosphate pathway (see Fig. 3.1). Although G6PDH deficiency is an uncommon cause of anaemia in the UK, it affects 130 million people worldwide, particularly in Africa, the Mediterranean, and South-East Asia. The inheritance of G6PDH deficiency is sex-linked, affecting males and being carried by females. Carriers have about half the normal G6PDH activity but have some degree of protection against *Plasmodium falciparum* which causes malaria, giving carriers an evolutionary advantage. Over 400 different mutations have been identified in the gene coding for G6PDH but only certain variants cause haemolytic anaemia.

Pathogenesis

The mechanism is that a decrease in G6PDH activity leads to decreased NADPH formation and therefore decreased production of reduced glutathione (see Fig. 12.7). RBCs are thus more susceptible to oxidative damage (see Chapter 3). Damage to the RBC membrane creates 'bite' or 'blister' cells. Damage to haemoglobin causes its oxidation to methaemoglobin and the globin chains are precipitated as Heinz bodies. Both can be observed on the blood film during a haemolytic crisis.

There are two types of G6PDH deficiency: type A is commonly found in Afro-Caribbeans. The G6PDH activity falls with increasing cell age, that is, when the cells are first made they have a normal enzyme activity. Type A is self-limiting and mild. Type B is commonly found in people of Mediterranean descent and is more serious. The enzyme activity is reduced throughout the life span of the cell. Any factor that causes oxidative stress leads to a large intravascular haemolysis.

The precipitating factors that cause oxidative stress and haemolysis are:

- Drugs: antibiotics (sulphamethoxazole), antimalarials (quinine, primaquine), and antipyretics (aspirin).
- Infection is the most common precipitating factor.
- Favism, only in type B. Consumption or even the inhalation of the pollen of fava beans (broad beans) leads to haemolysis.
- Neonatal jaundice.

Treatment is to avoid precipitants and, in severe cases, consider a blood transfusion.

Glycogen storage diseases

A full list of glycogen storage diseases can be found in Fig. 2.36. They are all rare.

Type I: von Gierke's disease

von Gierke's disease affects mainly the liver and the kidneys. It is caused by a deficiency of glucose-6-phosphatase, the gluconeogenic enzyme that catalyses the hydrolysis of glucose-6-phosphate in the liver, releasing free glucose into the blood (see Chapter 2).

The deficiency leads to an increased concentration of glucose-6-phosphate in the liver and kidneys, which in turn results in an increased amount of normal glycogen stored. It also means that the liver is unable to release glucose between meals to regulate and maintain the blood glucose in response to glucagon, leading to a fasting hypoglycaemia.

The main clinical features are: liver enlargement, severe fasting hypoglycaemia, failure to thrive, and ketosis as the body tries to use other fuels. Lots of treatments have been tried, for example:

- Drugs that inhibit the uptake of glucose by the liver leading to an increase in blood glucose.
- Frequent feeds or a carbohydrate infusion via a nasogastric tube to maintain the blood glucose.

Type V: McArdle's syndrome

McArdle's syndrome affects muscle. It is a deficiency of muscle glycogen phosphorylase; the liver enzyme is normal. Therefore, the muscle has a high level of normal glycogen because it cannot break it down. During exercise, the decreased level of muscle phosphorylase means that glycogen stores cannot be used as fuel. Increased blood lactate is not seen after exercise because of insufficient glycolysis. Therefore, these patients have a decreased exercise tolerance. Otherwise, they have a normal life span and development.

Errors of galactose metabolism

Galactose metabolism is covered fully in Chapter 2.

Galactosaemia

Galactosaemia is a rare, autosomal recessive disorder arising because of a deficiency in the enzyme galactose-1-phosphate uridyl transferase (see Fig. 2.40). Occasionally, it is caused by deficiency in galactokinase or UDP-hexose-4-epimerase. The formation of UDP-galactose is prevented, meaning that galactose cannot be converted into glucose-6-phosphate.

The disease presents in neonates when lactose-containing milk feeds are introduced. As galactose cannot be converted into glucose, the babies become hypoglycaemic. This results in galactosaemia, galactosuria, and a build-up of toxic metabolic by-products. This can lead to a high concentration of galactose in the lens of the eye where it is reduced by aldose reductase to galactitol, which is thought to facilitate cataract formation. An accumulation of galactitol also occurs in nerve tissue, liver, and kidneys leading to liver damage and mental retardation.

The clinical features are poor feeding, vomiting, jaundice, hypoglycaemia, and hepatosplenomegaly. Eventually, liver failure, cataracts, and severe mental

retardation occur if the condition is left untreated. The treatment is a lactose and galactose-free diet.

Errors of fructose metabolism

Errors of fructose metabolism are autosomal recessive disorders which occur as a result of a deficiency in one of the key enzymes involved in fructose metabolism; they are shown in Fig. 12.8 (see also Fig. 2.39).

Fructokinase deficiency: essential fructosuria

This is a benign, asymptomatic condition caused by an absence of fructokinase. All the fructose has to be metabolized by the hexokinase pathway, leading to a high concentration of fructose in the blood and fructose accumulation in the urine.

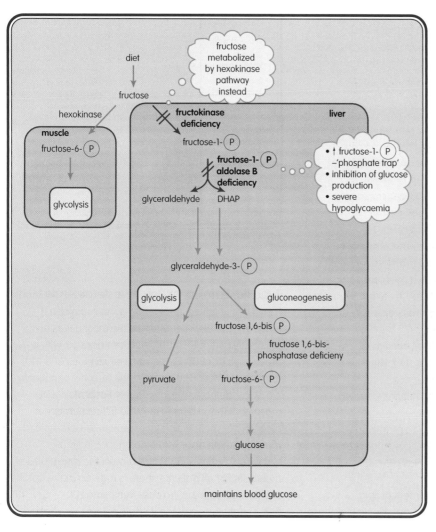

Fig. 12.8 Some errors of fructose metabolism.

Fructose-1-phosphate aldolase deficiency: hereditary fructose intolerance

Fructose-1-phosphate aldolase (aldolase B) cleaves fructose-1-phosphate to dihydroxyacetone phosphate and glyceraldehyde allowing the entry of fructose into glycolysis or gluconeogenesis (see Fig. 12.8). Deficiency leads to the accumulation of fructose-1-phosphate in the tissues, that is, phosphate is 'trapped' in fructose-1-phosphate, leading to a decrease in available phosphate. This leads to the inhibition of both glycogen phosphorylase (glycogenolysis) and aldolase A (glycolysis and gluconeogenesis) because they are normally activated by phosphorylation. This causes the inhibition of glucose production, leading to hypoglycaemia.

Clinically, fructose-1-phosphate aldolase deficiency presents as soon as a baby is weaned on to fructose-containing foods. Features include hypoglycaemia, vomiting, and eventually liver failure. Treatment is by the removal of fructose and sucrose from the diet.

- Discuss the aetiology and metabolic effects of the two main types of diabetes and describe the clinical features, diagnosis, and treatment of each.
- Describe the complications of diabetes, both acute and long term.
- Give two examples of RBC enzyme deficiencies and their mechanisms or pathogenesis.
- Describe galactosaemia and its effects.
- Give two examples of errors of fructose metabolism and their consequences.

METABOLISM

The hyperlipidaemias

This is a group of inherited disorders of lipid metabolism. Fig. 4.26 shows the classification of these disorders based on the Fredrickson classification. Here, the main clinical features of the more important hyperlipidaemias are considered.

Type I: Familial lipoprotein lipase or apolipoprotein-C2 deficiency

This is a rare, autosomal recessive disorder due to either a deficiency of the enzyme lipoprotein lipase (LPL), or apolipoprotein-C2 required for the activation of LPL. It results in a failure of the clearance of chylomicrons from the bloodstream, therefore it is also called familial chylomicronaemia. Its main clinical features, diagnosis and management are discussed in Fig. 12.9.

Clinical features and diagnosis of type I hyperlipidaemia		
Clinical features	**Diagnosis**	**Management**
presents in childhood with: • eruptive xanthomas • lipaemia retinalis and retinal vein thrombosis • recurrent abdominal pain • risk of pancreatitis • hepatospleno-megaly	based on the presence of high levels of chylo-microns in fasting sample of plasma stored overnight in morning, white layer at top of sample due to chylomicrons which float like cream N.B. plasma triacylglycerol is much greater than cholesterol	depends on serum triacylglycerol concentration: < 2.0 mmol/L = normal 2.0–6.0 mmol/L = minor problem; check other risk factors > 6.0 mmol/L = at risk; start low fat diet with medium chain fatty acids because these are absorbed directly from gut, i.e. not packaged as chylomicrons

Fig. 12.9 The clinical features and diagnosis of type I hyperlipidaemia, familial LPL deficiency.

Type IIa: Familial hypercholesterolaemia (FH)

Familial hypercholesterolaemia is the commonest inherited lipid disorder and has the most devastating results. It is an autosomal dominant disorder with a prevalence of 1:500 (0.2%) for heterozygotes and $1:10^6$ for homozygotes. The cause in the majority of patients (95%) is a defect in the low density lipoprotein (LDL) receptor: either a decrease in the actual number of receptors or malfunctioning receptors (for example, a mutation in the apo-B100 binding site). A smaller number of patients (5%) have a defective apo-B100 molecule. For all patients, there is a defect in the uptake of LDL, leading to an increase in plasma LDL concentration.

In homozygotes, no LDL receptors are present, leading to severely elevated plasma cholesterol levels, as high as 20 mmol/L. This causes a massive deposition of cholesterol in the arterial walls and skin. These patients usually develop coronary heart disease in childhood and, if untreated, rarely survive to adult life.

The clinical features, diagnosis, and management of familial hypercholesterolaemia are discussed in Fig. 12.10. The prognosis for homozygotes is poor. Plasmapheresis, if used regularly, is successful in the short term. Liver transplantation offers the possibility of a cure. For heterozygotes, the prognosis is reasonable; after treatment; patients tend to develop coronary heart disease about 20 years earlier than the normal population.

Do not confuse familial hypercholesterolaemia with the polygenic form, common hypercholesterolaemia.

Type IIb: Familial combined hyperlipidaemia

Familial combined hyperlipidaemia is relatively common with a prevalence of 1:300. The genetic basis is unclear but it is probably autosomal dominant. The abnormality is an overproduction of apolipoprotein-B leading to an increased very low density lipoprotein (VLDL) secretion from the liver which results in an increased plasma LDL. Usually, both plasma cholesterol and triacylglycerol are elevated (Fig. 12.11).

Type III: Remnant hyperlipidaemia (familial dysbetalipoproteinaemia)

Remnant hyperlipidaemia (familial dysbetalipoproteinaemia) is rare, with a prevalence of 1:10 000. It occurs due to inheritance of an abnormal apolipoprotein-E molecule (usually via the apo-E2 allele). It results in the increased accumulation of IDL remnants in the blood. Patients have an increased risk of coronary heart disease.

The clinical features are xanthomata in palmar creases (which are actually reasonably diagnostic) and tuberous xanthomata over the knees and elbows.

The diagnosis is made by measurement of a raised total cholesterol and triacylglycerol, and electrophoresis of the serum, showing a broad 'β-band' due to excess IDL remnants (see Fig. 11.13).

Type IV and V: Familial hypertriglyceridaemia

Type IV

This is the mild form of hypertriglyceridaemia. The prevalence is 1:600. It is an autosomal dominant disorder caused by an increased synthesis of VLDL by the liver, leading to a raised plasma VLDL.

Type V

This is the severe form of hypertriglyceridaemia. Other risk factors such as obesity and alcohol are also implicated in its aetiology, leading to an increase in plasma VLDL and chylomicrons.

Clinical features of FH	
Clinical Features	**Diagnosis and Management**
homozygotes: tendon xanthomata: thickening of Achilles tendon and xanthomata over extensor tendons of fingers xanthelasma: white yellow fatty deposits in skin of eyelid premature arcus senilis: thin white rim around iris of eye	**diagnosis:** fasting cholesterol > 16 mmol/L **management:** • diet: very low in cholesterol and saturated fat • drugs: statins, cholesterol binding resins, nicotinic acid (see Fig. 14.27) • low density lipoprotein removal by plasmapheresis • liver transplant • gene therapy: trials are underway
heterozygotes: • as above but not as severe • may have no physical signs	**diagnosis:** fasting cholesterol > 8 mmol/L **management:** • diet • drugs

Fig. 12.10 The clinical features of familial hypercholesterolaemia.

Clinical features and diagnosis of familial combined hyperlipidaemia	
Clinical features	**Diagnosis and management**
skin manifestations are usually present: • xanthelasma • arcus senilis N.B. ↑ risk of CHD	**diagnosis:** ↑ low density lipoprotein and ↑ triacylglycerol (TG) with a positive family history treatment is aimed at reducing cholesterol to < 6.5 mmol/L and TG to < 2.0 mmol/L **management:** • diet • fibrates reduce both cholesterol and TG and ↑ high density lipoprotein

Fig. 12.11 The clinical features and diagnosis of familial combined hyperlipidaemia.

Clinical features

Physical signs are only seen with the severe form, for example, eruptive xanthomata and lipaemia retinalis. Plasma triacylglycerol is vastly higher than the plasma cholesterol. The increased triacylglycerol results in an increased risk of pancreatitis.

Treatment

The treatment is diet, aiming to reduce body weight and to modify any co-existing factors, for example, alcohol, diabetes, or obesity. Drugs used include fibrates, nicotinic acid derivatives which decrease VLDL synthesis, and fish oils.

Common hypercholesterolaemia

This includes patients who have a raised serum cholesterol but do not have familial hypercholesterolaemia. It has a polygenic inheritance, that is, it is influenced by several genes. The plasma cholesterol is not as high as in familial hypercholesterolaemia and is influenced by the environment (e.g. diet). If plasma cholesterol levels are plotted for the population, they follow a normal distribution curve; patients with common hypercholesterolaemia have levels above the 95% confidence interval. Dietary treatment alone is often successful.

Errors of fatty acid metabolism

Medium chain fatty acyl CoA dehydrogenase deficiency

Medium chain fatty acyl CoA dehydrogenase deficiency has an incidence of 1:10 000 births. It is thought that the deficiency of this enzyme leads to a decreased oxidation of fatty acids and therefore an increase in and a greater reliance on glucose oxidation. When glycogen reserves become exhausted, severe hypoglycaemia occurs. It is believed that this is the cause of death in some cases of sudden infant death syndrome (cot death).

Jamaican vomiting sickness

This is believed to be caused by eating the unripe fruit of the ackee tree. The fruit contains a toxin, hypoglycin, which is in fact an unusual amino acid that inhibits both short and medium chain acyl CoA dehydrogenases. This results in the inhibition of β oxidation and therefore the oxidation of glucose takes place instead. Once glycogen reserves are depleted, hypoglycaemia occurs.

- What are the approximate prevalences and aetiologies of the main hyperlipidaemias?
- Describe the clinical features, diagnostic criteria, and management of type I–III hyperlipidaemias.
- What are the risk factors for coronary heart disease?
- Give two examples of errors in fatty acid metabolism.

Hyperlipidaemias lead to an increased risk of coronary heart disease. Other risk factors for coronary heart disease are:
- Modifiable: smoking, obesity, exercise, hypertension, diabetes mellitus, and stress.
- Non-modifiable: age (risk increases with age), sex (men are at a higher risk), family history.

These should always be taken into account when assessing risk.

DISORDERS OF AMINO ACID METABOLISM

Disorders of amino acid metabolism are rare inborn errors of metabolism that result in severe developmental abnormalities if left untreated.

Phenylketonuria

Phenylketonuria (PKU) is an autosomal recessive disorder that is caused by the deficiency of the enzyme phenylalanine hydroxylase. In a small number of patients it may be due to a deficiency in the enzymes that synthesize its co-factor tetrahydrobiopterin (see Fig. 5.3). The disease is characterized by an increased plasma phenylalanine level. It has a prevalence of 1:10 000–20 000 live births.

Mechanism

Normally, phenylalanine hydroxylase catalyses the hydroxylation of phenylalanine to tyrosine. Tyrosine is an extremely important amino acid: it is the precursor of dopamine, catecholamines, and melanin. In PKU, phenylalanine accumulates in the plasma and tissues and is converted into the phenylketones: phenylpyruvate, phenyllactate, and phenylacetate; these are not normally produced in significant amounts. High levels of phenylalanine may impair development and in the long-term can cause mental retardation (Fig. 12.12).

Treatment of phenylketonuria is by restriction of dietary phenylalanine. However, phenylalanine is an essential amino acid, therefore too much dietary restriction can also cause poor growth and neurological symptoms. Tyrosine cannot be made in patients with PKU and becomes an essential amino acid.

Pregnancy

In PKU patients, the restriction of dietary phenylalanine should be for life. It is particularly important during pregnancy when hyperphenylalaninaemia in the mother may damage the foetus, causing microcephaly, mental retardation, and heart defects.

Alkaptonuria

Alkaptonuria is a rare, autosomal recessive disorder with a prevalence of 1:100 000. It is caused by a deficiency of the enzyme homogentisic acid oxidase, normally involved in the breakdown of tyrosine to fumarate (Fig. 12.13). Unlike other amino acid disorders, it does not produce serious effects until adult life.

Mechanism

The enzyme deficiency leads to an accumulation of homogentisate, which polymerizes to produce a black–brown pigment that is deposited in cartilage and other connective tissue. This process is called ochronosis.

Clinical features

Joint damage and arthritis. Homogentisate is excreted in the urine; on standing, the urine turns black because of the formation of alkapton. Sweat may also be black. There is no specific treatment.

Clinical features and diagnosis of PKU	
Clinical features	**Diagnosis and management**
central nervous system symptoms: untreated, presents at 6–12 months with development delay, failure to thrive, and seizures	all neonates are screened for raised phenylalanine levels at 5–7 days, when milk feeding is established (so the phenylalanine levels are adequate); part of Guthrie test
hypopigmentation: many affected infants are fair-haired, blue eyed, and pale, since phenylalanine inhibits tyrosinase which converts tyrosine to melanin	**management:** • restriction of dietary phenylalanine • blood phenylalanine levels are monitored regularly and maintained in the normal range to allow normal growth and development

Fig. 12.12 Clinical features and diagnosis of phenylketonuria.

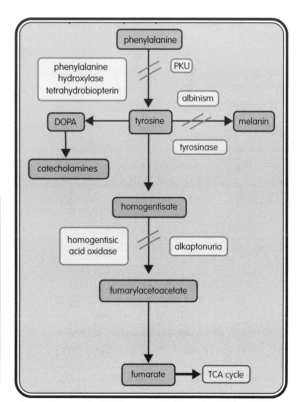

Fig. 12.13 Enzyme deficiencies in alkaptonuria, albinism, and phenylketonuria (PKU).

Albinism

Albinism is a deficiency of the enzyme tyrosinase which converts tyrosine into melanin. It has an incidence of 1:13 000. The clinical features and management of albinism are discussed in Fig. 12.14.

Disorders of amino acid metabolism are all rare autosomal recessive disorders, which mostly present in neonates with failure to thrive and developmental delay; the treatment is a restricted diet.

Clinical features and management of albinism	
Clinical features	**Management**
amelanosis: • whitish hair, pale skin, and grey–blue eyes • low pigment in iris and retina leads to failure to develop fixation reflex; resulting in nystagmus, photophobia, and constant frowning • pale skin leads to sunburn and skin cancer	tinted contact lenses from early infancy may allow development of normal fixation in some patients high sun protection long-term results in severe visual impairment

Fig. 12.14 Clinical features and management of albinism.

○ **Name the enzyme defect present in each amino acid disorder and describe the biochemical consequences of each.**
○ **Name the main clinical features and treatment of each amino acid disorder.**

Histidinaemia, homocystinuria, and maple syrup urine disease

These three diseases are described in Fig. 12.15.

Other amino acid disorders			
Disorder	**Enzyme defect**	**Biochemical feature**	**Clinical features**
histidinaemia 1:10 000	histidase	↑ histidine in blood and urine	mental retardation
homocystinuria (rare)	cystathionine synthetase (see Fig. 5.5)	↑ homocysteine in urine ↑ methionine in blood	failure to thrive, progressive mental retardation, and dislocation of lens in eye
maple syrup urine disease 1:200 000 (very rare)	branched chain α-ketoacid dehydrogenase (see Chapter 5)	↑ excretion of branched chain amino acids, valine, leucine and isoleucine and their α-ketoacids in plasma and urine; compounds smell like maple syrup	neonates present with metabolic acidosis, hypoglycaemia, and seizures delay in diagnosis leads to neurological problems

Fig. 12.15 Other amino acid disorders.

DISORDERS OF PURINE AND PYRIMIDINE METABOLISM

Lesch–Nyhan syndrome

Lesch–Nyhan syndrome is a very rare, X-linked disorder caused by an almost complete absence of the salvage enzyme hypoxanthine–guanine phosphoribosyl transferase (HGPRT). HGPRT catalyses the addition of 5-phosphoribosyl-1-pyrophosphate (PRPP) to the purine bases, guanine and hypoxanthine, in the salvage pathway, that is, it recycles free bases (see Fig. 6.10). In Lesch–Nyhan syndrome a decreased level of HGPRT results in:

- Increased guanine and hypoxanthine in excess of their requirements, which are broken down to form large amounts of uric acid leading to severe hyperuricaemia and gout.
- Increased levels of PRPP, which is therefore used for the de novo synthesis of purines, leading to purine overproduction and severe neurological disturbances.

The salvage pathway for adenine is normal. It is thought that the level of HGPRT activity is related to the severity of symptoms. For example:

- If HGPRT activity is less than 2%, moderate mental retardation is present.
- If HGPRT activity is less than 0.2%, severe mental retardation and self-mutilation occurs.

The prognosis is very poor; sufferers usually die by the age of 5 years. The clinical features and diagnosis of Lesch–Nyhan syndrome are discussed in Fig. 12.16.

Gout

The prevalence of gout varies from about 0.1–0.2% in Europe to as high as 10% in the Maori population of New Zealand. It is caused by an abnormality of uric acid metabolism resulting in hyperuricaemia and the deposition of sodium urate crystals in joints, soft tissues, and the kidney (Fig. 12.17).

The risk factors are that:

- Gout predominantly affects men in middle life. It does not occur before puberty (unless it is part of Lesch–Nyhan syndrome).
- In women, it only occurs after the menopause (the male to female ratio is 8:1).
- It is an obvious inherited condition in some families.
- Poor diet, alcohol, exercise, and stress all increase lactic acid levels, which increases the precipitation of uric acid (lactic acid competes with uric acid for excretion in the kidney).

Causes of gout

Genetic

- Decreased HGPRT levels; to 2–5% of normal. Similar to Lesch–Nyhan syndrome but not as severe.
- Overactive PRPP synthetase. The enzyme is involved in the regulation of purine biosynthesis (see Chapter 6). Overactivity causes the release from normal control leading to increased rates of de novo synthesis of purines.
- Insensitive PRPP amidotransferase, the rate-controlling enzyme of purine synthesis. A mutant form has full activity but no regulatory sites, therefore feedback control is lost, causing overproduction of purines.

Clinical features and treatment of Lesch–Nyhan syndrome	
Clinical features	**Diagnosis and treatment**
hyperuricaemia causing: • kidney stones • arthritis • gout severe neurological disturbances: • spasticity and mental retardation • self-mutilation (bite fingers and lips to the bone) symptoms begin at about 3 months	• orange nappy (urine) • hypoxanthine–guanine phosphoribosyl activity • symptoms **treatment:** • allopurinol lowers uric acid levels and helps to control gout and arthritis • with time, high purine levels result in worsening of neurological symptoms because no treatment is possible • boys usually die from kidney failure because of high sodium urate deposits causing kidney stones

Fig. 12.16 Clinical features and treatment of Lesch–Nyhan syndrome.

Clinical features and diagnosis of gout	
Clinical features	**Diagnosis**
hyperuricaemia recurrent attacks of acute arthritis caused by deposition of sodium urate crystals in joints; usually only one joint affected (big toe > 90%) kidney stones and ↑ chance of renal disease tophi under skin and around joints	synoval fluid examination: affected joint is aspirated and fluid examined under micro-scope for long, needle shaped, negatively birefringent crystals serum uric acid is not very reliable; hyperuricaemia does not necessarily cause gout

Fig. 12.17 Clinical features and diagnosis of gout.

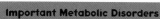
The excess purines produced in these conditions are broken down to uric acid, leading to hyperuricaemia and gout.

Secondary causes
- Increased purine turnover, for example, in leukaemia, myeloproliferative disorders, and due to the use of cytotoxic drugs in control of cancers.
- Decreased excretion of uric acid, for example, drug therapy (thiazides, aspirin), lead toxicity, excess alcohol.

Management of gout
Acute attacks are treated with anti-inflammatory drugs:
- Non-steroidal anti-inflammatory drugs (e.g. indomethacin) provide relief within 24–48 h.
- Colchicine works slowly and is rarely used. It inhibits the migration of neutrophils into the joint by its action on microtubules.
- Intramuscular adrenocorticotrophic hormone is effective in difficult cases.

Long-term prophylaxis is aimed at decreasing uric acid levels.
- Simple measures are weight reduction, decreased alcohol intake, and withdrawal of drugs such as salicylates and thiazides.
- Allopurinol is a xanthine oxidase inhibitor (see Chapter 6 for its mechanism of action). It is the main drug used for prophylaxis of gout.
- Probenecid, a uricosuric drug, is an alternative to allopurinol. It has a direct action on the renal tubule, preventing the re-absorption of uric acid in the kidney, causing it to be excreted.

Aspirin is absolutely contraindicated in gout because it impairs the excretion of uric acid by the renal tubules, aggravating hyperuricaemia.

- What are the causes and the main clinical features of Lesch–Nyhan syndrome?
- What are the main causes and risk factors for gout?
- Describe the main clinical features and management of the gout.

DISORDERS OF HAEM METABOLISM

The porphyrias
This is a group of rare, inherited disorders in which there is a partial deficiency of one of the enzymes of haem synthesis (see Fig. 6.21). This results in the inhibition of haem synthesis and thus the formation of excessive quantities of either porphyrin precursors, for example, δ-aminolevulinic acid (ALA) or porphobilinogen (PBG), or porphyrins themselves depending upon which enzyme is deficient (Fig. 12.18).

The inhibition of haem synthesis leads to decreased haem formation. The key, rate-controlling enzyme of haem synthesis is ALA synthase, which is normally inhibited by haem (see Fig. 6.22). In porphyrias, the absence of haem releases the inhibition (and thus the control) of ALA synthase, resulting in the increased formation of intermediates preceding the defective enzyme in each porphyria.

When porphyrin precursors are produced in excess (ALA and PBG), they cause mainly neuropsychiatric symptoms and abdominal pain (the precursors are neurotoxins). When porphyrins themselves are produced in excess, they cause photosensitive skin changes (that is, the skin burns and itches on exposure to light). This is because porphyrins absorb light, which excites them and induces the formation of free oxygen radicals. These can attack membranes, particularly lysosomal membranes, leading to the release of enzymes which damage underlying layers of skin, rendering it susceptible to the light.

Porphyrias are diagnosed on the basis of symptoms and the pattern of porphyrins and their precursors present in the blood and urine.

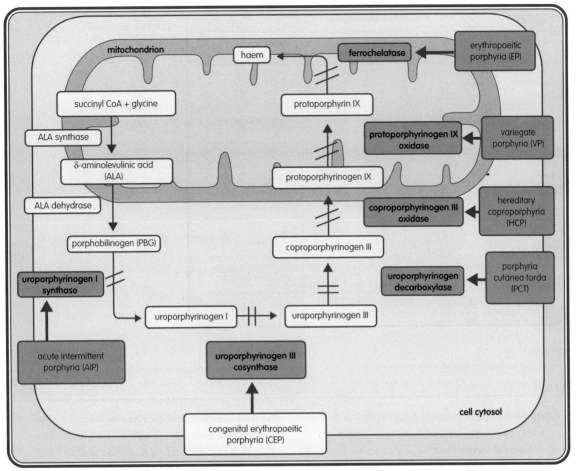

Fig. 12.18 Sites of enzyme deficiency in porphyrias.

Porphyrias are classified as either hepatic or erythropoeitic or acute and chronic (Fig. 12.19). They are all rare; the most common in the UK is acute intermittent porphyria. The major features of each porphyria are now considered.

Acute intermittent porphyria

Acute intermittent porphyria is an autosomal dominant disease with a prevalence in the UK of 1:100 000. The defect is a deficiency of uroporphyrinogen I synthase. Characteristically, acute attacks are separated by long periods of remission. The attacks are precipitated by various factors including alcohol, barbiturates, oral contraceptives, and certain antibiotics.

Clinical features
Presentation is usually in early adult life with a mixture of:

- Acute abdominal symptoms.
- Neuropathy.
- Neuropsychiatric symptoms: depression, anxiety, and even frank psychosis.

Biochemistry
Increased levels of PBG and ALA can be found in the urine of these patients. The urine also darkens to a port wine colour on exposure to air, due to the presence of PBG. The classic bedside test for excess PBG is to add Ehrlich's reagent to urine, which causes it to go pink; the colour persists when excess chloroform is added.

Management
The treatment is with fluids, pain relief, and a high carbohydrate diet, which inhibits the pathway. Avoid precipitants. Intravenous haemin can be given.

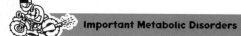

Summary of porphyrias				
Porphyria	Enzyme defect	Photo-sensitivity	Neurological symptoms	Biochemistry
acute intermittent (hepatic)	uroporphyrinogen I synthase		yes	urine: ↑ δ-aminolevulinic acid and porphobilinogen
congenital erythropoeitic	uroporphyrinogen III cosynthase	yes		red cell: ↑UROgen I urine: ↑UROgen I and COPROgen I
cutaneous (hepatic)	uroporphyrinogen decarboxylase	yes		urine: ↑UROgen I and III faeces: ↑COPROgen
hereditary coproporphyria (hepatic)	coproporphyrinogen III oxidase	yes	yes	urine: ↑ ALA, PBG and COPROgen III
variegate (hepatic)	protoporphyrinogen IX oxidase	yes	yes	urine: ↑ PBG and ALA faeces: ↑ PROTOgen IX, COPROgen III
erythropoeitic	ferrochelatase	yes		red cell: ↑ protoporphyrin

Fig. 12.19 A summary of porphyrias.

Congenital erythropoeitic porphyria

Congenital erythropoeitic porphyria is an extremely rare autosomal recessive disease that presents usually before 5 years of age. The defect is a deficiency of uroporphyrinogen III cosynthase. There are no neurological symptoms. In RBCs, increased levels of uroporphyrinogen I leads to severe photosensitivity. Increased levels of both uroporphyrinogen I and coproporphyrinogen I are found in the urine.

Porphyria cutanea tarda (cutaneous hepatic porphyria)

Porphyria cutanea tarda is an autosomal dominant condition. The defect is a deficiency of uroporphyrinogen decarboxylase. The condition has a high frequency in Europe and South America. There are no neurological symptoms.

Main clinical features are:
- Photosensitive rash
- Skin fragility.
- Hyperpigmentation.

Precipitants are alcohol, oestrogens, iron, and the autoimmune condition systemic lupus erythematosus.

The main biochemical changes include:
- Increased uroporphyrinogen I and III in the urine.
- Increased faecal coproporphyrinogen.
- Abnormal liver function tests.
- Mild iron overload.

Hereditary coproporphyria

Hereditary coproporphyria is a very rare autosomal dominant disease. The defect is a coproporphyrinogen III oxidase deficiency. It has an acute presentation with similar features to acute intermittent or variegate porphyria. However, patients may also be photosensitive. Increased levels of coproporphyrinogen III occur in both urine and faeces.

Variegate porphyria

Variegate porphyria is a rare autosomal dominant disease. The defect is a protoporphyrinogen oxidase deficiency. It presents acutely in the same way as acute intermittent porphyria but patients are also photosensitive. Increased levels of PBG and ALA are found in the urine. Increased levels of protoporphyringen IX and coproporphyrinogen III can be found in the faeces.

Erythropoeitic porphyria

Erythropoeitic porphyria is an autosomal dominant condition. The defect is a deficiency of ferrochelatase , the last enzyme of the pathway.

Clinical features.

These patients may present with either:
- Photosensitive rash.
- Gallstones.
- Liver disease.

Biochemistry

Diagnosis is made by fluorescence of peripheral RBCs because they contain free porphyrin. An increase in free protoporphyrin in RBCs, faeces, and bile is also observed and may lead to mild anaemia.

Overall management

The effects of all porphyrias can be decreased by intravenous haemin which inhibits ALA synthase, the rate-controlling enzyme, regaining the control of haem synthesis. An increased dietary intake of anti-oxidant vitamins A, C, and E also helps to protect against free radical damage.

Lead poisoning

The human body contains about 120 mg of lead. Excessive ingestion or inhalation can result from contaminated food, water, or air. Commonly in the UK the sources are old lead piping and petrol. As mentioned in Chapter 6, lead inhibits three key enzymes of haem synthesis, resulting in the accumulation of intermediates:
- ALA dehydrase leads to the accumulation of ALA,which can be measured in urine.
- Coproporphyrinogen III oxidase leads to the accumulation of coproporphyrinogen III.
- Ferrochelatase leads to the accumulation of protoporphyrin IX in RBCs, causing fluorescence.

The result is the inhibition of haem synthesis and anaemia. Lead also binds to bone. The main clinical features and diagnostic criteria are discussed in Fig. 12.20.

Treatment

Treatment is with lead chelators such as Ca-EDTA, D-penicillamine, or British Anti-Lewisite. They all bind lead, forming a complex which can be excreted in the urine.

Clinical features and diagnosis of lead poisoning	
Clinical features	**Diagnosis**
acute exposure: • severe weakness, vomiting, abdominal pain, anorexia, and constipation **chronic exposure:** • causes staining of teeth and bones, myopathy, peripheral neuropathy, renal damage, and sideroblastic anaemia • eventually causes lead enceph-alopathy and seizures • may cause mental retardation in children	blood lead levels > 800 mg/L are toxic urine: ↑ δ-aminolevulinic acid levels red cell: ↑ porphyrin levels and fluorescence blood film: anaemia with punctate basophilia; red cells may contain small, blue deposits

Fig. 12.20 Clinical features and diagnosis of lead poisoning.

Porphyrias are very rare. You will seldom see or be asked about them. Fig. 12.19 summarizes all you will ever need to know.

◦ **Name the types of porphyrias, the enzyme deficiency found in each, and how the deficiency influences the type of symptoms found.**
◦ **Give the diagnosis and biochemistry of each of the porphyrias.**
◦ **Name the three enzymes inhibited by lead.**
◦ **Describe the clinical features and treatment of lead poisoning.**

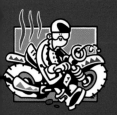

13. Important Nutritional Disorders

DISORDERS OF PROTEIN NUTRITION AND ENERGY BALANCE

Protein–energy malnutrition

Protein–energy malnutrition (PEM) occurs when the body's need for protein or energy, or both, is not met by the diet (see Chapter 8).

Causes of PEM

These can be one or a combination of the following
- Decreased dietary intake.
- Malabsorption.
- Increased requirement; for example, in preterm infants, infection (septic state increases catabolism), major trauma, or surgery.
- Psychological; for example, depression or anorexia nervosa.

In developing countries, PEM manifests as two conditions in children:
- Marasmus: lack of protein and energy.
- Kwashiorkor: lack of protein only—energy supply is adequate.

Incidence

In developing countries, 20–75% of children less than 5 years of age have some form of malnutrition. Five million children die every year because of malnutrition.

Aetiology and mechanisms of pathogenesis

Marasmus

Marasmus is the childhood form of starvation (Figs 13.1 and 13.2). Both protein and energy are limited leading to a low concentration of insulin but increased levels of glucagon and cortisol, that is, a starved state (see Chapter 7). As no fuel is available for the body, muscle and fat are broken down to provide energy, which leads to wasting. Muscle protein is broken down to amino acids which are used for the synthesis of albumin by the liver; therefore, there is no oedema.

Kwashiorkor

Translated this means the 'disease the first child gets

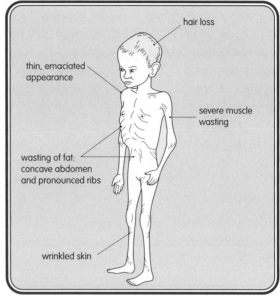

Fig. 13.1 Marasmus.

The features of marasmus	
Clinical features	Signs
very thin, wasted appearance	plasma albumin is usually **normal**
obvious muscle wasting and loss of body fat; < 60% normal body weight	diarrhoea and infection may be present
usually < 18 months old	electrolyte disturbances: low potassium and sodium common
no oedema	
wrinkled skin, hair loss, and apathy	anaemia

Fig. 13.2 The features and signs of marasmus.

when the second child is born'. In Kwashiorkor severe protein deficiency occurs but energy is maintained (Figs 13.3 and 13.4). It usually occurs when a young child is weaned from breast feeding because of the arrival of a new baby. The first child is fed a low protein, high starch diet instead. Kwashiorkor often develops after an acute infection, such as measles or gastroenteritis, when the demand for protein is increased.

As energy is not limiting, there is a high insulin to glucagon and cortisol ratio. Amino acids are taken up by muscle for protein synthesis. This diverts amino acids

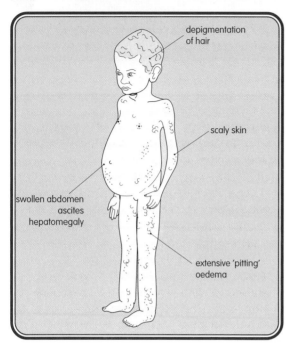

- depigmentation of hair
- scaly skin
- swollen abdomen
  ascites
  hepatomegaly
- extensive 'pitting' oedema

Fig. 13.3 Kwashiorkor.

The features of kwashiorkor	
Clinical features	**Signs**
oedema: 'hides' severe wasting of underlying tissues	**low plasma albumin**
usually 2–4 years of age	diarrhoea and infection usually present
scaly skin: 'flaky paint' rash with hyperkeratosis	low potassium, sodium, glucose, and other electrolyte disturbances
depigmentation of hair	
distended abdomen caused by ascites and enlarged fatty liver	anaemia: due to folate, iron, or copper disturbances
hypothermia and bradycardia	
apathy	

Fig. 13.4 The features of kwashiorkor.

from the liver so fewer are available for albumin synthesis: the resulting low albumin levels reduce the plasma oncotic pressure, causing oedema. The oedema causes a deceptively fat appearance and children are known as water or 'sugar' babies. It is possible there may also be some degree of energy loss in kwashiorkor and therefore other factors may contribute to or cause the oedema. For example:

- Excessive generation of free radicals causing membrane damage and oedema.
- Infection diverts protein synthesis from albumin to the synthesis of immunoglobulins and acute phase proteins (c-reactive protein).

A comparison of kwashiorkor and marasmus is given in Fig. 13.5.

Management and treatment of PEM
It is important to restore fluid and electrolyte balance first. Following this:

- Any infection, hypothermia or hypoglycaemia present can be treated.
- Re-feed initially, just enough to maintain a steady state that is to satisfy the normal daily requirement. Milk is often given with flour or maize slowly and regularly.
- Eventually, high energy foods are given to restore weight and also any necessary vitamin and mineral supplements.

Prognosis
Mortality rates for children with severe malnutrition are about 50%. The rate is so high because adequate treatment is usually not available.

Consequences of prolonged PEM
Malnourished children are less active and more apathetic; these behavioural abnormalities are usually reversed by re-feeding. However, severe, prolonged

A comparison of marasmus and kwashiorkor		
Feature	**Marasmus**	**Kwashiorkor**
deficiency	protein and energy	protein only
age	usually < 18 months	older: 1–5 years
oedema	absent	present
	severe wasting body protein and fat	hides wasting of body protein
body weight	< 60% normal	60–80% normal
cause	severe malnutrition	malnutrition
		free radical damage
		infection or anything which increases protein requirements
features	wrinkled skin	scaly skin and dermatitis
	hair loss	sparse, depigmented hair
	thin and emaciated	deceptively fat
		distended abdomen
		hepatomegaly

Fig. 13.5 A comparison of marasmus and kwashiorkor.

malnutrition causes much reduced brain growth and permanent damage to both physical and mental development. Immunity is impaired leading to delayed wound healing; protein loss from muscle may eventually include the diaphragm, leading to death. The physiological effects of severe prolonged malnutrition are listed in Fig. 8.6.

Prevention

Prevention of childhood malnutrition is a World Health Organization priority. The main targets are to provide:

- Food supplements and additional vitamins to 'at risk' groups.
- Family planning.
- Immunization programmes.

However, the occurrence of drought, famine, and war in affected countries makes these targets practically impossible to achieve.

Malnutrition in adults in developing countries has symptoms similar to those seen in children but the results are not as devastating. This is because adults are already physically and mentally mature and are thus more resilient.

Obesity

Obesity is defined as having a body mass index (BMI) of greater than 30 (see Chapter 8 for details). Most people as they get older develop some degree of obesity.

Aetiology

Fig. 8.5 discusses some of the proposed theories for obesity. Twin studies suggest a genetic factor and this is now backed up by recent evidence identifying a gene for obesity. However, genetic factors are clearly greatly influenced by environmental and socio-economic factors, for example, poor education, high alcohol intake, and less energy expenditure, all of which increase the incidence of obesity. The increase in obesity seen in the lower social classes may be related to the type of food consumed, which is largely governed by financial status. One conclusion that can be made is that obesity occurs when energy intake is much greater than energy expenditure. The reasons for overeating are usually complex and may be psychological in origin, for example, related to stress or a life event but, generally, not a metabolic cause.

Clinical consequences

The effects of obesity are clearly recognizable. In obese patients, there is an increased morbidity and mortality, mainly from heart disease, stroke, and diabetes. Therefore obesity is associated with an increased risk of:

- Coronary heart disease. There is a linear increase in morbidity and mortality caused by coronary heart disease with obesity.
- Hypertension.
- Non-insulin dependent diabetes mellitus (NIDDM). Obesity results in persistently high insulin levels, leading to a down-regulation of insulin receptors and thus insulin resistance by the tissues.
- Breathlessness and respiratory problems.
- Stroke.
- Gallstones. Especially if fat, female, forty, and fertile!
- Osteoarthritis and back pain.
- Gout.

Morbidity is the incidence of disease. Mortality is the number of deaths.

Treatment

Treatment of obesity is generally unsatisfactory. Possibilities include:

- Reduction of energy intake. The main treatment of an obese patient is an appropriate diet, with plenty of support and encouragement from a doctor. Most diets allow an intake of 1000 kcal/day. This must be a balanced intake of protein, carbohydrate, and fat (i.e. a mixed diet). The only way to lose weight is a prolonged moderation of intake and then a permanent change in eating habits to maintain the weight loss.
- Increase energy expenditure, provided there are no contraindications, for example, severe heart problems.
- Drug therapy is not generally recommended in the UK. Appetite suppressants such as fenfluramine (a

sympathomimetic) are occasionally used in severely obese patients, but usually they have very little effect. They are only licensed for use for a short period of time under supervision because they can cause serious side effects and dependence.

- Surgery. This is extreme and rarely performed now because of the complications involved. Examples include: jaw wiring, gastric plication (stapling the walls of the stomach together to form a smaller stomach), bypass of the small intestine, and gastric distension.

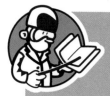

- ○ **Name the main causes of marasmus and kwashiorkor and at least five features of each.**
- ○ **Describe the management and consequences of protein–energy malnutrition.**
- ○ **What are the clinical consequences of obesity and its treatment?**

THE FAT-SOLUBLE VITAMINS: DEFICIENCY AND EXCESS

Vitamin A: retinol
Deficiency
Incidence
Vitamin A deficiency is rarely seen in developed countries because liver stores are sufficient to last 3–4 years. It is commonly found in children in developing countries such as India and parts of South-East Asia, where about 500 000 children each year are blinded as a result of vitamin A deficiency.

Causes
Vitamin A deficiency may be caused by a decreased dietary intake, however, this is usually only seen in very severe malnutrition. It may also occur secondary to fat malabsorption.

Clinical features
In the eye, the symptoms are progressive:
- Initially, deficiency causes impaired dark adaptation and night blindness. This is reversible.
- Severe prolonged deficiency results in

xerophthalmia: a dryness of the cornea and conjunctiva due to progressive epithelial keratinization. 'Bitot's spots' may be seen, which are white plaques of keratinized epithelial cells on the conjunctiva.

- If untreated, keratomalacia develops, causing corneal ulceration and the formation of opaque scar tissue (cataracts); this causes irreversible blindness.

In the skin, decreased epithelial cell turnover produces:
- Thickening and dryness of skin due to hyperkeratosis.
- Impaired mucosal function.

Diagnosis and treatment
Diagnosis and treatment is usually on the basis of the above clinical features. The following can also be measured:
- The plasma concentration of vitamin A and retinol binding protein.
- The response to replacement therapy.

Urgent treatment with vitamin A (as retinol palmitate) orally or intramuscularly prevents blindness. If the deficiency is severe and has already caused keratomalacia, eyesight cannot be restored. It is interesting to note that vitamin A is also used successfully to treat a number of skin problems, including acne (Fig. 13.6).

Uses of vitamin A in the treatment of skin disorders	
Condition	**Treatment**
moderate acne anti-ageing	topical retinoic acid (all *trans* retinoic acid)
severe disfiguring acne	isotretinoin (13-*cis* retinoic acid) orally
psoriasis	acitretin (both are contraindicated in pregnancy as they are teratogenic)

Fig. 13.6 Uses of vitamin A in the treatment of skin problems.

Toxicity
Hypervitaminosis A
Hypervitaminosis A is a serious toxic syndrome.

Excessive intake of vitamin A causes:
- Dry, itchy skin: dermatitis.
- Mucus membrane defects and hair loss.
- Hepatomegaly.
- Thinning and fracture of the long bones.
- Increased intracranial pressure.

Toxicity is very unlikely with normal sources but must be taken into account when prescribing high levels of retinoic acid for severe acne sufferers.

Teratogenicity
Pregnant women must not exceed 3.3 mg/day because vitamin A causes congenital defects. Therefore, they must avoid vitamin A supplements or eating liver because it contains about 13–40 mg of vitamin A per 100 g. Isotretinoin treatment for acne is absolutely contraindicated in pregnancy

Vitamin D: cholecalciferol
Vitamin D is involved in calcium homeostasis (see Fig. 8.9).

Deficiency
Causes
- Decreased dietary intake of vitamin D.
- Inadequate exposure to sunlight of the correct wavelength.
- Renal disease leads to inadequate formation of the active form 1,25-dihydroxycholecalciferol.
- Liver disease leads to decreased formation of 25-hydroxycholecalciferol (precursor to active form).
- Fat malabsorption, for example, due to coeliac disease or after surgery (gut resection).

Groups at risk of deficiency are:
- Children and women of Asian origin.
- Elderly and housebound individuals.
- Babies breast-fed in winter because light of the correct wavelength for production of vitamin D is not available for mothers.
- Vegans (vitamin D is not present in food of plant origin).

Clinical features and pathogenesis
Vitamin D deficiency disrupts calcium homeostasis and bone mineralization (Fig. 13.7). In children, this causes rickets; in adults, it causes osteomalacia. These disorders are covered later in this chapter with calcium deficiency.

The diagnosis and treatment of vitamin D deficiency	
Diagnosis	**Treatment**
low or normal serum calcium	exposure to sunlight
low phosphate	daily oral vitamin D supplements cures rickets and osteomalacia, continue until alkaline phosphatase returns to normal
increased serum alkaline phosphatase	
X-rays show defective mineralization	ensure adequate calcium intake

Fig. 13.7 Diagnosis and treatment of vitamin D deficiency.

A disruption of calcium homeostasis also causes hypocalcaemia and hypophosphataemia (low plasma calcium and phosphate). This may cause symptoms of neuromuscular irritability, numbness, parasthesiae, tetany and, eventually, seizures.

Toxicity
Vitamin D is the most toxic of all vitamins. It is fat soluble, stored in the body, and slowly metabolized. Normally, it is well tolerated but, in high doses, over a period of time, it can cause hypervitaminosis D. This condition presents with nausea, vomiting, and muscle weakness. Very high levels of vitamin D result in greatly increased rates of calcium absorption and bone resorption, causing hypercalcaemia and calcium deposition in tissues, particularly the arteries, heart, liver, kidneys, and pancreas. This is known as metastatic calcification and may interfere with the correct functioning of the organs, possibly causing renal stones, calcification of other arteries, and heart failure.

Vitamin E: tocopherol
Deficiency
Incidence
In humans, vitamin E deficiency is very rare and is seen virtually only in:
- Premature infants, causing haemolytic anaemia of the newborn. Vitamin E crosses the placenta in the last trimester of pregnancy; therefore, premature infants have only small vitamin E stores. Their red blood cell (RBC) membranes are fragile and are susceptible to free radical damage, leading to lysis of RBCs. Vitamin E supplements are given to pregnant mothers to prevent this.
- Children and adults, secondary to severe fat malabsorption, for example, biliary atresia, cholestatic liver disease, or a lipoprotein deficiency (e.g. abetalipoproteinaemia).

Clinical features

Vitamin E deficiency causes muscle weakness, peripheral neuropathy, ataxia, and nystagmus. In children with abetalipoproteinaemia, vitamin E therapy can prevent severe spinocerebellar degeneration and gross ataxia occurring. Animal studies with rats have shown that vitamin E deficiency causes muscular dystrophy and sterility; this is not true in humans.

Toxicity

Vitamin E is the least toxic of all the fat-soluble vitamins. The use of vitamin E supplements helps to protect against the development of heart disease by protecting low density lipoproteins (LDL) from oxidation by free radicals. Oxidized LDL is taken up more readily by macrophages, forming foam cells which initiate the formation of atherosclerotic plaques.

Vitamin K

Vitamin K is a co-enzyme required for the γ-carboxylation of clotting factors II, VII, IX, and X, activating them and thus the clotting cascade.

Deficiency

A true deficiency is rare because most of the body's vitamin K is synthesized by bacteria in the gut.

Causes

The main causes of vitamin K deficiency are:

- A decreased level of bacteria in the gut, for example, due to long-term antibiotic therapy.
- A decrease in dietary intake.
- Newborn babies have sterile guts and therefore cannot initially make vitamin K.
- Oral anticoagulant drugs (e.g. warfarin) are vitamin K antagonists (Fig. 13.8).

Mechanism

A deficiency of vitamin K results in low levels of the vitamin K-dependent clotting factors II, VII, IX, and X and thus inhibition of the clotting cascade. Patients will have an increased tendency to bleed and to bruise.

Diagnosis and treatment

The diagnosis and treatment of vitamin K deficiency is covered in Fig. 13.9.

Deficiency in newborn babies

Newborn babies have sterile guts and thus have no

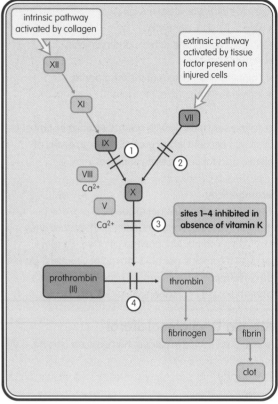

Fig. 13.8 Vitamin K deficiency: inhibition of the clotting cascade.

The diagnosis and treatment of vitamin K deficiency	
Diagnosis	**Treatment**
clinical features: bruising and bleeding, e.g. in urine or from GI tract increased prothrombin time increased APTT (activated partial thromboplastin time)	vitamin K supplements

Fig. 13.9 Diagnosis and treatment of vitamin K deficiency.

bacteria to make vitamin K. Since human milk is a very poor source, babies are particularly susceptible to deficiency. Vitamin K deficiency causes **haemorrhagic disease of the newborn**, which can occur either in the first week of life or between weeks 1 and 8. Usually, the bleeding is minor but it can result in major bleeds, leading to intracranial haemorrhage. About 50% of children with major bleeds end up permanently disabled or die. Therefore, every newborn baby in the UK is given prophylactic intramuscular or oral vitamin K.

For each fat-soluble vitamin describe:
- The main causes and clinical features of their deficiency disease.
- A basic idea of the diagnosis and the treatment available.
- The effects and problems of toxicity.

THE WATER-SOLUBLE VITAMINS: EFFECTS OF DEFICIENCY

Vitamin B₁: thiamin deficiency
Beriberi
Incidence
Beriberi (Fig. 13.10) is now seen only in the poorest areas of South-East Asia where the staple food is polished rice, that is, the husk which contains most of the vitamins, including thiamin, has been removed.

Diagnosis
Diagnosis is by measurement of the transketolase activity in RBCs, before and after the addition of thiamin pyrophosphate (TPP). A greater than 30% increase in activity with TPP, indicates a deficiency.

Treatment
Treatment is initially by intramuscular injections of thiamin for approximately 3 days (varies according to severity) followed by daily, oral supplements of thiamin. For wet beriberi, treatment results in a dramatic decrease in oedema and a quick improvement of symptoms. For dry beriberi, there is a slower improvement.

Wernicke–Korsakoff syndrome
Incidence
As thiamin is present in most foods, a dietary deficiency is rare in developed countries. The deficiency manifests itself as Wernicke's encephalopathy (Fig. 13.11). In the UK, a low thiamin intake is seen in:
- Chronic alcoholics: alcohol inhibits the uptake of thiamin.
- The elderly.
- People with diseases of the upper gastrointestinal tract (e.g. gastric cancer).

Types of beriberi		
	Clinical features	Signs
wet beriberi	oedema: spreads to involve the whole body → ascites and pleural effusions congestive heart failure	raised JVP tachycardia and tachypnoea
infantile beriberi	a form of wet beriberi that occurs in breastfed babies whose mothers are thiamin deficient	acute onset: anorexia and oedema that can involve the larynx → aphonia tachycardia and tachypnoea develop → death
dry beriberi	gradual, symmetrical, ascending peripheral neuropathy resulting in progressive paralysis	initially, stiffness of legs → weakness, numbness, and 'pins and needles' ascends to involve trunk, arms and eventually brain

Fig. 13.10 Types of beriberi.

Wernicke's encephalapathy and Korsakoff's psychosis	
Clinical features	Causes
Wernickes' encephalopathy: • acute confusional state • ataxia; cerebellar signs • ophthalmoplegia and nystagmus • peripheral neuropathy diagnosis: made on clinical assessment; condition is reversible with immediate thiamin therapy	alcohol ischaemic damage to brainstem and connections may be genetic element major cause of dementia in developed countries
if untreated it may develop into Korsakoff's psychosis: a severe irreversible amnesic syndrome characterized by loss of short-term memory	progresion from untreated Wernicke's encephalopathy

Fig. 13.11 Clinical features of Wernicke's encephalopathy and Korsakoff's psychosis.

Niacin deficiency
Pellagra: a disease of the skin, gastro-intestinal tract, and central nervous system
Incidence
Pellagra is rare and is found in areas where maize is the staple food. It is now seen only in certain parts of Africa. Maize contains niacin in a biologically unavailable form, niacytin. Niacin can only be removed from the maize by alkali treatment (Mexicans soak maize in lime juice to release the niacin). Pellagra (Fig. 13.12) can also occur in conditions in which large amounts of tryptophan are metabolized for example, carcinoid syndrome, which is also rare.

Causes
The causes of pellegra are:
- A dietary deficiency of niacin.
- A deficiency of protein (as niacin is made from tryptophan, see Chapter 8).
- Vitamin B_6 and thus pyridoxal phosphate deficiency (pyridoxal phosphate is a co-factor for niacin synthesis from tryptophan).
- Hartnup's disease: a failure to absorb tryptophan from the diet (Fig. 5.23).
- Isoniazid treatment for tuberculosis inhibits vitamin B_6, causing a decrease in tryptophan synthesis.

Clinical features of pellagra	
Clinical features	**Symptoms**
3Ds: **dermatitis**; deficiency of NAD, inhibits DNA repair of sun-damaged skin (Fig. 8.17)	photosensitive symmetrical skin rash occurs when skin is exposed to sunlight: • skin may crack and ulcerate • on neck, called Casal's necklace; extent depends on area of skin exposed
diarrhoea	may also see glossitis and angular stomatitis
dementia	dementia occurs in chronic disease and is usually irreversible; may develop tremor and encephalopathy

Fig. 13.12 Clinical features and symptoms of pellagra.

Diagnosis
Diagnosis is by the measurement of niacin or its metabolites (N-methylnicotinamide or 2-pyridone) in the urine.

Treatment
As niacin can be formed from tryptophan, treatment involves:
- High-dose niacin supplements.
- A high protein diet.

Mild cases are reversible, dementia usually is not and may lead to death.

Vitamin B_6: pyridoxine deficiency
Causes
A dietary deficiency is extremely rare but may be seen in:
- Newborn babies fed formula milk.
- Elderly people and alcoholics.
- Women taking oral contraceptives.
- Patients on isoniazid therapy for treatment of tuberculosis.

Isoniazid binds to pyridoxal phosphate to form an inactive hydrazone derivative, which is rapidly excreted thus causing the deficiency.

Clinical features
The main features include:
- Hypochromic, microcytic anaemia.
- Secondary pellagra.
- Convulsions and depression.

Treatment
Vitamin B_6 supplements are given to all patients on isoniazid therapy. A deficiency caused by an increased requirement due to either a physiological or pathological state or due to the action of an antagonistic compound (e.g. isoniazid) is called a 'vitamin dependency state'.

Vitamin B_{12}: cobalamin deficiency
Causes of deficiency
Reduced intake, for example, by vegans because vitamin B_{12} is only found in animal-derived foods. Reduced absorption caused by:
- A lack of intrinsic factor, for example in pernicious anaemia.
- Diseases of the terminal ileum (the site of B_{12} absorption), for example, Crohn's disease or tuberculosis.
- Bypass of the B_{12} absorption site, for example, fistulae or surgical resection of gut.
- Blind-loop syndrome: parasites compete for B_{12}.

Body stores (mainly in the liver) are large relative to the daily requirement, therefore a reduced intake alone takes about 2–3 years to cause a deficiency.

Pernicious anaemia
Pernicious anaemia is the commonest cause of vitamin B_{12} deficiency.

Incidence
It is commoner in older women and is often associated with fair-haired and blue-eyed individuals, and also the presence of other auto-immune disorders, for example, thyroid and Addison's disease.

Pathogenesis
Pernicious anaemia is an auto-immune disorder where antibodies are made to either:
- Gastric parietal cells, causing atrophy or wasting of the cells thus preventing the production of intrinsic factor and stomach acid (Fig. 13.13a).
- Intrinsic factor itself (Fig. 13.13b); the antibodies bind to the intrinsic factor preventing it from either binding to vitamin B_{12} (blocking antibodies) or binding to the receptors in the terminal ileum (binding antibodies). A lack of intrinsic factor leads to a decreased uptake of vitamin B_{12}. The clinical features of pernicious anaemia are discussed in Fig. 13.14.

Diagnosis
Diagnosis is performed by analysis of the blood film and bone marrow specimens and by the Schilling test which measures the absorption of vitamin B_{12}.
- Radioactive vitamin B_{12} is given orally.
- A 24-h urine collection is performed to measure the percentage of radioactive vitamin B_{12} excreted in the urine.
- If the subject is vitamin B_{12} deficient, less than 10% will be excreted because the vitamin B_{12} is being used to replenish depleted stores.
- If the result is abnormal, the test is repeated with the addition of intrinsic factor.
- If excretion is now normal, the diagnosis is pernicious anaemia.

Treatment
The treatment of vitamin B_{12} deficiency is 3-monthly intramuscular injections of hydroxycobalamin for life. Initially, these are more frequent to fill the stores.

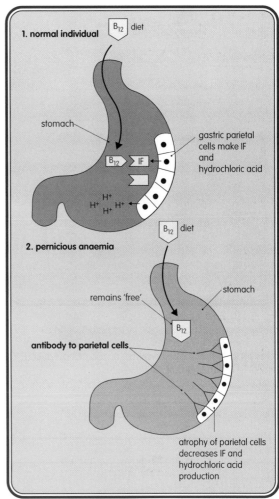

Fig. 13.13a Antibodies in pernicious anaemia. **1.** In normal individuals, vitamin B_{12} released from food in the stomach becomes bound to intrinsic factor (IF) produced by gastric parietal cells. **2.** In individuals with pernicious anaemia antibodies to the gastric parietal cells cause wasting of the cells and thus prevent production of intrinisc factor by them. Vitamin B_{12} is therefore not absorbed resulting in B_{12} deficiency.

Pernicious anaemia carries a slightly increased risk of carcinoma of the stomach.

Folate deficiency
The stores of folate are small relative to the daily requirement therefore a deficiency state can develop in only weeks, particularly if it is associated with a period of rapid growth.

Causes
Decreased intake
A poor diet is the commonest cause, for example, in slimmers, elderly people, and alcoholics.

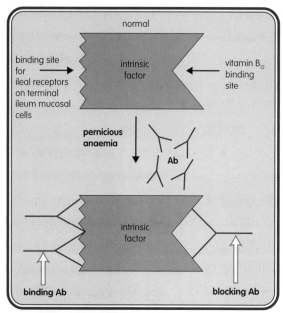

Fig. 13.13b Antibodies to intrinsic factor. Intrinsic factor contains two binding sites; one for vitamin B_{12} and a second one for ileal receptors in terminal ileum, its site of absorption. In pernicious anaemia, antibodies produced may bind to either or both of these sites.

The clinical features and mechanism of pernicious anaemia	
Clinical features	**Mechanism**
megablastic anaemia: blood film: macrocytes (MCV >100 fL) bone marrow: megaloblasts (developing red cells where nuclei mature more slowly than the cytoplasm)	B_{12} deficiency causes secondary folate deficiency, which leads to decreased production of DNA and defective cell division
neurological abnormalities peripheral neuropathy affecting sensory neurons of posterior and lateral columns of spinal cord; leads to subacute combined degeneration of spinal cord	inadequate fatty acid and myelin synthesis caused by B_{12} deficiency alone severe irreversible damage
lemon yellow colour	combination of jaundice from red cell lysis and pallor because of anaemia
glossitis, diarrhoea, and weight loss	
gastric atrophy and achlorhydria (↓ hydrochloric acid production)	antibodies to gastric parietal cells

Fig. 13.14 Clinical features and mechanism of pernicious anaemia.

Increased requirement
During periods of rapid cell growth such as:
- Pregnancy, infancy, or adolescence.
- Cancer, inflammatory states, or recovery from illness.
- Haemolytic anaemias.

Malabsorption
Malabsorption occurs, for example, in coeliac disease or gut resection.

Drugs
- Anticonvulsants (e.g. phenytoin and phenobarbitone)—impair absorption.
- Dihydrofolate reductase inhibitors (e.g. methotrexate).
- Antimalarial drugs (e.g. pyrimethamine).

Secondary to B_{12} deficiency
Vitamin B_{12} is essential to maintain an adequate supply of the active form of folate, that is 5,6,7,8-tetrahydrofolate. Specifically it regenerates THF from N^5-methyl-THF in the methionine salvage pathway (Fig. 6.2). Even if there are adequate amounts of folate in the diet, in the absence of vitamin B_{12}, folate deficiency arises.

Clinical features and diagnosis of folate deficiency
The clinical features and diagnosis of folate deficiency are covered in Fig. 13.15.

Treatment
The treatment of folate deficiency is daily, oral folate supplements.

The clinical features and diagnosis of folate deficiency	
Clinical features	**Diagnosis**
megablastic anaemia: this is identical to vitamin B_{12} deficiency (see Fig. 13.14)	blood film: macrocytes (MCV >100 fL) megaloblasts in bone marrow
growth failure	low serum folate
N.B. peripheral neuropathy and neurological symptoms do not occur in folate deficiency	red cell folate is a better test of folate stores normal = 135–750 mg/mL
	must always consider and eliminate vitamin B_{12} deficiency and malignancy

Fig. 13.15 Clinical features and diagnosis of folate deficiency.

Folate deficiency in pregnancy

It is known that the development of the neural tube in the foetus is dependent on the presence of folic acid. All women planning a pregnancy should take prophylactic folate supplements to reduce the risk of neural tube defects such as spina bifida or anencephaly. The critical time is the first few weeks after conception: women should therefore start supplements before conception to cover this period. A woman who has already had a baby with a neural tube defect has about a 1:20 risk of a second affected baby; the use of folate supplements has been shown to reduce this risk.

A comparison of folate and vitamin B$_{12}$ deficiencies

A comparison of folate and vitamin B$_{12}$ deficiencies is given in Fig. 13.16. A deficiency of either can cause a macrocytic, megaloblastic anaemia. Patients suspected of having either deficiency, must always be investigated for both folate and B$_{12}$ deficiency since the administration of folic acid corrects the anaemia but masks a B$_{12}$ deficiency. Therefore, folate should never be given alone in treatment of pernicious anaemia and other B$_{12}$ deficiency states because it may precipitate an irreversible, peripheral neuropathy.

Vitamin C deficiency: scurvy

This used to be common among sailors who spent weeks at sea without any fresh fruit or vegetables.

Causes

Scurvy is caused by a poor dietary intake of fresh fruit and vegetables. In the UK, it is seen in elderly people, alcoholics, and smokers. Smokers require twice the normal intake of vitamin C (80 mg/day). Humans have about 6 months' store of vitamin C in the body.

Clinical features

The clinical features of scurvy are described in Fig. 13.17.

Treatment

The treatment of vitamin C deficiency is 1 g daily of ascorbate and lots of fresh fruit and vegetables in the diet.

The megadose hypothesis

Some people believe that large doses of vitamin C cure many illnesses, such as the common cold and certain immune-mediated diseases, and even help in cancer prevention and promote fertility. The benefits of large doses are unresolved and under review. It is thought that 1–4 g/day of vitamin C can decrease the severity of symptoms of colds but not decrease the incidence. However, vitamin C is an anti-oxidant and, along with vitamins A and E, is thought to decrease the incidence of coronary heart disease and certain cancers by scavenging free radicals thus preventing oxidative damage to cells and their components.

Vitamin B$_{12}$ deficiency compared with folate deficiency		
Characteristics	Vitamin B$_{12}$	Folate
most common cause	pernicious anaemia	↓ dietary intake
onset	slow, 2–3 years	develops over weeks
neurological symptoms	frequent + severe	never
drug-related	no: vitamin B$_{12}$ deficiency usually causes secondary folate deficiency	yes: anticonvulsants, dihydrofolate reductase inhibitors

folate deficiency occurs frequently on its own because of ↓ intake or ↑ demand |

Fig. 13.16 A comparison of vitamin B$_{12}$ and folate deficiency; main differences.

Clinical features of scurvy	
Clinical features	Diagnosis
• swollen, sore, spongy gums with bleeding; loose teeth • spontaneous bruising and petechial haemorrhages • anaemia • poor wound healing • swollen joints and muscle pain	hypochromic, microcytic anaemia caused by secondary iron deficiency

low plasma ascorbate level (not very accurate)

concentration of ascorbate in white blood cells provides an accurate assessment of tissue stores of ascorbate (usually measure buffy layer ascorbate concentration instead as this provides a reasonable estimation) |

Fig. 13.17 Clinical features of scurvy.

You must know about Wernicke–Korsakoff syndrome, pernicious anaemia, folate deficiency, and scurvy because these are commonly examined.

For each deficiency disease describe:
- The incidence, where in the world they still occur, and two or three causes of each.
- The main clinical features, relating them to the functions of the vitamin concerned (see Chapter 8).
- The main diagnostic criteria and the treatment.

DISORDERS OF MINERAL NUTRITION

The main functions of minerals and trace elements have already been covered in Chapter 8.

Iron deficiency anaemia

Bioavailability
Haem iron, present in meat, is readily absorbed. Inorganic (non-haem) iron, present in vegetables and cereals, is mostly in the oxidized (Fe^{3+}) state and must be reduced for absorption.

Factors affecting bioavailability
- Absorption is favoured in the ferrous (Fe^{2+}) as opposed to the ferric (Fe^{3+}) form.
- Stomach acid and ascorbic acid both favour absorption by reducing iron to the ferrous form.
- Increased erythropoietic activity, for example, due to bleeding, haemolysis, or high altitude, increases absorption.
- Alcohol increases absorption.
- Phosphates and phytates (plants) form insoluble complexes with iron and prevent absorption.

Causes of deficiency

Inadequate intake
This is probably the most common cause of iron deficiency, particularly, in a vegan diet.

Increased requirement:
- In premature babies, because iron is transferred to the fetus during the last trimester of pregnancy.
- During infancy, adolescence, and pregnancy, that is, during periods of increased growth.

Blood loss
1 mL of blood contains 0.5 mg of iron. Therefore, a small blood loss of 3–4 mL/day over a period of weeks to months can cause a chronic iron deficiency. Losses can be from:
- The gut for example, due to peptic ulcers, hiatus hernias, cancer of the stomach or caecum, ulcerative colitis, and so on.
- Menstrual loss, if periods are particularly heavy.

Malabsorption
For example, due to high levels of phytates in the diet; secondary to vitamin C deficiency; or after surgery (partial or total gastrectomy).

Often, there is more than one cause, for example, a poor quality diet and heavy periods in an adolescent.

Groups in the population at risk of deficiency
Infants, toddlers, adolescents, pregnant women, menstruating women, and elderly people are all at risk of iron deficiency.

Clinical features and diagnosis of iron deficiency anaemia
The clinical features and diagnosis of iron deficiency anaemia are covered in Fig. 13.18.

Management and treatment
The treatment for iron deficiency anaemia is oral iron supplements, for example, ferrous sulphate or gluconate. If malabsorption is suspected, use intramuscular or intravenous iron. Iron supplements should be given for long enough to correct the haemoglobin level; when this is normal, iron must then be continued for 3–6 months to replenish stores.

Prognosis
Pathological changes are reversed by adequate replacement therapy.

Clinical features and diagnosis of iron deficiency anaemia	
Signs and symptoms	**Diagnosis**
↓ **production of haemoglobin**: less oxygen reaches the tissues especially the brain and heart muscle causing **pallor, tiredness, giddiness, and heart failure**	**blood tests:** • ↓ haemoglobin, serum ferritin, and iron • ↑ total iron-binding capacity (TIBC) (due to increase in 'free' transferrin
symptoms usually show when haemoglobin < 8 g/dL	
epithelial abnormalities: angular stomatitis (cracked corners of mouth)	**gold standard** for diagnosis of iron deficiency is the absence of iron stores in the bone marrow
glossitis (sore tongue)	**blood film:** microcytic, hypochromic red blood cells (RBC), i.e. small, pale RBCs where: • MCV (mean cellular volume) < 80 fL • MCH (mean cell Hb) < 27 pg
koilonychia (spoon shaped nails)	
	N.B. normal haemoglobin concentration is 13 g/dL in men, 12 g/dL in women

Fig. 13.18 Clinical features and diagnosis of iron deficiency anaemia.

Iron overload
Causes
There are two principal causes of iron overload. There is an inherited form called idiopathic primary haemochromatosis which has a prevalence in the population of 0.5% for homozygotes. Iron overload may also be acquired, where it occurs secondary to an increased administration of iron. This is called transfusional iron overload.

Idiopathic primary haemochromatosis
Pathogenesis
Idiopathic primary haemochromatosis is an autosomal recessive disorder characterized by the excessive absorption of iron in the small intestine. The gene defect is located on chromosome 6. Only homozygotes manifest clinical features; the accumulation of iron is gradual. It usually presents in the fifth decade when levels of iron are about 40–60 g compared with 3–5 g in a normal person. The disease is clinically manifested more commonly in men because women can compensate a certain amount for excessive absorption by menstrual bleeding. The course of the disease depends on the amount of dietary iron and the presence of other dietary factors such as vitamin C or alcohol.

Clinical consequences
Iron is deposited as insoluble haemosiderin forming yellow granules in tissues (Fig. 13.19), which eventually interferes with tissue function. Ultimately, increased iron leads to the increased formation of free radicals, especially the hydroxyl radical (see Chapter 8). This results in the oxidation and destruction of cell membranes and tissues.

Sites of iron deposition	
Tissue	**Effect**
liver	liver fibrosis and pigmentation resulting in cirrhosis and eventually liver failure; may progress to hepatocellular carcinoma (30%)
pancreas	'bronze diabetes': iron damages islet cells causing diabetes mellitus
heart	heart failure
skin	grey/bronze skin colour because of increased production of melanin
testes	impotence
joints	arthropathy

Fig. 13.19 Sites of iron deposition in iron overload.

Treatment and management
The treatment for idiopathic primary haemochromatosis is regular venesection (i.e. removal of blood) to reduce the iron load. Usually about 500 ml are removed, once or twice a week for about 2 years (there are 250 mg of iron in one unit of blood). Plasma iron and ferritin levels are used to monitor the treatment. Once the excess iron is removed, the frequency of venesection is reduced.

Transfusional iron overload: transfusion siderosis
Causes
Repeated blood transfusions over a long period of time can cause iron overload. The ability of the reticuloendothelial cells (spleen, liver, and bone marrow) to store iron is exceeded and iron is deposited at other sites. As with primary iron overload, iron is deposited mainly in the skin, heart, liver, and pancreas. Patients with any condition requiring regular blood transfusions are regarded as 'at risk' (e.g. thalassemia major, aplastic anaemia).

Treatment
Chelation therapy with desferrioxamine is highly effective in chelating the iron, thus enabling its excretion.

Zinc deficiency
Acrodermatitis enteropathica
Acrodermatitis enteropathica is an extremely rare, autosomal recessive disorder that leads to the malabsorption of zinc in the small intestine. It presents in infancy with a severe symmetrical, eczematous rash around orifices and on the hands and feet. Frequently, the lesions become severely infected with *Candida* or bacterial infections, leading to death. Infants may also develop growth retardation, hypogonadism, and poor wound healing.

Treatment
The condition is completely cured by zinc therapy. Zinc deficiency is also a well-recognized complication of parenteral nutrition when insufficient supplementation is given.

Calcium deficiency
In children, calcium deficiency causes rickets (derived from the old English word 'wrickken' meaning to twist). In adults, calcium deficiency causes osteomalacia. They both may occur:
- From dietary deficiency of calcium, seen particularly in developing countries.
- Secondary to vitamin D deficiency. Vitamin D is necessary for the intestinal absorption of calcium and phosphate (Fig. 8.9).
- From malabsorption, for example, due to coeliac disease.

Pathogenesis
Both rickets and osteomalacia are the result of inadequate mineralization of bone, resulting in a reduction in its normal strength, leading to soft, easily deformed bones. The difference is that they occur at different stages of bone development. In rickets the production of underminerulized bone results in a failure of adequate growth, whereas in osteomalacia, demineralization of existing bones leads to an increased risk of fractures.

Rickets
The characteristics of rickets are listed in Figs 13.20 and 13.21.

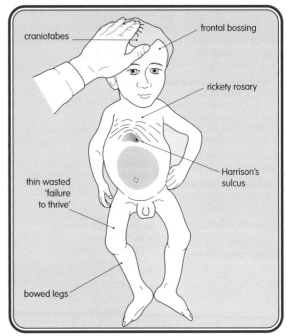

Fig. 13.20 Characteristic deformities of rickets.

Clinical features of rickets	
Clinical features	**Diagnosis**
bowed legs, short stature and failure to thrive	↓ serum calcium and phosphorus
craniotabes: skull bones easily indented by finger pressure	↑ alkaline phosphatase: secreted by osteoblasts to compensate and ↑ bone formation
rickety rosary: expansion or swelling at costochondral junctions	X-rays show defective mineralization of pelvis, long bones and ribs
Harrison sulcus: indrawing of softened ribs along attachment of diaphragm→ 'hollowing'	N.B. low calcium results in ↓ neuromuscular transmission; therefore infant may present with seizures
expansion of metaphyses especially at wrist	
delayed dentition	

Fig. 13.21 The clinical features and diagnosis of rickets.

Treatment is with calcium supplements and education about a balanced diet. Vitamin D supplements may also be required.

Osteomalacia
This disease of adults is seen particularly in elderly people and is usually secondary to vitamin D deficiency. The characteristics of osteomalacia are listed in Fig. 13.22.

Clinical features of osteomalacia	
Clinical features	Diagnosis
spontaneous, incomplete (sub-clinical) fractures often in long bones or pelvis bone pain weakness of proximal muscles causing a proximal myopathy with a characteristic waddling gait	low serum calcium bone biopsy shows increase in non-mineralized bone matrix X-rays show defective mineralization of long bones and pelvis

Fig. 13.22 Clinical features of osteomalacia.

Osteoporosis

This is the progressive reduction of total bone mass usually due to the effects of oestrogen deficiency post-menopause. It is prevented by the use of hormone replacement therapy but calcium is also thought to have a role in its prevention. It is thought that adequate calcium nutrition when young, helps to achieve a peak bone mass and this decreases the effects of loss and osteoporosis in later life. Calcium supplements both before and after menopause, usually with vitamin D, are recommended.

Calcium overload: hypercalcaemia
Causes

The major causes of hypercalcaemia are primary hyperparathyroidism and malignant disease and have nothing to do with nutrition and are therefore beyond the scope of this book. Very rarely, hypercalcaemia is associated with the excessive ingestion of milk and antacids for the control of indigestion. This decreases the renal excretion of calcium: milk–alkali syndrome.

Clinical features

Calcium ions are normally found in cells but calcium salts are restricted to bones and teeth. In overload, calcium salts are deposited in normal tissues leading to tissue 'metastatic calcification' and impaired function. This may cause renal stones, arrhythmias, heart failure, and calcification of the arteries. Muscle weakness, tiredness, anorexia, constipation, and a sluggish nervous response may also be seen.

Copper deficiency
Menkes' kinky hair syndrome

Menkes' kinky hair syndrome is a rare, X-linked disease with an incidence of 1 in 50 000–100 000. It is caused by the defective absorption of copper from the intestine

leading to a decreased synthesis of copper-containing enzymes (Fig. 13.23).

Treatment
Copper therapy has no significant effect. The life expectancy is less than 2 years.

Clinical features of copper deficiency	
Clinical features	Explanation
depigmentation of hair 'steely hair'	↓ tyrosinase and melanin production
arterial degeneration	↓ lysyl oxidase resulting in defective collagen and elastin
neuronal degeneration and mental retardation	↓ catecholamine neurotransmitters
growth failure and anaemia	↓ caeruloplasmin

Fig. 13.23 Clinical features of copper deficiency (refer back to Fig. 8.34 also).

Copper overload
Wilson's disease
Aetiology
Wilson's disease is a rare, autosomal recessive disorder (incidence of 1 in 100 000). The defect has been identified on chromosome 13 and results in failure of the liver to excrete copper in the bile. Copper incorporation into caeruloplasmin is also impaired. Copper accumulates and is deposited in the liver, basal ganglia of the brain, kidneys, and the eyes, causing damage (Fig. 13.24).

Clinical features of copper overload	
Clinical effects of copper accumulation	Diagnosis
liver: chronic hepatitis → cirrhosis **brain**: severe, progressive neurological disability including tremor, mental deterioration and loss of coordination **eyes**: characteristic yellow–brown Kayser–Fleischer rings around corneal limbus	low serum concentration of caeruloplasmin ↑ urinary copper excess copper in liver biopsy

Fig. 13.24 Clinical features of copper overload.

Treatment
Wilson's disease is treated by daily chelation therapy with D-penicillamine. This is very effective at binding copper and eliminating it in the urine. The resulting liver and neurological damage however, is permanent.

Iodine
The human body contains only about 15–20 mg of iodine, most of which is in the thyroid gland. It is essential for the synthesis of the thyroid hormones thyroxine and triiodothyronine.

Deficiency
Endemic goitre: generalized enlargement of the thyroid gland
Endemic goitre occurs in areas where the soil and water lack iodine such that the daily intake is less than 70 µg (usually mountainous areas). In the UK, it used to be found in people in Derby, causing the so-called Derbyshire neck. The problem has now been eliminated in most countries by the addition of iodine to table salt and its prevalence is mostly restricted to developing countries.

Pathogenesis of goitre
Normally, iodine is used to make thyroxine and triiodothyronine. Increased levels of these hormones exert a negative feedback effect on the hypothalamus and anterior pituitary, inhibiting the further release of thyroid-releasing hormone and thyroid-stimulating hormone (Fig. 13.25), resulting in a decrease in their synthesis. However, low levels of iodine decrease thyroxine formation by the thyroid gland. This releases the negative feedback on the hypothalamic-pituitary axis, causing an 'uncontrolled' increase in thyroid-stimulating hormone secretion. High levels of TSH overstimulate the thyroid gland causing hyperplasia of the thyroid epithelium and generalized enlargement (Fig. 13.26). The addition of iodine to the diet should reverse this effect.

Cretinism
Pregnant mothers who are deficient in iodine may give birth to babies who are hypothyroid. Growth and mental development in these babies are severely impaired, sometimes irreversibly so. The diagnosis is made by a neonatal screening test, called the Guthrie test which is performed on all newborn babies and looks for raised thyroid-stimulating hormone levels. Treatment is lifelong oral replacement of thyroxine.

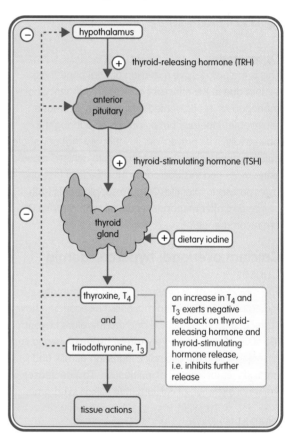

Fig. 13.25 The hypothalamic–pituitary–thyroid feedback system: normal status. In the presence of dietary iodine, thyroid hormones are produced which exert a negative feedback effect on hypothalamus and pituitary, inhibiting release of TRH and TSH.

Cretinism can be prevented by the iodination of salt in the maternal diet.

Iodine overload

Excessive dietary iodine may cause the symptoms of hyperthyroidism, that is, an overactive thyroid.

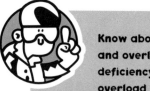
Know about iron deficiency and overload, calcium deficiency, and copper overload because they are commonly asked about.

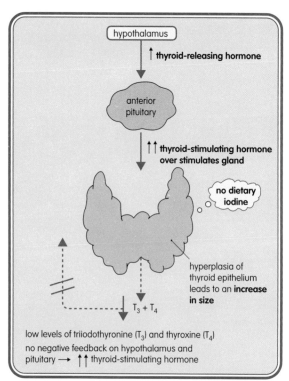

Fig. 13.26 The hypothalamic–pituitary–thyroid feedback system: dietary iodine limiting. Decreased production of thyroid hormones releases negative feedback on hypothalamus and anterior pituitary.

For each mineral disorder describe:
- **The main causes, clinical features, and criteria for diagnosis and treatment.**
- **The differences between iron-deficiency anaemia and pernicious anaemia—this is very important.**

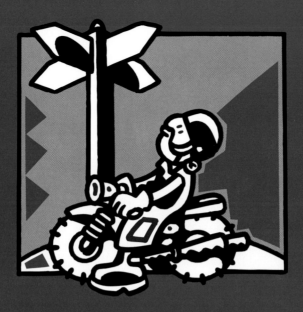

SELF-ASSESSMENT

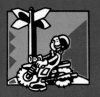

Multiple-choice Questions

Indicate whether each answer is true or false.

1. Glycolysis:

(a) Occurs in the cell cytosol.
(b) Can operate under both aerobic and anaerobic conditions.
(c) Does not occur in red blood cells.
(d) Contains three essentially irreversible reactions.
(e) Under aerobic conditions, generates the net production of 12 molecules of ATP.

2. The reaction catalysed by phosphofructokinase-1 (PFK-1):

(a) Is an example of an isomerization reaction.
(b) Catalyses the phosphorylation of fructose-6-phosphate.
(c) Is the rate-limiting reaction of the glycolytic pathway.
(d) Is allosterically inhibited by fructose 2,6-bisphosphate.
(e) Is allosterically inhibited by ATP and citrate.

3. Regarding glucose metabolism:

(a) Under anaerobic conditions pyruvate is reduced to lactate, regenerating NAD^+.
(b) The malate–aspartate shuttle has a role in the regeneration of NAD^+.
(c) Net ATP yield from anaerobic glycolysis is two ATP.
(d) Pyruvate kinase is regulated by reversible phosphorylation.
(e) A deficiency of pyruvate kinase may result in a haemolytic anaemia

4. The conversion of pyruvate to acetyl CoA:

(a) Is reversible.
(b) Requires lipoate as a co-factor.
(c) Occurs in the cytosol.
(d) Requires the co-enzyme biotin.
(e) Is inhibited in vitamin B_1 (thiamin) deficiency.

5. Acetyl CoA:

(a) Serves as a donor of acetyl groups in fatty acid synthesis.
(b) Cannot be formed from protein.
(c) Is used to make cholesterol and ketone bodies.
(d) Allosterically activates pyruvate dehydrogenase.
(e) Is carboxylated by pyruvate carboxylase to form malonyl CoA.

6. The following enzyme activities would be decreased in thiamin deficiency.

(a) Pyruvate carboxylase.
(b) Isocitrate dehydrogenase.
(c) α-ketoglutarate dehydrogenase.
(d) Lactate dehydrogenase.
(e) Transketolase.

7. The TCA cycle:

(a) Operates under aerobic and anaerobic conditions.
(b) Occurs in the mitochondrial matrix.
(c) Does not occur in red blood cells.
(d) Is an amphibolic pathway.
(e) Each turn of the cycle produces three molecules of $FADH_2$ and one molecule of NADH per mole of acetyl CoA oxidized.

8. α-Ketoglutarate dehydrogenase:

(a) Catalyses the oxidative decarboxylation of citrate.
(b) Requires thiamin pyrophosphate as a co-factor.
(c) Is activated by ATP.
(d) Has activity measured in red blood cells in thiamin deficiency.
(e) Requires pyridoxal phosphate as a co-factor.

9. Oxidative phosphorylation:

(a) Occurs in the inner mitochondrial space.
(b) Involves the transfer of electrons from NADH or $FADH_2$ down a series of electron carriers to molecular oxygen.
(c) The oxidation of NADH by the et chain produces 1.5 ATP.
(d) The oxidation of $FADH_2$ by the et chain produces 1.5 ATP.
(e) Is the process in which electron transport is coupled to the transport of protons across the inner mitochondrial membrane.

10. 2,4-Dinitrophenol:

(a) Inhibits electron transport and ATP synthesis.
(b) Allows electron transport to occur without ATP synthesis.
(c) Inhibits electron transport without the impairment of ATP synthesis.
(d) Specifically inhibits cytochrome c.
(e) Is a competitive inhibitor of NAD^+-requiring reactions in mitochondria

11. Regarding the components of the electron transport chain:

(a) Proton pumping occurs at complex I–NADH dehydrogenase.
(b) Proton pumping occurs at complex II–succinate ubiquinone reductase.
(c) Antimycin A inhibits electron transport at complex II.
(d) Cyanide inhibits electron flow in complex IV–cytochrome oxidase.
(e) Oligomycin is an uncoupler of the chain.

12. The following enzymes catalyse substrate-level phosphorylation reactions.

(a) Phosphoglycerate kinase.
(b) Isocitrate dehydrogenase.
(c) Phosphofructokinase-1.
(d) Succinyl CoA synthetase.
(e) Pyruvate kinase.

13. Gluconeogenesis:

(a) Occurs exclusively in the cell cytosol.
(b) Usually occurs in muscle.
(c) Is important in maintaining blood glucose concentration during early starvation.
(d) Is activated by fructose 2,6-bisphosphate.
(e) Allows fatty acids to be converted into glucose in net amounts.

14. The following reactions are unique to gluconeogenesis.

(a) Lactate $\rightarrow$ Pyruvate.
(b) Fructose-6-phosphate $\rightarrow$ Glucose-6-phosphate.
(c) Glucose-6-phosphate $\rightarrow$ Fructose-6-phosphate.
(d) 1,3-Bisphosphoglycerate $\rightarrow$ Glyceraldehyde-3-phosphate.
(e) Pyruvate $\rightarrow$ Phosphoenolpyruvate.

15. Glycogen:

(a) Contains α–1,4 linkages that enable it to form branches.
(b) Muscle glycogen is vital to the maintenance of the blood glucose concentration.
(c) During fasting, liver glycogen stores last only between 12 and 24 h.
(d) Glucagon promotes glycogen breakdown in muscle.
(e) Insulin promotes glycogen synthesis in both liver and muscle.

16. Glycogen storage disorders:

(a) Are all inherited as autosomal dominant disorders.
(b) Type I disorder is caused by a deficiency of glucose-6-phosphatase in the liver.
(c) In McArdle's disease, patients tend to have an increased exercise tolerance.
(d) Are only seen in boys.
(e) In Pompe's disease, glycogen accumulates in lysosomes and is usually fatal before the age of 2 years.

17. Fructose:

(a) Entry into cells is insulin dependent.
(b) Most dietary fructose is metabolized by the muscle.
(c) In the liver, the first step of its metabolism is phosphorylation by fructokinase.
(d) Is metabolized at a greater rate than glucose because it is a smaller molecule.
(e) Excessive ingestion of fructose can result in lactic acidosis.

18. Sorbitol:

(a) Can be used as a sweetener in diabetic foods.
(b) Is synthesized from glucose in the lens, liver, kidney, and Schwann cells.
(c) In the lens of the eye, sorbitol dehydrogenase oxidizes sorbitol to fructose.
(d) May accumulate in diabetic patients and contribute to the formation of cataracts.
(e) Is metabolized by the enzyme catalase in peroxisomes.

19. Regarding the pentose phosphate pathway:

(a) The net ATP yield from the pathway is six ATP.
(b) It is located in mitochondria.
(c) It generates reducing power as NADPH.
(d) Glucose-6-phosphate dehydrogenase catalyses the rate-limiting step.
(e) It produces five-carbon ribose sugars which can be used for nucleotide synthesis.

20. Which of the following is a function of NADPH?

(a) Provides reducing power for lipid synthesis.
(b) Regeneration of active glutathione.
(c) Anti-oxidant.
(d) Oxidized by the electron transport chain to make ATP.
(e) May be generated during oxidative deamination of glutamate.

21. Glucose-6-phosphate dehydrogenase deficiency:

(a) Is inherited as an autosomal recessive disorder.
(b) Results in a haemolytic anaemia.
(c) Carriers have some protection against malaria.
(d) May be precipitated by certain drugs such as antibiotics or aspirin.
(e) Type B; Mediterranean variant can be precipitated by the ingestion of broad beans.

22. Galactosaemia:

(a) Is always caused by a deficiency of galactose-1-phosphate uridyl transferase.
(b) Can be caused by a deficiency of galactokinase.
(c) Presents in adults.
(d) Patients may become hypoglycaemic because galactose cannot be metabolized to glucose.
(e) May result in cataract formation because of the high levels of galactose.

23. Fatty acid synthesis:

(a) Occurs in the mitochondrial matrix.
(b) Requires NADPH.
(c) Is catalysed by fatty acid synthase, an enzyme complex that requires biotin as a co-factor.
(d) Is activated by glucagon.
(e) Requires specific enzymes found in the endoplasmic reticulum and mitochondria to form fatty acids longer than 18 carbon atoms.

24. Acetyl CoA carboxylase:

(a) Catalyses the rate-limiting reaction of fatty acid synthesis.
(b) Requires pyridoxal phosphate as a co-factor.
(c) Is inhibited by citrate and palmitoyl CoA.
(d) Is activated by reversible phosphorylation.
(e) Is activated by insulin.

25. 3-Hydroxy-3-methylglutaryl CoA (HMG-CoA) reductase:

(a) Is the rate-limiting enzyme of cholesterol synthesis.
(b) Is inhibited by cholesterol.
(c) Is activated by reversible phosphorylation.
(d) High intracellular levels of cholesterol cause repression of transcription of both HMG-CoA reductase and the LDL receptor gene.
(e) Is inhibited by lovastatin.

26. About plasma lipoproteins are correct:

(a) They provide an efficient transport system for lipids.
(b) Chylomicrons transport endogenously synthesized triacylglycerol and cholesterol from the liver to the tissues.
(c) HDL particles are produced from LDL particles in the circulation by the action of lipoprotein lipase.
(d) HDL removes 'used' cholesterol from tissues and takes it to the liver.
(e) LDL formed from VLDL in the circulation, binds to receptors on cells, to be taken up by receptor-mediated endocytosis.

27. Familial hypercholesterolaemia:

(a) Is inherited as an autosomal dominant disorder.
(b) Is caused by a deficiency of the enzyme lipoprotein lipase.
(c) Homozygotes may exhibit tendon xanthomata, xanthelasma, and arcus senilis.
(d) Patients are able to metabolize chylomicrons normally.
(e) Homozygotes are treated very effectively using fish oils.

28. Ketone bodies are:

(a) Only produced in starvation or in poorly controlled diabetes.
(b) Used by the brain in the fed state in preference to glucose.
(c) Formed from acetyl CoA in mitochondria.
(d) Not used as a fuel by the liver because it lacks 3-ketoacyl CoA transferase.
(e) The principal fuel for red blood cells.

29. The following are essential amino acids:

(a) Phenylalanine.
(b) Leucine.
(c) Lysine.
(d) Tyrosine.
(e) Tryptophan.

30. Glutamate dehydrogenase:

(a) Occurs in mitochondria.
(b) Catalyses the removal of amino groups from most amino acids.
(c) Uses either NAD^+ or $NADP^+$ as a co-factor.
(d) Requires pyridoxal phosphate (PLP) as a co-factor.
(e) Is activated by ADP.

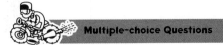

31. Protein degradation:

(a) Can be influenced by the nature of the *N*-terminal amino acid.
(b) Is rapid if the protein contains a [Pro-Glu-Ser-Thr] region.
(c) For abnormal or cytosolic proteins occurs mainly in lysosomes.
(d) Can be influenced by the attachment of ubiquitin to proteins.
(e) Is regulated by the rate of the urea cycle.

32. The urea cycle:

(a) Occurs mainly in liver hepatocytes.
(b) All reactions occur in the cell cytosol.
(c) Rate-limiting step is catalysed by a cytosolic enzyme, carbamoyl phosphate synthase II.
(d) Net ATP consumption is four ATP.
(e) The urea formed is insoluble and must be converted into uric acid for excretion.

33. About amino acid disorders:

(a) Phenylketonuria is always caused by a deficiency of the enzyme phenylalanine hydroxylase.
(b) Alkaptonuria is usually caused by a deficiency of homogentisic acid oxidase.
(c) Histidinaemia is usually caused by a deficiency of cystathionine synthetase.
(d) In albinism, patients have low levels of pigment in the iris and retina and are prone to skin cancer.
(e) The treatment of phenylketonuria involves life-long restriction of dietary phenylalanine.

34. 5,6,7,8-Tetrahydrofolate (THF):

(a) Is formed from folate by the action of dihydrofolate reductase.
(b) Is a carrier of one-carbon units in purine synthesis.
(c) Certain anti-cancer drugs, for example, methotrexate, inhibit its synthesis.
(d) The methionine salvage pathway is essential for maintaining a continual supply of THF.
(e) Folate deficiency can occur secondary to vitamin B_{12} deficiency.

35. Lesch–Nyhan syndrome:

(a) Is caused by a deficiency of the salvage enzyme, adenine phosphoribosyl transferase (APRT).
(b) Is often seen in girls.
(c) Causes patients to develop severe mental retardation and to self-mutilate.
(d) The salvage pathway for guanine and hypoxanthine is virtually inactive.
(e) Increased levels of guanine and hypoxanthine result in hyperuricaemia and gout.

36. Gout:

(a) Predominantly affects men.
(b) May be caused by low levels of hypoxanthine–guanine phosphoribosyl transferase (HGPRT).
(c) Clinical features include recurrent, acute arthritic attacks, kidney stones, and tophi.
(d) Acute attacks are treated with xanthine oxidase inhibitors.
(e) Is very effectively treated using aspirin.

37. Insulin usually stimulates:

(a) Glycogen synthesis.
(b) Lipolysis.
(c) Gluconeogenesis.
(d) The uptake of glucose by peripheral tissues.
(e) The uptake of amino acids by most tissues.

38. The main metabolic effects found in diabetes mellitus are:

(a) Hyperglycaemia.
(b) An increase in the rate of gluconeogenesis.
(c) A decrease in ketone body synthesis.
(d) Hypertriglyceridaemia.
(e) An increase of lipolysis.

39. In NIDDM:

(a) There is usually an absolute deficiency of insulin.
(b) Patients are often obese.
(c) Patients frequently develop ketoacidosis.
(d) Genetic factors are not implicated.
(e) Patients can present with polyuria and polydipsia.

40. Zinc:

(a) Is a co-factor for the enzyme superoxide dismutase.
(b) Absorption is increased in the presence of vitamin C.
(c) Deficiency causes acrodermatitis enteropathica.
(d) Deficiency is often seen in patients on parenteral nutrition.
(e) Overload causes liver cirrhosis.

41. Iron:

(a) Its absorption is favoured in the ferrous state (Fe^{2+}).
(b) Is stored in the body as transferrin.
(c) Deficiency results in a macrocytic anaemia.
(d) Overload can result in diabetes mellitus.
(e) Overload can be treated with desferrioxamine.

42. Vitamin C:

(a) Is a co-factor for proline and lysine hydroxylases involved in collagen synthesis.
(b) Is an anti-oxidant.
(c) Is a powerful oxidizing agent.
(d) Deficiency results in pellagra, characterized by swollen sore gums and poor wound healing.
(e) Deficiency can lead to anaemia.

43. Vitamin A:

(a) Is a fat-soluble vitamin.
(b) Can increase epithelial cell turnover.
(c) Deficiency results in impaired dark adaptation and night blindness.
(d) Can be used in the treatment of severe acne.
(e) Is safe to use in pregnancy, even in excess.

44. Regarding niacin:

(a) It can be synthesized from the amino acid tryptophan.
(b) Deficiency results in beriberi.
(c) The nutritional requirement for niacin is decreased when the diet contains large amounts of protein.
(d) The clinical features of niacin deficiency include dermatitis, diarrhoea, and dementia.
(e) Nicotinic acid can be used in the treatment of hyperlipidaemias.

45. Biotin:

(a) Is synthesized by bacteria in the gut.
(b) Is the co-enzyme for the aminotransferases.
(c) Deficiency can be induced by eating lots of raw egg whites.
(d) Deficiency results in night blindness.
(e) Deficiency may result in defective fatty acid synthesis.

46. Vitamin B_{12}:

(a) Is only found in food of animal origin.
(b) Is the co-factor for methylmalonyl CoA mutase, involved in the breakdown of odd-numbered fatty acids.
(c) Intrinsic factor released by gastric parietal cells is required for its absorption.
(d) The stores of vitamin B_{12} are very small.
(e) Deficiency results in both neurological symptoms and megaloblastic anaemia.

47. Vitamin D:

(a) Can be synthesized by the body in sufficient amounts to satisfy the daily requirement.
(b) Active form is 25-hydroxycholecalciferol.
(c) Principal role is in calcium homeostasis.
(d) Is a recognized teratogen.
(e) Is an anti-oxidant.

48. The following statements are correct:

(a) A deficiency of vitamin A or D, or calcium causes rickets in children.
(b) Vitamins B_{12}, C, and E are all anti-oxidants.
(c) Vitamins A, D, E, and C are all fat-soluble vitamins.
(d) A deficiency of vitamin B_{12} or C, or folate or iron results in anaemia.
(e) Both vitamin K and vitamin B_{12} are synthesized by intestinal bacteria.

49. Calcium:

(a) Is the most abundant mineral in the human body.
(b) Deficiency can occur secondary to vitamin D deficiency.
(c) Deficiency in children causes rickets.
(d) Deficiency in adults results in osteomalacia, characterized by a reduction in the total bone mass.
(e) In overload, is deposited in the eyes producing yellow–brown, Kayser–Fleischer rings on the cornea.

50. Kwashiorkor:

(a) Is an example of protein–energy malnutrition.
(b) Is always caused by a lack of protein and energy.
(c) Is often seen in the UK.
(d) Children are usually oedematous with scaly skin.
(e) Usually occurs when a child is weaned from breast feeding because of the arrival of a second child.

Short-answer Questions

1. Define 'catabolism' and 'anabolism' and give an example of each process.

2. Define 'substrate-level phosphorylation' and give an example to illustrate your answer.

3. NADH formed in glycolysis must be re-oxidized to NAD^+ for glycolysis to continue. Give two examples of how NAD^+ is regenerated.

4. Answer the following questions about the conversion of pyruvate to acetyl CoA.

    (a) Name the enzyme that catalyses this reaction and three co-factors that it requires.
    (b) What type of reaction is involved?
    (c) Where in the cell does this occur?
    (d) What product other than acetyl CoA is formed?
    (e) What is the significance of this reaction to carbohydrate and fat metabolism?

5. What is the main difference between the action of an inhibitor and that of an uncoupler on the electron transport chain? Give a named example of each.

6. Look at the reaction shown in Fig. 1.

    (a) Name substrate A and product B.
    (b) Where in the cell does this reaction occur?
    (c) What enzyme catalyses this reaction?
    (d) Name an important co-factor of this enzyme.
    (e) Name one activator and one inhibitor of this reaction.

7. (a) Name the two essential fatty acids.
    (b) Why are these substances important to humans?

8. Why is allopurinol used to treat gout?

9. What is transdeamination? Name the two enzymes involved.

10. Explain how the hormone glucagon activates glycogen breakdown in the liver.

11. Name three mechanisms by which enzymes are regulated and give an example of each.

12. What are the main fuels that supply blood glucose during the fed, fasted, and early and late starved states? Give an approximate time period for each state.

13. What is the effect of lead on haem synthesis and what treatments are available for lead poisoning?

14. Why are statins used in the treatment of patients with hypercholesterolaemia?

15. Name a disorder in which the following can be found in increased quantities in the urine:

    (a) Porphobilinogen and δ-aminolevulinic acid.
    (b) Valine.
    (c) Fructose.
    (d) Acetoacetate.

16. The deficiency of a number of vitamins and minerals can cause anaemia. Name four and state the type of anaemia observed in each.

17. Discuss the effects of a vitamin K deficiency in newborn babies. How is it prevented?

18. What is bioavailability? Discuss the absorption of iron from the diet and name three substances that affect it.

19. What is the main function of vitamin B_1 and explain why its deficiency results in neurological disorders.

20. Discuss the principal effects of a deficiency of vitamin B_6 on metabolism.

Fig. 1.

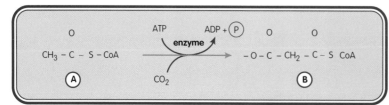

Essay Questions

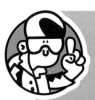

It is vital that for any exam question you answer only what is asked. For example, in Question 4 below, they are not asking you to say all you know about the vitamins A, C, and E, only about their functions. Do not waste your time because it does not get you any extra marks!

1. Acetyl CoA is often said to have a central place in metabolism. Discuss this statement illustrating your answer with examples from protein, carbohydrate, and fat metabolism.

2. Discuss the transport of both dietary and endogenously synthesized cholesterol and its removal from the blood.

3. Discuss the roles of gluconeogenesis and ketogenesis in the starved state and their contribution to the maintenance of the blood glucose concentration.

4. Give a brief account of the functions of vitamins A, C, and E and discuss their common role as anti-oxidants.

5. Outline the main reactions of the urea cycle in mammals, indicating their site within the cell. How is the cycle regulated? What are the consequences of a deficiency in any one of the enzymes of this pathway?

6. Make short notes on the following:

   (i). 'Uncouplers' and 'inhibitors' of the electron transport chain.
   (ii). The sources of NADPH for fatty acid synthesis.
   (iii).The ATP yield from aerobic and anaerobic glycosis.

7. Discuss the main features of marasmus and kwashiorkor. What are the long-term physiological effects of severe malnutrition in infancy?

8. Discuss the main functions of vitamin B_{12} and folate in metabolism. What are the effects of their deficiency?

9. Discuss the effect of a low insulin to glucagon ratio on the metabolic processes in insulin-dependent diabetes mellitus (IDDM).

10. Make short notes on three of the following:

   (i). Haemochromatosis.
   (ii). Zinc deficiency.
   (iii).Wernicke's encephalopathy.
   (iv).   Scurvy.

1.	(a) T,	(b) T,	(c) F,	(d) T,	(e) F.	**26.**	(a) T,	(b) F,	(c) F,	(d) T,	(e) T.
2.	(a) F,	(b) T,	(c) T,	(d) F,	(e) T.	**27.**	(a) T,	(b) F,	(c) T,	(d) T,	(e) F.
3.	(a) T,	(b) T,	(c) T,	(d) T,	(e) T.	**28.**	(a) F,	(b) F,	(c) T,	(d) T,	(e) F.
4.	(a) F,	(b) T,	(c) F,	(d) F,	(e) T.	**29.**	(a) T,	(b) T,	(c) T,	(d) F,	(e) T.
5.	(a) T,	(b) F,	(c) T,	(d) F,	(e) F.	**30.**	(a) T,	(b) F,	(c) T,	(d) F,	(e) T.
6.	(a) F,	(b) F,	(c) T,	(d) F,	(e) T.	**31.**	(a) T,	(b) T,	(c) F,	(d) T,	(e) F.
7.	(a) F,	(b) T,	(c) T,	(d) T,	(e) F.	**32.**	(a) T,	(b) F,	(c) F,	(d) F,	(e) F.
8.	(a) F,	(b) T,	(c) F,	(d) F,	(e) F.	**33.**	(a) F,	(b) T,	(c) F,	(d) T,	(e) T.
9.	(a) F,	(b) T,	(c) F,	(d) T,	(e) T.	**34.**	(a) T,	(b) T,	(c) T,	(d) T,	(e) T.
10.	(a) F,	(b) T,	(c) F,	(d) F,	(e) F.	**35.**	(a) F,	(b) F,	(c) T,	(d) T,	(e) T.
11.	(a) T,	(b) F,	(c) F,	(d) T,	(e) F.	**36.**	(a) T,	(b) T,	(c) T,	(d) F,	(e) F.
12.	(a) T,	(b) F,	(c) F,	(d) T,	(e) T.	**37.**	(a) T,	(b) F,	(c) F,	(d) T,	(e) T.
13.	(a) F,	(b) F,	(c) T,	(d) F,	(e) F.	**38.**	(a) T,	(b) T,	(c) F,	(d) T,	(e) T.
14.	(a) F,	(b) F,	(c) F,	(d) F,	(e) T.	**39.**	(a) F,	(b) T,	(c) F,	(d) F,	(e) T.
15.	(a) F,	(b) F,	(c) T,	(d) F,	(e) T.	**40.**	(a) T,	(b) F,	(c) T,	(d) T,	(e) F.
16.	(a) F,	(b) T,	(c) F,	(d) F,	(e) T.	**41.**	(a) T,	(b) F,	(c) F,	(d) T,	(e) T.
17.	(a) F,	(d) F,	(c) T,	(d) F,	(e) T.	**42.**	(a) T,	(b) T,	(c) F,	(d) F,	(e) T.
18.	(a) T,	(b) T,	(c) F,	(d) T,	(e) F.	**43.**	(a) T,	(b) T,	(c) T,	(d) T,	(e) F.
19.	(a) F,	(b) F,	(c) T,	(d) T,	(e) T.	**44.**	(a) T,	(b) F,	(c) T,	(d) T,	(e) T.
20.	(a) T,	(b) T,	(c) F,	(d) F,	(e) T.	**45.**	(a) T,	(b) F,	(c) T,	(d) F,	(e) T.
21.	(a) F,	(b) T,	(c) T,	(d) T,	(e) T.	**46.**	(a) T,	(b) T,	(c) T,	(d) F,	(e) T.
22.	(a) F,	(b) T,	(c) F,	(d) T,	(e) T.	**47.**	(a) T,	(b) F,	(c) T,	(d) F,	(e) F.
23.	(a) F,	(b) T,	(c) F,	(d) F,	(e) T.	**48.**	(a) F,	(b) F,	(c) F,	(d) T,	(e) T.
24.	(a) T,	(b) F,	(c) F,	(d) F,	(e) T.	**49.**	(a) T,	(b) T,	(c) T,	(d) F,	(e) F.
25.	(a) T,	(b) T,	(c) F,	(d) T,	(e) T.	**50.**	(a) T,	(b) F,	(c) F,	(d) T,	(e) T.

1. Catabolism is the process where energy-rich complex molecules such as protein, carbohydrate, and fat are broken down or oxidized to their simpler constituent molecules. The energy released is 'captured' as ATP and stored for use in synthetic reactions.

    Example: The β oxidation of fatty acids in which a molecule of fatty acid is completely oxidized to CO_2 and H_2O. Other examples you could have chosen are glycogen breakdown (glycogenolysis) or glycolysis (see Table 1.1).

    Anabolism is the synthesis of complex molecules from simpler ones, that is, amino acids to proteins, or glucose to glycogen. Synthetic reactions require energy from hydrolysis of ATP.

    Example: Glycogen synthesis (glycogenesis) in which amolecule of glycogen is synthesized or 'built up' from glucose residues.

2. Substrate-level phosphorylation is defined as the formation of ATP by the direct phosphorylation of ADP. Therefore ATP is produced directly from the metabolites by the transfer of a phosphoryl group from a 'high-energy' intermediate to ADP to form ATP. It does not require oxygen and therefore is important for generating ATP in tissues short of oxygen, e.g. active skeletal muscle.

    Example: The formation of pyruvate from phosphoenolpyruvate (last reaction of glycolysis) by pyruvate kinase (Fig.2).

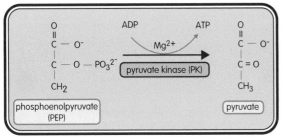

Fig. 2.

3. (a) Under anaerobic conditions, pyruvate is reduced to lactate by lactate dehydrogenase (LDH) with the simultaneous oxidation of NADH to NAD^+. The reaction occurs in the cell cytosol and is important in red blood cells (no mitochondria) because it is their only pathway for NAD^+ regeneration; it is also important in active skeletal muscle when oxygen is limiting. N.B. It's always best to illustrate your answers wherever possible with the relevant equation or a quick sketch of a pathway.

(b) Under aerobic conditions, NADH is oxidized to NAD^+ via the electron transport chain in mitochondria, generating energy. NADH first has to enter the mitochondria. The inner mitochondrial membrane is impermeable to NADH and therefore only its two 'high energy' electrons are transported into the mitochondria by either the glycerol-3-phosphate shuttle or the malate–aspartate shuttle.

    In the malate–aspartate shuttle, NADH is used to reduce oxaloacetate to malate, regenerating cytosolic NAD^+. In the glycerol-3-phosphate shuttle, NADH is used to reduce dihydroxyacetone-3-phosphate to glycerol-3-phosphate, regenerating NAD^+. The answer to this part is best illustrated with a simple sketch of both shuttles as shown in Figs 2.6 and 2.7.

4. (a) Pyruvate dehydrogenase complex (PHD). The three co-factors required are thiamine pyrophosphate, FAD, and lipoate.
   (b) Oxidative decarboxylation.
   (c) Mitochondrial matrix.
   (d) CO_2.
   (e) The reaction is completely irreversible such that pyruvate cannot be formed from acetyl CoA. Therefore, carbohydrates can form fats but not vice versa, meaning there can be no net synthesis of glucose from fatty acids!

5. This answer is best illustrated with a quick sketch of the electron transport chain showing the action of inhibitors and uncouplers.

    Inhibitors of the electron transport chain bind to specific components of the chain, blocking the transfer of electrons at that site. For example, rotenone and amytal bind to and inhibit electron transfer within NADH dehydrogenase (complex 1), causing inhibition of the chain. Normally electron transport is accompanied by pumping of protons across the inner mitochondrial membrane into the inner mitochondrial space. The inhibition of electron transport results in the inhibition of the proton pump and thus of ATP synthesis.

    Uncouplers (e.g. 2,4-dinitrophenol) increase the permeability of the inner mitochondrial membrane to protons, so that they can re-enter the matrix at sites other than ATP synthase. This dissipates the proton gradient without ATP production. Normally, the proton gradient 'couples' electron transport to oxidative phosphorylation (ATP synthesis). Uncouplers dissipate the proton gradient so that electron transport still occurs normally but without ATP production.

6. (a) A = acetyl CoA. B = malonyl CoA.
   (b) The cell cytosol.
   (c) Acetyl CoA carboxylase.
   (d) Biotin.

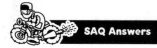
(e) Activators are either citrate (allosteric activator) or insulin (causes reversible dephosphorylation). Inhibitors are either palmitoyl CoA or glucagon (causes reversible phosphorylation).

7. (a) Linoleic acid (C18:2), a member of the ω6 series of fatty acids and α-linolenic acid (C18:3), ω3 series.
   (b) Essential fatty acids cannot be synthesized by the body and therefore must be obtained from the diet. This is because mammals do not possess the correct enzymes (desaturases) to insert double bonds beyond the C9 position, which enable these polyunsaturated fatty acids to be formed. Essential fatty acids are necessary to form other important unsaturated fatty acids, for example, arachidonic acid, the precursor molecule of prostaglandins, leukotrienes, and thromboxane molecules.

8. In gout, high levels of insoluble uric acid can precipitate out to form sodium urate crystals, which may become deposited in joints and tissues causing damage. Treatment is aimed at reducing uric acid levels. Allopurinol, an analogue of hypoxanthine, inhibits xanthine oxidase, the key enzyme involved in controlling the amount of uric acid produced. Treatment with allopurinol decreases the amount of insoluble uric acid formed and increases the amounts of the soluble precursors hypoxanthine and xanthine, which are easily excreted in the urine (Fig. 6.11). Other actions of allopurinol:
   - Salvage enzyme (HGPRT) catalyses addition of ribose-5-phosphate to allopurinol, forming allopurinol ribonucleotide which can inhibit PRPP amidotransferase, the rate-limiting enzyme of purine synthesis.
   - Allopurinol can be metabolized by xanthine oxidase to oxypurinol, an even stronger inhibitor of xanthine oxidase.

9. Transdeamination is transamination followed by oxidative deamination by glutamate dehydrogenase. The best way to answer this is to draw the reactions (see Figs 5.1 and 5.2).
   (a) Transamination: aminotransferases catalyse the transfer of the amino group (NH_3^+) from all amino acids to α-ketoglutarate, forming glutamate. Enzymes require pyridoxal phosphate as a co-factor and can be found in both the cytosol and mitochondria. The reaction 'funnels' amino groups of amino acids to glutamate, which can then undergo oxidative deamination.
   (b) Oxidative deamination: glutamate dehydrogenase removes the amino group from glutamate in mitochondria. The amino group then enters the urea cycle. Glutamate dehydrogenase is specific for glutamate.

10. The easiest and quickest way to do this is to draw it. (see Fig. 3). N.B. refer back also to Fig. 2.34 for details.

11. (a) **Allosteric control**
    (i). Product inhibition: may be positive or negative. For example, the glycolytic enzyme hexokinase

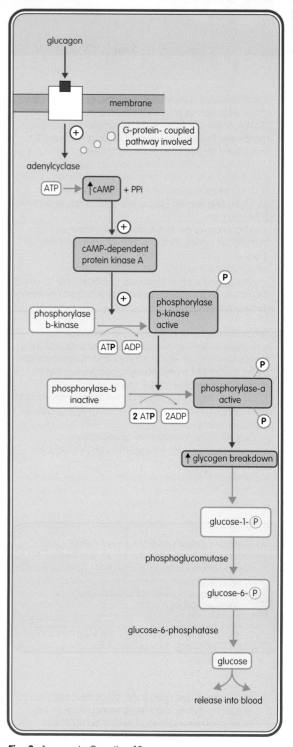

Fig. 3 Answer to Question 10.

is allosterically inhibited by high levels of glucose-6-phosphate.

(ii). By the production of allosteric effectors that bind to regulatory sites on the enzyme distinct from the catalytic site; they may either increase or decrease the enzyme activity. For example, fructose 2,6-bisphosphate is a potent allosteric activator of phosphofructokinase-1.

(b) **Reversible phosphorylation**
This may either activate or inhibit the enzyme. For example, glucagon activates a reaction cascade that brings about the phosphorylation of both glycogen synthase (inhibiting it) and glycogen phosphorylase (activating it). This ensures glycogen synthesis and breakdown are not active at the same time.

(c) **Change in the total quantity of enzyme**
This is usually via a change in the rate of transcription. Hormones can either increase the amount of enzyme synthesized (induction) or decrease synthesis (repression). For example, glucagon increases the rate of transcription and thus synthesis of the gluconeogenic enzyme PEP-carboxykinase.

12. (a) Fed state (0–4 h after a meal): Exogenous glucose (carbohydrate in the diet) provides the main fuel.
(b) Fasted state (4–12 h after a meal): The breakdown of liver glycogen stores provides glucose for oxidation mainly by the brain. Stores are only sufficient to last between 12 and 24 h.
(c) Early starved (12 h to 16 days): Once most of the liver glycogen has been used up, glucose is formed from non-carbohydrate precursors via gluco-neogenesis. Protein breakdown in muscle releases amino acids, mainly alanine and glutamine, and the hydrolysis of triacylglycerol in liver and adipose tissue releases glycerol. Along with lactate formed in muscle, they are all used to form glucose. The rate of gluconeogenesis is at its greatest after about 2–6 days of fasting and then starts to fall off.
(d) Late starved (longer than 16 days): In prolonged starvation, the breakdown of muscle protein and thus gluconeogenesis slows down. There is less need for glucose because the brain adapts to using more ketone bodies, namely acetoacetate, and β-hydroxybutyrate.

13. Lead inhibits three key enzymes involved in haem synthesis, resulting in an accumulation of intermediates, namely:
(i). ALA dehydrase leading to the accumulation of ALA, which can be measured in urine.
(ii). Coproporphyrinogen III oxidase leading to the accumulation of coproporphyrinogen III.
(iii). Ferrochelatase leading to the accumulation of protoporphyrin IX in RBCs, causing fluorescence.

The result is the inhibition of haem synthesis and thus of haemoglobin production. This leads to anaemia unless treated. Treatment is with lead chelators such as Ca-EDTA, D-penicillamine or British Anti-Lewisite.

They bind lead forming a complex that can be excreted in the urine.

14. Statins, for example, simvastatin or lovastatin help to reduce plasma cholesterol. They reversibly inhibit HMG-CoA reductase, the rate-limiting enzyme of cholesterol synthesis, resulting in a decreased rate of cholesterol synthesis by cells. The resulting low intracellular cholesterol concentration stimulates transcription of the LDL-receptor gene resulting in an increased number of LDL-cholesterol receptors on cells. This increases cholesterol uptake by cells thus lowering plasma cholesterol. This is illustrated in Fig. 4.

15. (a) Acute porphyrias (either acute intermittent, variegate, or hereditary coproporphyria).
(b) Maple syrup urine disease (branched chain α-ketoacid dehydrogenase deficiency).
(c) Fructokinase deficiency (essential fructosuria).
(d) Acetoacetate is a ketone body and can be found in the urine in poorly controlled IDDM.

16. (a) Iron deficiency causes a decrease in haemoglobin production leading to a microcytic, hypochromic anaemia.
(b) Vitamin B_{12} deficiency, due to either a dietary deficiency or an auto-immune condition (pernicious anaemia) causes a megaloblastic anaemia.
(c) Folate deficiency causes a macrocytic, megaloblastic anaemia.
(d) Vitamin C deficiency: vitamin C is required for reduction of dietary Fe^{3+} to Fe^{2+} in the gut, allowing its absorption. Therefore vitamin C deficiency causes a secondary iron deficiency, leading to microcytic, hypochromic cells (minor importance only).

17. In adults, vitamin K deficiency is rare because most of our vitamin K is synthesized by bacteria in the gut. However, newborn babies have sterile guts and therefore cannot initially make vitamin K and human milk is a very poor source. Newborn babies may develop a vitamin K deficiency, resulting in a condition called 'haemorrhagic disease of the newborn'. They have low levels of vitamin K-dependent clotting factors (II, VII, IX, and X) and thus an increased bleeding tendency. Bleeding is usually minor but in some cases this can lead to major bleeds, causing intracranial haemorrhage and death. Therefore, every newborn baby in the UK is given prophylactic intramuscular or oral vitamin K shortly after birth to prevent haemorrhagic disease.

18. Bioavailability is the (percentage) efficiency with which any dietary nutrient is absorbed and used in the body. A number of factors influence the absorption and use of nutrients such as:
(a) Chemical form of nutrient.
(b) Antagonistic or facilitatory ligands.
(c) Breakdown of nutrient.
(d) pH and redox state.
Dietary iron exists in two forms, haem and non-haem iron. These are derived from haemoglobin or

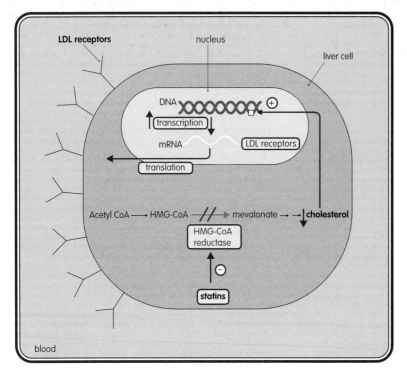

Fig. 4 Part of answer to Question 14.

myoglobin present in meat and are rapidly absorbed. Inorganic, non-haem iron is present in vegetables and cereals and is absorbed slowly. Iron is more readily absorbed in the ferrous (Fe^{2+}) rather than ferric (Fe^{3+}) state. Inorganic iron present in vegetables is in the ferric state and must be reduced for absorption.

(a) Gastric acid and ascorbic acid favour absorption by reducing iron to Fe^{2+}.

(b) Phosphates and phytates (plants) form insoluble complexes with iron and prevent absorption.

(c) Alcohol also increases absorption.

19. Vitamin B_1 (thiamin) is a co-factor for four key enzymes in the form of thiamine pyrophosphate (TPP).

(a) Pyruvate dehydrogenase which converts pyruvate into acetyl CoA.

(b) α-ketoglutarate dehydrogenase (TCA cycle).

(c) Branched chain amino acid α-ketoacid dehydrogenase.

(d) Transketolase, an enzyme of the pentose phosphate pathway (PPP).

In thiamin deficiency, the activity of all four enzymes is reduced. The decreased activity of pyruvate dehydrogenase and α-ketoglutarate dehydrogenase result in a decrease of acetyl CoA and ATP formation and thus a fall in acetylcholine. Decreased activity of transketolase results in decreased activity of the PPP, leading to a decrease in the NADPH necessary for fatty acid synthesis. This results in decreased fatty acid synthesis of the myelin causing a peripheral neuropathy.

Neurological disorders caused by thiamin deficiency include:

(i). Dry beriberi, characterized by gradual, symmetrical, ascending peripheral neuropathy.

(ii). Wernicke's encephalopathy which, untreated, may progress to Korsakoff's psychosis, a severe irreversible amnesic syndrome.

20. Vitamin B_6 (pyridoxine), is a co-factor for a number of enzymes in the form of pyridoxal phosphate (PLP):

(i). Aminotransferases: In vitamin B_6 deficiency, a decreased activity of aminotransferases would result in the inhibition of protein metabolism and possibly eventual protein deficiency. The neurotransmitters serotonin and noradrenaline are derived from amino acids, therefore, PLP deficiency could cause a secondary deficiency of these.

(ii). δ-Aminolevulinic acid (ALA) synthase, which catalyses the rate-limiting step of haem synthesis. A vitamin B_6 deficiency could cause hypochromic, microcytic anaemia.

(iii). Glycogen phosphorylase, which catalyses glycogen breakdown. A pyridoxine deficiency would result in the accumulation of normal glycogen in liver and muscle. This could cause hypoglycaemia because liver glycogen stores could not be mobilized easily during fasting.

(iv). PLP is a co-factor for the enzyme which synthesizes niacin from tryptophan. A PLP deficiency could cause niacin deficiency and secondary pellagra.

A

abdominal distension, 166
abdominal examination, 166–8
abdominal pain, 168
absorptive state *see* fed state
acetaldehyde, 41, 42
acetoacetic acid (acetoacetate), 74, 75
acetoacetyl-acyl carrier protein (ACP), 54, 55
acetoacetyl CoA, 52, 66, 91, 92
acetone, 74
acetyl CoA, 15–17, 19, 22
   in amino acid catabolism, 91, 92
   carboxylation to malonyl CoA, 52, 53
   central role, 16
   in cholesterol synthesis, 66
   control of gluconeogenesis, 93–4
   in fatty acid breakdown, 62
   in fatty acid synthesis, 52, 53, 54, 55–6
   in ketogenesis, 74, 75, 76
   in pyrimidine breakdown, 111
   in pyruvate–malate cycle, 47, 48
   structure, 15–16
   synthesis from pyruvate, 16–17, 51, 53
   transport to cytosol, 51, 52, 53
acetyl CoA carboxylase, 53, 56, 64
acetyl transacylase, 54
aconitase, 19
acrodermatitis enteropathica, 212
acycloguanosine, 112
acyclovir, 112
acyl carrier protein (ACP), 54
acyl CoA: cholesterol acyl transferase (ACAT), 68, 69, 72
adenine, 101–2
adenine phosphoribosyl transferase (APRT), 106
adenosine, 101
adenosine diphosphate *see* ADP
adenosine monophosphate *see* AMP
adenosine triphosphate *see* ATP
adenylsuccinate lyase, 105
adenylsuccinate synthase, 104, 105
adipose tissue, brown, 28
ADP
   ATP hydrolysis to, 24
   control of ATP synthesis, 21, 28
   oxidative phosphorylation, 24–6
   substrate level phosphorylation, 9–10, 24, 25
ADP:ATP ratio, 21, 22, 28
adrenaline, 121
   in exercise, 122

adrenaline *continued*
   in glycogen metabolism, 34–5
   in lipid breakdown, 64
adrenocorticotrophic hormone (ACTH), 64, 93
aerobic respiration (glycolysis), 7, 10–11
ALA *see* δ-aminolevulinic acid
alanine, 77
   in absorptive state, 95, 96
   biosynthesis, 80, 82
   breakdown, 91, 92
   in gluconeogenesis, 89
   in post-absorptive state, 96, 97
   in starvation, 119, 120
   see also glucose–alanine cycle
alanine aminotransferase, 77
albinism, 191, 192
albumin, plasma, 170, 177
alcohol *see* ethanol
alcohol dehydrogenase, 41, 42
alcoholic fermentation, 11
aldehyde dehydrogenase, 41, 42
aldolase, 9
aldolase B *see* fructose-1-phosphate aldolase
aldose reductase, 42, 43
alkaptonuria, 191
allantion, 107
allergies, 150
allopurinol, 107, 194
allosteric control, 4
altitude acclimatization, 38
amino acids, 77–81
   biosynthesis, 22, 23, 78–81, 82
   branched chain (BCAA), 93
   breakdown (catabolism), 91–4
   deamination, 85–6
   essential, 77
   glucogenic, 91
   ketogenic, 91
   limiting, 130
   metabolism
      disorders of, 94, 153, 190–2
      to glucose/fat, 89–94
      in individual tissues, 95–8
   non-essential, 77
   one-carbon pool and, 100
   oxidative deamination, 78, 85
   pool, 82, 83
   transamination, 77–8, 85–86, 87
   transdeamination, 85

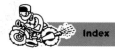

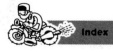

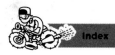

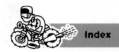